*The publisher and the University of California Press Foundation grate-
fully acknowledge the generous support of the Anne G. Lipow Endowment
Fund in Social Justice and Human Rights.*

Remaking a Life

Remaking a Life

HOW WOMEN LIVING WITH HIV/AIDS
CONFRONT INEQUALITY

Celeste Watkins-Hayes

UNIVERSITY OF CALIFORNIA PRESS

University of California Press, one of the most distinguished university presses in the United States, enriches lives around the world by advancing scholarship in the humanities, social sciences, and natural sciences. Its activities are supported by the UC Press Foundation and by philanthropic contributions from individuals and institutions. For more information, visit www.ucpress.edu.

University of California Press
Oakland, California

Library of Congress Cataloging-in-Publication Data

Names: Watkins-Hayes, Celeste, author.
Title: Remaking a life : how women living with HIV/AIDS confront inequality / Celeste Watkins-Hayes.
Description: Oakland, California : University of California Press, [2019] | Includes bibliographical references and index. |
Identifiers: LCCN 2018061419 (print) | LCCN 2019001371 (ebook) | ISBN 9780520968738 (Epub) | ISBN 9780520296022 (cloth : alk. paper) | ISBN 9780520296039 (pbk. : alk. paper)
Subjects: LCSH: HIV-positive women—United States. | AIDS (Disease) in women—United States. | Equality—Health aspects—United States. | HIV-positive women—Medical care—United States.
Classification: LCC RA643.83 (ebook) | LCC RA643.83 .W38 2019 (print) | DDC 362.19697/920082--dc23
LC record available at https://lccn.loc.gov/2018061419

28   27   26   25   24   23   22   21   20   19
10   9   8   7   6   5   4   3   2   1

I am so grateful to every single woman,
and everyone who loved her,
who we've had to say goodbye to.
Who we've had to bury.
Who we've had to hold,
whether physically or in our hearts,
for the rest of our lives.
And we continue to say their names
and hold them dear
and appreciate and love them
for being the ancestral guidance that we need.

—Dázon Dixon Diallo, Founder of SisterLove
  Women Now! 2016 Summit
  Durban, South Africa

Contents

Figures and Tables

Key Abbreviations

ACT UP—AIDS Coalition to Unleash Power

ADAP—AIDS Drug Assistance Program

AIDS—acquired immunodeficiency syndrome

ART—antiretroviral therapy

AZT—azidothymidine

CDC—Centers for Disease Control and Prevention

GMHC—Gay Men's Health Crisis

HIV—human immunodeficiency virus

HSN—HIV/AIDS safety net

MMWR—*Morbidity and Mortality Weekly Report* (CDC)

MSM—men who have sex with men

NBLCA—National Black Leadership Commission on AIDS

PACHA—Presidential Advisory Council on HIV/AIDS

PEPFAR—President's Emergency Plan for AIDS Relief

PLWHA—people living with HIV/AIDS

PWID—people who inject drugs

PWN—Positive Women's Network

SFAF—San Francisco AIDS Foundation

UNAIDS—Joint United Nations Programme on HIV/AIDS

WHO—World Health Organization

WLWHA—women living with HIV/AIDS

WORLD—Women Organized to Respond to Life-Threatening Diseases

Injuries of Inequality
and the Transformative
Project

"If it weren't for HIV, I'd probably be dead." The first time Dawn Stevens was diagnosed with HIV, it was 1985. Then only 24 years old, Dawn brought her six-month-old daughter Chyna to the emergency room with a high fever that would not break. The doctors were puzzled. After hours of tests, one physician thought to ask Dawn about her own health history. With little subterfuge, she disclosed her history of intravenous drug use. The doctor, convinced that he had solved the mystery, recommended that they test Dawn and her daughter for something called "H-I-V." Chyna's test came back negative, and doctors eventually diagnosed her with a treatable virus. Dawn, however, received the sobering news that she had in fact tested positive for HIV. The epidemic was still in its early stages, when information was limited and medical providers had few plans or protocols in place to guide the newly diagnosed. Dawn left the hospital with a life-threatening illness and little understanding of what it meant.

In many ways, the seeds of that fateful diagnosis had been planted years before. Dawn grew up in the 1970s and 1980s in a black working-class community on Chicago's west side that was precariously situated near several high-poverty areas. She matured to adulthood at a time of massive change in neighborhoods like hers. De facto racial and economic residential segregation and lack of investment by government and private businesses limited upward mobility for residents, including young adults.[1] Given the increasing availability of illegal drugs, the drug trade offered many in Dawn's cohort fast money and emotional escape from the blight that surrounded them. Rising intracommunity violence, declining funding for healthcare and other community services, and a precipitous rise in mass incarceration that warehoused many friends, family members, and neighbors made the barrier between life and death increasingly porous for young people like Dawn.[2]

When the sexual trauma of Dawn's childhood collided with the structural blows and deteriorating safety net afflicting her community, the effects were combustible. The first instances of molestation at the hands of two family members, including her stepfather, occurred when she was just five years old and would continue intermittently until she was 16. "My village wasn't safe," Dawn tearfully recalled as I interviewed her. She told no one about the sexual abuse, convinced that her mother wouldn't believe her and her biological father would retaliate violently against the perpetrators and she would lose him to prison. But she acted out in other ways. She snuck sips of her father's drinks at house parties and began smoking marijuana and cigarettes in the eighth grade. By sophomore year of high school, she was drinking regularly. By the time she was a 16-year-old junior, her rebellion intensified, tensions with both her parents escalated, and she ran away from home. "I had been sexually molested for years. So, when I left home, I was crazy," Dawn reflected.

Dawn moved in for a few weeks with the person she most idolized, her 19-year-old stepsister Jackie. Jackie had already graduated to the fast life, shooting drugs intravenously and dating the neighborhood dealers who maintained her supply. When those relationships dried up, Jackie began to "turn dates," selling sex for money or drugs. Dawn followed suit, learning how to inject by observing Jackie and trading sex for the next high. Her habits became a source of deep disappointment and sadness for her parents, who knew nothing about the molestation. Their lack of awareness fueled Dawn's sense of anger and betrayal, and she continued to distance herself.

DEATH AND LIFE IN THE EYE OF A SYNDEMIC

The environmental and personal turmoil in Dawn's life was occurring precisely when the AIDS epidemic was gaining an early and strong foothold in vulnerable communities, quietly taking up residence in neighborhoods and networks and weaving itself into the epidemiological fabric. Human immunodeficiency virus (HIV) attacks specific cells of the immune system, known as CD4 cells or T-cells, and reduces the body's ability to fight infections and diseases. It is communicable, transmitted through infected blood, semen, breast milk, or vaginal fluids.[3] HIV progresses to acquired immunodeficiency syndrome (AIDS) when too many T-cells have been destroyed, and it can be fatal if left untreated.[4] Worldwide, 36.7 million people live with HIV/AIDS; approximately 1.1 million live with it in the United States, with an estimated 40,000 new infections each year.[5]

From its early stages, HIV has had a disproportionate impact on black communities, and it would be years before the threat was fully understood and aggressively fought with prevention and treatment services.[6] Despite making up only 12 percent of the US population, blacks comprised 45 percent of both new HIV infections and people living with HIV/AIDS (PLWHA) in 2015. Medical anthropologist Merrill Singer introduced the concept of syndemics to describe overlapping and mutually reinforcing epidemics of drug addiction, violence, and HIV that accompany severe health and social disparities.[7] Although Dawn's associates in addiction were beginning to talk about AIDS with a note of concern in the 1980s, its early public association with a group that seemed far different from hers prevented Dawn from recognizing the growing syndemic in her midst. "I had no reason to get tested. HIV was a gay white man's disease," she stated. "I was in an all-black community. It didn't affect us. Now the majority of the people that I hung out with are dead."

Ironically, the only HIV prevention message that Dawn recalled from those days was one delivered by a self-appointed public health advocate, an ex-pimp whom she knew who began distributing clean needles to his friends, restocking his supply during appointments at the free clinic. "'I don't want y'all to get AIDS,' he'd say. We really didn't know what he was saying; we just knew he didn't want us to have it. We didn't really know what AIDS was. Again, it was a gay white man's disease. So we shared syringes on a regular basis."

Dawn's drug use continued and escalated after that 1985 visit to the hospital with Chyna, but it did not go unnoticed. Having recently come to terms with her sexuality, her first serious girlfriend asked Dawn to leave their shared apartment, insisting that Chyna remain in the girlfriend's care. Dawn agreed, knowing that she was in a deep downward spiral. This would be Dawn's third child to leave her custody. Several years prior, her grandmother, exasperated by Dawn's hard-partying ways, demanded that the son she bore at age 17 live with her. A second son was born three years later in 1981, and Dawn's first cousin offered to raise him. In 1991, yet another daughter would be born and immediately taken by the foster care system. Frustrated and fed up, her family stopped speaking to her, beginning a silence that would last for 16 years.

After exhausting all of her invitations to sleep on the couches of various family members and friends, Dawn ended up on the streets. She became an active trader in a drug and sex market patronized by individuals of every race and class, from the city to the suburbs, but located squarely in the poor black neighborhoods on the south and west sides of Chicago that Dawn called home. "There were a lot of white guys who came through," she recalled, "and a lot of them were looking for dates and to get high." Although Dawn's most meaningful intimate relationships were with women, sex with men proved to be an important economic survival strategy. Encounters with those who wanted to buy both sex and drugs from her were especially lucrative.

Abandoned buildings and hallways became Dawn's temporary homes, and jail served as her way station when she needed a break from the streets: "I could actually tell people when I was coming [to jail], and that was usually when I got tired of living somewhere else. So I'd do something to get arrested." This was a striking testament to how dire things had become: Dawn sometimes saw the brutality and vulnerability awaiting her in jail as a marginal improvement over the brutality and vulnerability that she both experienced and witnessed on the street:

I saw a woman get dragged by a car. I've seen women get beaten and raped. While I was out there, I refused to be one of those women. I fought. When I was in a car with someone, and I saw him pulling up next to a wall of a building where I couldn't open my passenger door, trapping me inside the car, I'm like, "This is getting ready to get real interesting." And I would just look for any little break, any moment where I could pull out my knife and say, "Okay, now what're we gonna to do? 'Cause I have my knife . . . and I'm going to cut it off. So you get one chance to open the door and step out."

Suffering through a life of mental, physical, economic, and social deterioration, Dawn estimates that she experienced more than 50 residential moves after turning 18 years old, driven by "addiction, bad relationships, in and out of jail, stuff like that." Confrontations with fellow members of the underground economy also shaped the patterns of her movements:

> I'm originally from the west side, but in my addiction I changed sides of town and changed to the suburbs. [I lived] wherever it was conducive to my well-being at that time. In addiction you have many variables that would initiate you leaving a certain side of town. Running off with people's [drug] packages, owing people money, fighting. So sometimes I had to leave a side of town, and I'd stay gone basically until I figured those people were in jail, and then I'd go back. It was different . . . just everything that went with addiction.

For years, Dawn lived in this brutal cycle of drug addiction, survival sex, incarceration, and sometimes sincere, sometimes half-hearted, attempts at avoiding drugs. Shifting in and out of sobriety reflected a desire to stay clean, but the emotional scars of childhood sexual trauma and the toll of life on the streets could be papered over only so long before the pain required numbing.

Old News Becomes New Again

In 1992, seven years after her initial diagnosis, Dawn was arrested for knifing a customer who attempted to sexually assault her. It was a sad irony that the incident that finally led this survivor of childhood sexual abuse into extended incarceration had to do with her forceful resolve to fight back against a subsequent violation—her girlhood experience setting the stage for how she interpreted, experienced, and attempted to resist sexual violence later in life.[8] Instead of one of her relatively short stints in the Cook County Jail, she was sent to prison, where she experienced her second HIV diagnosis:

> In the penitentiary, when I went in they asked me, "Have you ever had tuberculosis?" . . . I've had TB. And the nurse goes, "Well, we've got to test you for HIV." I'm like, "Okay." And it didn't register that I'd already had this test. I didn't know what HIV was, what it meant to be HIV positive. So when they called me back to the clinic, she goes, "Ms. Stevens, you have HIV." I'm like, "Okay." And she goes, "Is there anything you need?" "No." And, again, that was the end of it. There was no explanation. I still didn't know any more than I did the first time I got tested. So . . . now two tests with no information.

Dawn served her time, aware of her status but unaware of its seriousness. She told no one. "I didn't know *what* to tell anybody," she shrugged. Upon her release three years later, Dawn completed a county-sponsored HIV education program, a requirement for being granted visitation rights with Chyna, who had been living in foster care since Dawn's ex-girlfriend died. A whopping ten years after her first HIV diagnosis, the county program served as Dawn's first substantive orientation to her condition. By this time, AIDS was the leading cause of death for all Americans aged 25 to 44.[9] The program initiated Dawn's efforts to grapple with the meaning and significance of her diagnosis. As she explained in her characteristically frank style, Dawn felt a sense of resignation, even acceptance: "When I finally began learning about HIV, I was surprised, but not really, because I did everything you could do to get it. I had unprotected sex. I was an intravenous drug user. I did everything possible to get it. . . . I don't question where it came from. I mean, there were so many people that I got high with, it's hard to say."

The program facilitators informed Dawn about the practical implications of living with HIV. "[They told me] that I was going to have it for the rest of my life, and that there were things that I had to do, such as start sleeping again. I needed to take better care of myself." Dawn knew this would be easier said than done. Homeless, estranged from family, struggling with drug addiction, and embedded in a world of criminal activity with few opportunities for second chances—just living, let alone living with HIV, would be a feat. "They're not supposed to release you to the streets, but they do," she commented about her post-incarceration experience. "I ended up at a shelter, and they had no idea what HIV was. They had no idea what to do with an HIV-positive person, especially someone who was out about their status."

Dawn stayed clean for stretches, securing a spot in a transitional housing facility run by Catholic nuns, regaining custody of Chyna, and celebrating almost two years of sobriety by the late 1990s. But she struggled to fully escape the uncompromising grip of the drugs. She started using again, pawning everything she owned to support her habit. She lost her job at a small nonprofit, her apartment, and custody of her daughter within a span of six months. Chyna, Dawn explained, "was smart enough at 12 to tell a teacher that I was using, so [Child Protective Services] came and got her."

This time when Dawn returned to life on the streets, she understood that she was also living with HIV. Negotiating that status as a sex worker in the drug economy would prove to be difficult:

> In that life, the men have the power. Because the men have the money, very few women who are out there are going to say no when the guy doesn't want to use a condom. You know the risk to yourself, "But right now, I need that money." So, okay, [he doesn't] want to use a condom, that's on him. It's easier to let him do what he's going to do without the condom and be gone. And you get high and don't even think about it anymore, 'cause you gave him an opportunity to protect himself and he chose not to. . . . And you don't want to argue about condom use. [If you do], first thing they go, "Why? You got something?" That's the last thing you need, a rumor in the neighborhood that you got something. So you go along with it. And knowing that I have HIV, and you're not ready to use a condom may in some way also give me some satisfaction for you berating me, "Yep come on, let's do this, I got ya," you know. Sometimes that in itself is a high for the woman. It's about who holds the power.

Dawn's health suffered grievously over this period as she was entangled in what I term the sexualized drug economy. She ignored the advice she had received in the county program. She barely slept. "In addiction, nobody thinks about health. When you don't feel good, you get high and you feel better. The depression comes when you're coming off the drugs. So you take another hit and you feel better. I was smoking crack all day, every day." She became a frequent patient in emergency rooms with fevers and opportunistic infections. During a particularly low moment, Dawn attempted suicide by washing down an overdose of antidepressants with tequila, feeling hopeless about the tailspin that she was in and physically worn down. At this point in time, Dawn had so few T-cells that she was diagnosed with AIDS.

As the Bottom Drops Away, Caught by a Safety Net

Dawn's 1999 stint in St. Mary's, a housing facility for women struggling with both HIV/AIDS and drug and alcohol addiction, helped her turn things around. At 38 years old, and 14 years after her initial HIV diagnosis, Dawn knew that she desperately needed another chance to change course. It was perhaps nothing short of a miracle that she had made it this far, her body bruised, somehow managing to survive on a steady diet of illegal drugs and no consistent HIV medication regimen. When she was released from the hospital after overdosing, she begged St. Mary's to take her, having previously used it as one of her temporary way stations when she was deep in her addiction.

This time, Dawn actually took her time, staying at St. Mary's for two full years to get strong enough to make it in the world without numbing herself with drugs. She began systematically gathering the tools she would need to change her life's course. She finally absorbed and accepted the incompatibility between abusing drugs and alcohol and managing HIV and got clean: "I realized that doing drugs was killing my body more [than HIV]. I decided that I wasn't ready to die. I didn't want HIV to take me out. So I had to stop getting high."

Further radical changes would be necessary. Dawn became a proactive advocate for her health, approaching the healthcare system with a new mindset: "I paid my physician a visit. I did my research and had this list of unacceptable HIV medications [those that people were saying were the most toxic]. It just so happened that my doctor and I were on the same page. She recommended the same medications that I was thinking about trying out. So that was a good beginning for us because she had just become my doctor."

Her stay at St. Mary's also enabled Dawn to meet a fellow resident named Raquel. "[I had a lot of] jailhouse relationships, a lot of relationships in my addiction. I guess my best relationship was with cocaine. So nobody else had a chance with that," Dawn reflected. Raquel represented something different and soon became Dawn's romantic partner: "She was in recovery, I was in recovery. The relationship didn't initiate in jail, it didn't initiate in my addiction." Meeting at a transitional facility for women living with HIV/AIDS also eliminated the challenging work of HIV status disclosure. "I guess my mind told me that it was time to actually look for a long-term relationship," Dawn explained. "I wanted to stop doing things the way I used to do them."

Putting the Pieces Together

Dawn's decision to "stop doing things the way she used to do them" applies to many aspects of her life, not just her romantic partnerships. When in 2005 Dawn enrolled in the research study for this book, just six years from living on the streets, the distance between her former and new life was vast. Up most days at 6:30 a.m., Dawn now concentrated on family and her extensive work in the HIV advocacy community. Dawn and Raquel had moved out of the St. Mary's facility in 2001 and remained in a deep and loving partnership, two souls who counted on each other as they created new ways of existing in the world. Like any couple, they had their pet peeves. Raquel found it endlessly frustrating that Dawn so often turned off her cell phone or refused to answer it. "But then Raquel will answer my phone for me and go, 'Here, it's for you.' Well, no shit, it's *my* cell phone!" Dawn laughed. But Dawn saw this period, with Raquel by her side, as one of the best of her life. There was someone in her life who cared about her, who "kept her in line," and who wouldn't allow her to withdraw into herself. Perhaps that was at the root of their tiffs over the phone. Part of their new life was reminding each other that they had obligations that mattered and loved ones to whom they were accountable.

While in the throes of addiction, Dawn's four children were taken away one by one. When our research team met her, she and Raquel were the trusted caretakers of a four-year-old girl named Daisy, whose teenage mother had asked Dawn and Raquel to care for her when Daisy was just six months old—the same age Chyna had been when Dawn was first diagnosed. This time things would be different. "I did the potty training, I got her out of diapers, all the shots, the doctor visits. We read together. Raquel likes to let Daisy help her cook. When we got her, she was rocking and pulling her hair out. She's stable now, mentally, physically, and emotionally."

Dawn's personal story also led her into political work. After leaving St. Mary's and throughout the decade during which my research team followed her, Dawn has been a prominent voice in the HIV community, a trusted leader. She has traveled the country speaking about HIV prevention, met with politicians to advocate for increased funding for AIDS programs and services, and served on the boards of some of the most prominent national and local HIV organizations. "I think my real work comes from being an activist and an advocate," she commented. "The only risky behavior that I do now is telling a politician what I really think of him."

As her political engagement built up both her confidence and her network, Dawn parlayed her volunteer work into paid employment in several human service organizations, addressing issues ranging from domestic violence to homelessness to HIV. She has worked as the assistant director of a small housing program, a case manager, and a personal assistant for other PLWHA.

Over the course of ten years, my research assistants and I would interview Dawn more than half a dozen times, tracing her health, social, economic, and political transformation.[10] When we met, her graying hair reflected a 20-year journey with HIV, which evolved into a 30-year journey by the time we conducted our last interviews with her in 2015. As of this writing, Daisy is 14 and thriving under Dawn's care. Sixteen years free of alcohol and illegal drugs, Dawn still bears the scars of her previous life, walking with a cane and struggling with a variety of old injuries. However, she has an undetectable viral load, indicating minimal presence of HIV in her bloodstream, which she controls with only one prescribed pill daily, a far cry from her once 25 -pill daily regimen.

Since the turning point that she experienced at St. Mary's, Dawn has embarked upon an extensive process of learning how to live with HIV, reluctantly but successfully weaving it into the fabric of her life. During one of our conversations, Dawn offered this challenging assessment: "If it weren't for HIV, I'd probably be dead."

REMAKING A LIFE AS A TRANSFORMATIVE PROJECT

Dawn's statement represents the fundamental puzzle at the center of this book. The admission may sound shocking, fodder for those who would use Dawn's words to dismiss or pathologize her. But it would be a mistake to interpret her comment as evidence of intrinsic deviance or as romanticizing or downplaying the devastation of AIDS. Her statement calls for a nuanced analysis that reveals what underlies such a challenging assertion, contextualizes it, and gleans important lessons. Her words are also deeply ironic: how can a life-threatening illness, responsible for the deaths of millions around the world, actually help *prevent* a death?

In Dawn's assertion, she is reflecting on the asphyxiating chokehold of drugs. Addiction, with its roots in her history of childhood sexual abuse, was shaping every aspect of Dawn's life, from her tools of economic survival to her residential choices to how she formulated, sustained, or damaged relationships with friends, family, and intimate partners. Dawn's broader environment, lacking many opportunities and resources, also posed obstacles that she addressed through a variety of coping and survival strategies that were destroying her health. Over time Dawn came to see that HIV would require her to manage her health differently if she had any chance of surviving. But addressing the diagnosis would also demand new ways to navigate the economic, psychological, and social hurdles that had previously hobbled her. HIV rendered Dawn's prior coping and survival strategies untenable. Acknowledging her past, Dawn nevertheless chose to create a future for herself by living another kind of life.

Talking with women living with HIV/AIDS (WLWHA) for more than a decade, I heard countless stories like Dawn's, the trauma and struggle perhaps not surprising given the devastation wrought by AIDS and the dynamics that fuel the epidemic. But I also heard stories of transformation. Women in my research talked about following a trajectory that began with *dying from* HIV/AIDS and took them to *living with* and even *thriving despite* HIV.[11] I became deeply curious as the number of transformation accounts grew. Were the women simply offering rationalizations and positive thinking to combat this potentially terminal disease? Was this merely a story about the effectiveness of highly active antiretroviral therapy (ART) and other medical discoveries? Or was something else happening—something that would shed light on the larger question of what it might take for us to ameliorate the wounds produced by social and economic disadvantage and psychological trauma?

Explaining transformation—what supports it, what obstructs it, and what happens when people are able to achieve it under difficult conditions—is the central goal of this book. We will bear witness to women's transitions from severe and compounding crises—the body blow of a health diagnosis that is at once life-threatening and highly stigmatizing, sexual trauma, chronic unemployment, homelessness, and drug addiction—to major successes such as dramatic improvements in health, the rebuilding of familial ties, hard-won economic stability, civic engagement, and leadership that speaks truth to power. We will compare and contrast these stories against a broader array of experiences among WLWHA to consider how social and economic marginalization (and privilege) cast a unique frame around an HIV diagnosis. Notably, the HIV diagnosis on its own was seldom the direct catalyst for radical life changes and transformation: a surrounding set of social processes drove the more profound shift that Dawn and others experienced.

Alongside the women's stories of transformation, this book therefore presents a second, equally important narrative of change. The companion story to the remarkable life transformations experienced by many of the women I follow in this book is the transformation, over the same period, of the epidemic that threatened their lives. The extraordinary conversion of HIV/AIDS from an inevitable death sentence to a manageable chronic illness in well-resourced countries like the United States is not only one of the most noteworthy medical achievements of the past 35 years, it is also a significant social achievement. AIDS activists and advocates on the front lines of the domestic and global response have confronted a deadly disease and battled a political climate that ranged from unequivocally hostile to dangerously complacent. They pushed the medical community and governments around the world to invest significant dollars in research and shaped a public dialogue that increased awareness and pushed HIV/ AIDS high up the list of societal concerns during some of the epidemic's most destructive periods.[12] Activists, advocates, and government officials drove important bipartisan policy gains, such as the Ryan White CARE Act, the AIDS Drug Assistance Program (ADAP), expansions of the Americans with Disabilities Act, the President's Emergency Plan for AIDS Relief (PEPFAR), and the National HIV/AIDS Strategy (NHAS). Perhaps one of the most important but under-recognized outcomes of this mobilization was the emergence of an extensive HIV safety net (HSN) of human service providers and other entities who would prove vital for individuals confronting difficult circumstances by offering four things: access to healthcare, modest economic assistance, extensive social support, and a path to political and civic engagement.

"If it weren't for HIV, I'd probably be dead." In fact, what undergirds Dawn's provocative comment is the community and infrastructure that afforded her the opportunities—and perhaps more importantly, the resources—to personally heal from, economically and socially navigate, and politically confront inequality, trauma, and their associated wounds. Dawn and many women like her had sustained so many blows throughout their lives that they were dying from their cumulative effects even before they were diagnosed with HIV. Rarely, if ever, had they been offered the kinds of openings that would give them the chance to repair these wounds. In the HIV/AIDS community, Dawn and others would find an unexpected place to create their lives anew.

Confronting Injuries of Inequality

Injuries of inequality—big and small wounds to personal, familial, and community well-being—represent the mental, physical, and social toll of acute inequity. They are the cumulative markers and scars of economic and social marginalization, the visible and invisible evidence of disadvantage.[13] Injuries of inequality have dimensions shaped by gender, race, class, and sexuality, as the likelihood of occurrence is not random but shaped by where we are on the social hierarchy. The brutal truth deserves emphasis: *Injuries of inequality produce, and are produced by, a compromised ability to protect oneself from harm.*

Scholars of social inequality have extensively analyzed the mechanisms that inflict injuries on disadvantaged groups through processes such as mass incarceration, residential segregation, and chronic unemployment. We document the injuries themselves and their short- and long-term implications by examining experiences and outcomes related to education, health, housing, and economic well-being. Researchers also consider how individuals and communities respond to these injuries, identifying processes of identity formation, everyday survival, struggles for mobility, and political resistance in a context of constraint and confinement.

But how do women remake, not simply rebuild, their lives after traumas produced by injuries of inequality? Rebuilding suggests a return to a prior state. Remaking, however, is much more dramatic; it is transformational. We often think of significant life transformations as highly personal and perhaps even spiritual experiences. In this book I argue that life transformations are also deeply *social* events—negotiated processes influenced by the people, places, and public policies that we encounter.

By analyzing the lives of women living with HIV/AIDS as they grapple with their pasts while creating a future, this book delineates what I term the *transformative project*. I define the transformative project as a multidimensional process by which individuals *fundamentally shift how they interpret, strategize around, and tactically address struggles related to complex inequalities that affect their everyday lives*. It entails adopting a radically different set of approaches to negotiating questions of physical, social, economic, and political survival. To remake their lives, women alter how they engage in interpersonal interactions, with institutions and communities, and even with public policy, to create meaningful change over time. The transformative project typically incorporates several meaningful changes in multiple arenas of life and thereby generates a new modus operandi. The transformative project represents one's active and purposeful physical, psychic, economic, and social restructuring after being pummeled by some of the harshest blows of racism, poverty, sexism, and homophobia.

At its core, the transformative project does not target personal transformation as an end in itself, what we commonly think of as "self-help." It is not about "fixing" alleged deficiencies. Nor is the transformative project a repackaged elixir of "bootstrapping" personal responsibility. Rather, the transformative project is about the integration of individual agency with environmental networks, institutions, and public policies. By charting that sociological process, including the resources women leverage and the barriers they confront, my work explicitly challenges the highly individualistic personal responsibility frame that dominates discourse about both HIV/AIDS and social/economic disadvantage. Therefore, this book analyzes how marginalized or stigmatized individuals use their power, however limited, to create dramatic and positive personal and social change while simultaneously engaging with the social, political, and economic conditions they seek to escape or alter.

The Launch of a Transformative Project

How did Dawn effect such a radical and dramatic change in the trajectory of her life? What accounts for her movement from *dying from*—a state of extreme physical, emotional, economic, and social distress—to *living with* and even *thriving despite,* in which she is taking a leadership role in her community, building a strong family, and significantly improving her physical and mental health? It would be tempting to say that once Dawn decided to change, her circumstances improved, but this explanation would be incomplete. Her story points instead to clear relationships among the cognitive shift that determined for Dawn that "something had to change," a set of institutional relationships and public policies that anchored and supported that shift, and a fresh modus operandi comprised of newly adopted economic, social, and health strategies that are sustained over time. These factors together appear to have been necessary conditions for the success of Dawn's transformative project, illustrated in figure 1.

Dawn suffered daunting injuries of inequality, from childhood sexual abuse to the frustrations and stresses of operating in a resource-deprived context in which her health, social incorporation, and economic prospects deteriorated with each dramatic turn of events. Life's traumas had become embodied, coursing through Dawn's mind, body, and spirit. Her cognitive shift came when she acknowledged that her coping and survival strategies— self-medicating and living on the streets—were killing her. Managing the pain and stress of living in a context of unrelenting injury had become exhausting:

> I wanted to do something different. Drugs were flowing freely in the neighborhood when I started getting high. At some point, they stopped flowing as freely, and I had to get out and hustle for them. And that got old. I guess if I had not had the mindset to want to do better, I'd probably either be dead or still locked there in my addiction. Because there's a lot of women who couldn't handle the frustration or the pressure that being in a sober environment 24/7 would put on them, and they would just disappear. So you definitely have to have your mind made up.

Nevertheless, it took more than a change in mindset to transform Dawn's situation. Along with the medical and pharmacological discoveries that evolved in the decades since Dawn's initial HIV diagnosis, a safety net

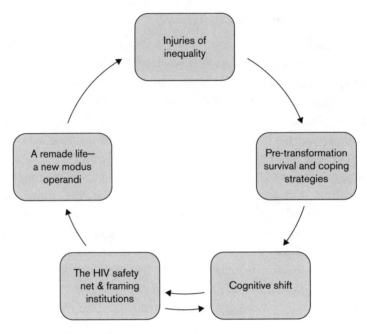

Figure 1. The transformative project.

emerged that offered Dawn new strategies and tools for confronting the deadly triad of sexual trauma, poverty, and HIV/AIDS that illegal drugs no longer helped her escape. Perhaps the deadly risk of AIDS created the final spark of urgency, but it was the institutional infrastructure that supported the change.

As a part of the HIV safety net, St. Mary's provided a roof over Dawn's head for two years as she embarked on her transformative project and reconstituted the pieces of her life. It surrounded her with people who were struggling through transformations of their own, allowing her to meet Raquel, who would become a major source of support. As an institutional broker, St. Mary's also connected Dawn with a network of HIV service providers who would help her survive physically by introducing her to a physician who perfected her HIV medication regimen, survive economically by assigning her a case manager who helped her access financial resources, and survive socially by connecting her to HIV support groups.[14] Those relationships then facilitated her entrée into the city's

AIDS activist and advocate network, which she used to achieve a measure of political influence and economic opportunities.

Support from those institutional relationships gave Dawn the freedom she needed to explore different pathways, validate her newfound operating approach, and sustain it over time as her new modus operandi. Consider that when they left St. Mary's in 2001, Dawn and Raquel had to find a place to live. A local AIDS organization provided Raquel with a subsidized housing voucher via lottery and renewed the assistance for more than a decade, reducing their rent in 2015 from $750 to $375 per month. Dawn's case manager helped them find an apartment on the north side of Chicago, a short train ride from Boystown, home to many in Chicago's LGBTQ community and a cluster of AIDS service organizations. Residential migration from the far south and west sides of Chicago to the north and near south side of town occurs fairly commonly among the WLWHA in this book, as they gravitate toward their institutional support services.[15] Dawn's relocation from her former neighborhoods would unfortunately take her away from her community just as she was beginning to thrive, yet it also meant moving away from memories of her life as an addict and those who did not necessarily support her new path.

After settling the issue of long-term housing, Dawn adopted additional health-management strategies. From their new apartment she and Raquel were able to move throughout the city using free bus and subway cards courtesy of Dawn's case manager at St. Mary's. This helped Dawn and Raquel make doctor's appointments, attend support group meetings, and buy groceries. The physician who prescribed a viable medication regimen when Dawn was at St. Mary's referred her to specialists to address some of her other health concerns, all of which were covered by Medicaid. Dawn then began seeing a therapist, working hard to repair the emotional injuries and process the sexual violence she had experienced.

As former participants in the drug economy, Dawn and Raquel next had to fashion less risky economic survival strategies. Raquel's health challenges qualified her for Social Security disability assistance. Dawn worked in several nonprofits until chronic and severe back and hip pain qualified her for Social Security disability benefits as well, albeit after a long fight to demonstrate her eligibility. Like many women we will meet in this book, Dawn also leveraged her experiential capital. She utilized the knowledge and wisdom derived from traumatic events to lend her voice to the HIV/AIDS advocacy community, generating speaking engagements and volunteering to participate in research studies that offered stipends.

To be sure, Dawn describes her family even now as living "barely above the federal poverty level," and life is by no means easy. Nevertheless, Dawn's new financial strategies offered greater physical safety and a fundamentally new approach to managing economic stress:

> It's like my sponsor says, the devil tries everything to get you to come back to his way, but he doesn't have any new tricks. I had my car repossessed last night. . . . That's an old trick, I'm not falling for it. [Back then], I didn't have money for rent, credit cards, light, gas, car note, any of that, and I just gave it all up to get high. Wander the streets and be homeless, but at least I had no responsibilities. But I also had very little contact with my children. So it's just not worth it. I'm just not there today . . . been there, done that.

Notably we are not observing socioeconomic mobility here, marked by substantial gains in education, income, or wealth that sociologists typically count as legitimate mobility. Rather, Dawn's mobility is animated by a transition from *dying from* to *living with* injuries of inequality, including HIV. The transformation enhanced Dawn's social status through her community work. Most importantly, however, it generated improvements in well-being, with better housing, a consistent source of income, improved physical and psychological health, and socially supportive relationships. Once she reached this level of stability, Dawn was much better equipped not simply to cope with but also to confront injuries of inequality by supporting other marginalized women and by becoming politically active.

The area of Dawn's life that seems the hardest to repair and remake, a place where her transformative project has its limits, involves her relationships with her biological children. She worked hard to reconnect with them after getting clean. Chyna, now 28, played an important role, serving as the family's anchor by keeping in touch with her siblings while their mother struggled for all those years. As the child who had the most extensive contact with Dawn growing up, Chyna "saw a lot of stuff, and I had to explain a lot of stuff," Dawn lamented. The family is just beginning to talk about the trauma—sexual and otherwise—that Dawn's children experienced as they were moved from home to home as children. Dawn cannot discuss the pain and guilt of that reality without becoming emotional.

Dawn's sons, now 35 and 33 years old, and her other daughter, now 22, each engage with her very differently. None of Dawn's children is HIV positive. When her oldest son Damon learned of Dawn's status from a gossiping relative, he dismissively told his mother that he could have gone his entire life without finding out. Her youngest son Devon is also unwilling to talk about it, but he will occasionally check in to ask if Dawn is taking her meds and will visit to see how she's feeling. Twenty-two-year-old Delisha lives in another state. During one of our last interviews in 2015, Dawn had just returned from visiting Delisha, who allowed her daughter Talia to travel with Dawn back to Chicago to visit the rest of the family in the city, an encouraging show of trust.

Dawn did not glean positive results from all of her institutional relationships. In some instances, institutions failed. For example, the prison where Dawn spent years knowing that she was HIV positive gave her little information about the illness, and the homeless shelter appeared to have no protocols in place to assist clients with HIV/AIDS. Later in the book we will explore how institutional failings threaten to undermine transformative projects.

We see in Dawn's case, however, many more instances in which institutions played pivotal and positive roles in her transformation. I once asked Dawn to recall a time in her life when she felt most accepted as a WLWHA. She described being elected to the city's HIV Planning Council, a federally mandated advisory group of service providers, public health officials, and affected community members that establishes service priorities for allocating Ryan White CARE Act Title I funds.[16] These dollars provide medical and social support services for PLWHA: "With the planning council, it didn't really matter that I was HIV positive," she explained. "It was important, obviously, but not as important as who I was and what my capabilities were. Plus you get elected by the other people that are on that body, and they've got to think a lot about you to make you one of the spokespersons on HIV for the entire city." After surviving sexual abuse, homelessness, drug addiction, and sex work in a community struggling with its own trauma, Dawn has remade her life.

TOWARD A SOCIOLOGY OF THE
TRANSFORMATIVE PROJECT

Many narratives of the lives of the "truly disadvantaged" adopt the metaphor of being "stuck," which is understandable given the massive structural forces that conspire against economic and social mobility for these individuals.[17] The dynamic changes in life trajectory that people seek are not, however, confined to gains in education or income. What do we miss when we fail to account for other kinds of major shifts in the lives of those who have suffered massive injuries of inequality? The movement from *dying from* to *living with*, which entails radically reconfiguring physical, emotional, economic, political, and social survival strategies to grow and achieve a new level of stability, is not limited to WLWHA. Such a framework can help us understand how many individuals resist marginalization.

A growing body of social science literature captures life transformations in disadvantaged contexts, such as Edward Orozco Flores's *God's Gangs*, Laurence Ralph's *Renegade Dreams*, Rob Sampson and John Laub's "Desistance from Crime over the Life Course," and Sharon Oselin's *Leaving Prostitution*.[18] While not yet explicitly advancing what I term a sociology of transformative projects, these texts nevertheless share several features that contribute to my framework. First, they identify significant environmental challenges that constrain everyday life and long-term opportunity and demonstrate how those forces inflict injuries of inequality upon those in their path. Next, they explicate the adaptations of individuals living under these conditions and explain how their adopted strategies further undermine quality of life and life opportunities. Some behaviors, such as gun violence and drug dealing, are illegal. Others, such as certain sexual behaviors, are not illegal but are high risk.[19] These strategies prove threatening to individual health as well as to the overall health of families and communities.

This scholarship diverges from much of the urban poverty and inequality literature by focusing on the social processes through which these same individuals later seek out alternative strategies and ways of being after previously adopted practices become problematic. Orozco Flores documents, for example, the processes by which young Latino gang members—immigrants or the descendants of immigrants struggling to make it in postindustrial Los Angeles—exit gang life by cultivating a reformed barrio masculinity through religiously oriented recovery programs. The men advance "redemption scripts," describing their transformations in their own terms and carving out new spaces of legitimacy in a social context that often pushes them to the margins. To be sure, texts that document what I am calling transformative projects explicitly and implicitly challenge explanations that posit a pathology that must be "fixed." Through nuanced ethnographic work, these authors show how transformation efforts—like the originally adopted strategies—are deeply embedded in context, and the authors emphasize both policies and conditions that marginalize and those that facilitate positive movement.

These studies documenting life transformations offer valuable evidence of their potential to improve lives, but we lack an overarching theory or conceptual framework that captures this process of transformation across injuries of inequality. Although the "crisis points" may differ—an HIV diagnosis, incarceration, a life-threatening gunshot wound—the similarities between the underlying causes and the dynamic process of dramatically changing one's strategies after a life-altering and traumatic event beg for a more systematic explanation. More specifically, we must shift away from life transformation narratives that focus solely on the individual. From the truly disadvantaged to the "one percent," the structural scaffolding on which transformations are built is too often masked, providing the false impression that the individual is the sole architect of the change we witness.

I believe that the transformative project framework can help us understand many situations in which individuals radically restructure their lives. These undertakings represent the integration of agency—beliefs, strategies, and action to inspire radical life change—with environmental networks, institutions, and public policies that support these efforts. Yet we can distinguish transformative projects from other major life shifts insofar as the restructuring alters how one responds to and navigates complex inequality. The framework is therefore a theory about power relations, revealing how individuals shift their responses to social marginalization at the societal, institutional, and interpersonal levels.

Is a life-threatening condition a necessary antecedent to a transformative project? No, as any individual who embarks on a deliberate effort to improve upon the strategies they have used in the past to confront inequality is engaged in a transformative project as long as we see evidence of a cognitive shift; engagement with people, institutions, and policies that provide new strategies, networks, and resources; and a fresh modus operandi. It is likely, however, that a life-threatening issue heightens the urgency and stakes involved in such a transformation.

Remaking a Life therefore addresses central questions in sociology, public policy studies, public health, African American Studies, social work, and gender and sexuality studies by exploring the complex relationship between social, economic, and political inequality and health; the emergence of effective safety nets in sometimes unexpected places; and the radical possibility that those suffering from marginalization might imagine and experience their lives anew after devastating and multiplicative injury. It is often through this reimagining and reshaping process that some of the most effective organizers, thoughtful critics, and energized community leaders emerge.

As I explicate the sociology of transformative projects and unpack the mechanisms that drive this process, I use an intersectional lens.[20] Black feminist and legal scholar Kimberlé Crenshaw is widely credited with coining the term *intersectionality*, building on the work of feminists of color who challenged single-category thinking about identity and group status and emphasized how race, class, gender, sexuality, and other social identities operate simultaneously to shape individual social experiences and large-scale societal dynamics.[21] An intersectional approach reveals interlocking power dynamics and demonstrates how they are shaped by our societal approach to sameness (embrace) and difference (hostility).[22]

Scholars have conceptualized intersectionality as a theory of power relations, a methodological imperative to uncover interlocking inequalities, and a political perspective that resists oppression in all forms.[23] With its roots in black feminist scholarship and activism, intersectionality allows us to present robust theoretical and empirical analyses of identity, representation, and narrative, especially as they manifest in the lives of marginalized populations.[24] These three themes will arise often here, as a common goal of intersectional work is to critique powerful public discourses and stereotypes that limit and distort the realities of women, people of color, LGBTQ individuals, low-income people, PLWHA, and any others who inhabit multiple marginalized statuses. The concept operates in several disciplines, including legal studies, sociology, public health, ethnic studies, gender studies, queer studies, history, psychology, social work, and anthropology. It is also a driving principle of feminism and other forms of activism and will emerge in this book as an important value and tension point within AIDS mobilization.

While this book documents and analyzes several impressive transformative projects, it also highlights the hurdles and obstacles associated with these transformations. In spite of the agency that the women with whom I spoke exercised, racism, sexism, poverty, homophobia, and HIV stigma remain powerful forces, shaping their opportunities and experiences. Women's progress in transforming their lives does not inoculate them from the punishing hurdles that continue to confront them. Moreover, they continue to cope with a serious health issue that can kill them if not appropriately managed. For all these reasons, the process of remaking a life is not rapid or linear. Rather, it is best characterized by fits and starts, periods of marked improvement followed by crushing setbacks. In this book, I demonstrate the hard work involved in testing and struggling with new strategies. Moreover, some women we will meet were unable to move beyond the shock of diagnosis and other traumas to launch successful transformative projects. In those cases, I attempt to explain why they remained locked in destructive and heart-wrenching patterns.

Notably, therefore, *Remaking a Life* is not a story about upward mobility, a well-trod area in sociology and other disciplines. The women in this book by and large do not experience major leaps in socioeconomic status. But many *do* experience a noteworthy and radical movement from social, and in many cases almost physical, *death* to a *life* in which they are much more stable and better positioned to confront structural barriers in their paths. Their survival represents a form of resistance as they have cheated a presumed "death sentence" and withstood additional traumas that threatened to destroy them. Such movements in life trajectories are grossly under-analyzed in the sociological literature despite their fairly frequent occurrence. With my theory I therefore attempt to recognize the agency of social actors living in difficult contexts, highlight and account for the possibility of dynamic and significant change in the lives of stigmatized individuals that disrupts the narrative of stasis, and analyze the policy and institutional infrastructure that facilitates (and sometimes undermines) these transformations.

STUDYING THE HIV/AIDS EPIDEMIC

For years, I have been intellectually and socially engaged in the continuing struggle against the AIDS epidemic. In the late 1990s, I was working on a project exploring the effects of the 1996 welfare reform legislation on the lives of low-income women, and one of the women whom I interviewed several times was living with HIV. Although I would develop the terminology to describe what I was observing later, I immediately understood HIV/AIDS as an injury of inequality, as those most affected were often already marginalized. But I was also struck by how her social networks, institutional ties, and access to resources differed so markedly from those of other low-income women in our sample. The seed was planted that I might be observing a safety net in action that was very different from the weakening welfare system, one that represented an alternative approach to offering support to vulnerable populations.

In 2005, while completing my book on the welfare system (*The New Welfare Bureaucrats*), I began conducting interviews and participant observation with black cisgender women living with HIV/AIDS (WLWHA) in Chicago. Over the course of a decade, my research team and I expanded this work, culminating in interviews with over 100 WLWHA of diverse racial, ethnic, class, and sexual identities and backgrounds in Chicago. We also conducted interviews with over 75 AIDS activists, advocates, policy officials, and service providers working at both the local and national levels.

By analyzing a series of transformative projects, this book captures how women have fought for survival in the epidemic and claimed their space in the organized AIDS response. Although the virus was understood in the beginning as a "gay man's disease" in places like the US, women constitute *more than half* of all adults living with HIV/AIDS worldwide.[25] Yet, historically, they have not been centered in global research, prevention and treatment initiatives, or AIDS policy. This is especially so in the United States, where women currently account for one in five new HIV diagnoses and deaths caused by AIDS.[26] I focus on women to highlight and analyze their role and significance, not only as PLWHA but also as steadfast and effective (but largely unacknowledged) advocates, activists, policy officials, and service providers in the epidemic from the earliest recognition of the disease.

Black women have been disproportionately affected by the HIV/AIDS epidemic. In January 1983, when the Centers for Disease Control and Prevention (CDC) documented the first two cases of AIDS in women, one woman was black and the other was Latinx.[27] When I began this research in 2005, black women comprised 37 percent of Chicago's female population, but they accounted for 80 percent of female HIV diagnoses; and HIV/AIDS was the number-one cause of death for black women aged 25 to 34.[28]

More than a decade later, racial disparities persist. Among all US women with HIV diagnoses in 2015, 61 percent (4,524) were African American, 19 percent (1,431) were white, and 15 percent (1,131) were Latinx. That year, HIV/AIDS was the fourth leading cause of death among black women ages 35 to 44, before diabetes, stroke, and homicide. Younger generations of black women continue to be affected, as HIV/AIDS remains one of the leading causes of death among those in their twenties and early thirties, while women from other racial backgrounds have fortunately seen the illness drop below their top ten leading causes of death.[29] Black women have also been unsung leaders and foot soldiers in HIV/AIDS activist and advocacy work. For these reasons, their experiences constitute a central part of this analysis. *Remaking a Life* takes readers deep into the lives of four black women to trace the what, why, and how of transformative projects using data collected through more than ten years of engagement, from 2005 into 2015. Dawn's story is presented in this chapter; in subsequent chapters I present the stories of Keisha, Beverly, and Yvette.

Many women living with HIV/AIDS have experienced multiple injuries of inequality. For them, the diagnosis was unceremoniously added to a long list of urgent concerns. For other women, the HIV diagnosis is a stunning setback, an experience that contradicts the relatively smooth trajectory they believed they were following. They come from a range of racial and ethnic backgrounds. Many do not have histories of drug use or sex work. Some are quite well-off economically, with high levels of education and white-collar jobs. Others contend with the added dimension of immigration status as they seek assistance to address health concerns. Hearing from a diverse group of women enables us to consider what it means to confront HIV and other difficult life events from multiple vantage points.

Therefore, in addition to Keisha, Beverly, and Yvette, we will also follow Trisha, a white Canadian immigrant who launched a transformative project after the trauma of childhood sexual abuse, and Rosario, a Latina whose experiences were also shaped by her engagement with the HIV safety net. Alongside these central storytellers, I present the words of other interviewed women throughout the book. I also offer my observations as I accompanied some interviewees to medical appointments and support group meetings, sat in the audience during speaking engagements when they told their stories, and visited them in their homes. All of these women had to consider whether and how to transition from believing and behaving as though they have been given a death sentence at diagnosis to interpreting and coping with HIV as a chronic but manageable illness. As they reflect on the physical, social, economic, and political impact of HIV/AIDS on their lives, we will see how the disease's imprint extends well beyond the issue of health.

Remaking a Life uses the case of HIV/AIDS to advance a conceptual and policy framework for improving women's social well-being. The creation of what I call the HIV safety net, as a political and institutional response to human crisis, is noteworthy for the lessons that it offers. The HIV safety net funnels medical care, social services, and opportunities for political engagement to people living with HIV/AIDS and those at higher risk of contracting the disease. Undergirded by the initial mobilization and support of activists, the HIV safety net now functions through a three-sector partnership (public, private, and nonprofit) and provides a supportive infrastructure to combat the disease. My research therefore would not be complete without talking to some of the people who constitute the safety net, with a special focus on those fighting the epidemic among women. In addition to their interviews, I also conducted participant observation by attending HIV/AIDS conferences, meetings, and public presentations in which members of this community were actively discussing and shaping the AIDS policy agenda. These interviews and observations locate the experiences of WLWHA within a broader institutional and policy context. I regret that I could not speak to every activist, advocate, policy official, and service provider who played a crucial role in the development and growth of the HIV safety net.[30] My hope is, however, that this book, through the stories represented, offers a sense of the collective that built the AIDS response. Further, while the HIV safety net operates all over the world as part of the global fight against the epidemic, this book focuses on the US context, with its unique political, social, and economic specificities.

It is important to note that both cisgender and transgender women have historically struggled to have their voices and needs included in the AIDS response. Cisgender women are women whose sense of personal identity and gender corresponds with their birth sex. Transgender women are women whose sense of personal identity and gender does not correspond with their birth sex. Estimates suggest that transgender women have an overall HIV seroprevalence rate of 28 percent, with extremely high occurrence rates (56 percent) among black transgender women.[31] Transgender women, when included, have often been grouped with gay men in the research, service provision, and political activism related to the epidemic.[32] This approach clearly suffers from limitations, as it does not address the unique struggles of transgender women and conflates sexual and gender identity. This can elide the ways in which the benefits of advances in AIDS services, information, and treatments have eluded transgender women as compared with gay men.

In recent years, we have witnessed a seismic shift in societal understandings of transgender individuals, due in no small part to their growing media presence and political activism.[33] For example, when I began this project in 2005, it was not uncommon to focus a study of women living with HIV/AIDS exclusively on cisgender women. I followed that convention when I conducted interviews with Chicago WLWHA. However, during the later stages of my data collection, I interviewed transgender activists to ask whether and how the HIV/AIDS safety net has evolved to become more responsive to the needs of transgender women.

My multilayered approach enables us to examine women's stories of transformation (with their successes and limitations) against the backdrop of the transformation of the AIDS epidemic and the organized AIDS response (with its successes and limitations). To preserve confidentiality, I use pseudonyms for all Chicago WLWHA and the people who appear in their narratives, but in discussions of the social history of the AIDS response, I use real names to reference the activists, advocates, policy officials, and service providers with national profiles in the AIDS community. I present additional methodological details in appendix A. Tables capturing the book's featured storytellers and additional demographic information about the Chicago women can be found in appendix B. Photos of several referenced activists and advocates are at remakingalife.org

OVERVIEW

The chapters of *Remaking a Life* move between the perspectives and personal lives of the Chicago women and those of advocates, activists, policy-makers, and service providers who work on the issue of HIV/AIDS at the national, state, and local levels. In chapter 1, I explain the context that creates the impetus for women's transformative projects, the state of extreme distress that I have termed *dying from*. Women with this status are destabilized in multiple areas of their lives—physical and mental health, family, finances, housing, intimate relationships, self-esteem, and so on—and have suffered to the point that these life domains are interdependently undermining one another. An HIV diagnosis can both initiate and serve as an indicator of this state of *dying from*, and WLWHA believe and behave as though they have death sentences.

In this chapter, I also trace the epidemiological history of the AIDS epidemic in the United States to help us understand the women's health risks. The women in my study describe a variety of events that might have exposed them to HIV, including sexual activity, intravenous drug use, and blood transfusions that were received before the advent of protocols for screening the nation's blood supply for HIV. For an alarming number of women, experiences with early sexual trauma likely contributed to pathways that later increased their risk for HIV infection. I also examine HIV's continuing devastating and disproportionate impact on women entangled in, or in close geographic or social proximity to, the sexualized drug economy. Legal and illegal drugs, in conjunction with an unevenly applied spike in incarceration, increase women's exposure to sexual and social networks that put them at higher risk for contracting HIV. In Chicago, the sexualized drug economy has arguably had the most devastating and visible impact on black and Latinx communities; however, a growing opioid drug epidemic in the United States, including and especially within white rural and suburban communities, demonstrates that economically depressed communities in general are especially vulnerable to this threat.

Chapter 2 charts the rise of the safety net that emerged in response to the AIDS epidemic in the 1980s. I consider how multiple stakeholders eventually coalesced after initial conflicts to create an infrastructure targeted toward HIV/AIDS prevention and treatment. Adopting an intersectional approach in chapter 2 helps to explain why the institutional response to HIV has taken form as it has. In light of the growing economic, cultural, and political clout of white, middle-class gay men, I point to how the AIDS response was powerfully fueled by both the privilege and marginalization experienced by this group. They passionately demanded and received resources, with their status as white men bolstering their claims and opening doors that were clearly shut to black and brown people suffering from the same disease. Simultaneously, the need to offer safe spaces that provided respite from crushing homophobia and other forms of stigmatization was programmed into the DNA of many institutions that emerged from AIDS activism, and this ethos would prove extremely attractive to many women seeking to address their own injuries. Challenges facing women, poor people, gay men of color, and transgender individuals pushed the ethos surrounding AIDS mobilization even further as these segments of the community demanded racial, gender, and class diversity, inclusivity, and parity in the plans, policies, practices, and spokespeople that constituted the growing safety net. I therefore argue that part of the success and the struggle of the AIDS response is that social privilege and marginalization are embedded in the movement in a constant collaborative tension. Emerging from these contests and confrontations, the AIDS community has produced a structure and culture of care that differs markedly from many other models of human service delivery and creates a space for women to remake their lives.

Chapter 3 returns to the Chicago women and begins to chart the specific components of the transformative projects that my research team and I observed. I illustrate how framing institutions within the HIV safety net are vital to the process of remaking a life.[34] These organizations can positively or negatively frame what it means to live with HIV by offering critical information about HIV as a medical diagnosis and social status; language with which to talk about HIV and its implications for women's lives; and resources and networks that help or hinder women in restructuring post-diagnosis life. As institutional brokers, framing institutions are often invisible to those who do not rely on them but critically important to those who do. In addition to implementing programs, distributing resources, and facilitating everyday social encounters that may not otherwise occur, the most effective institutional interactions help women generate new thinking about their lives, a cognitive shift that helps them realize that "something has to change."

I capture how the women then begin to generate alternative strategies for navigating the entrenched environmental hurdles and widening social inequalities that initially put them at risk for acquiring HIV. This chapter and the next also consider which characteristics, of both individuals and organizations, are more likely to anchor (or undermine) a transformative project.

In chapter 3 I also address the limitations of framing institutions within the HIV safety net. For example, engaging with the HIV/AIDS community has varying class-based implications for women, as public association often improves the social status of impoverished and working-class women while diminishing that of middle-class women, who are deeply concerned about the stigma of identification. Overall, middle-class women report less engagement with the HIV safety net, and they possess fewer social ties with service providers and other PLWHA on whom they can rely for HIV-related information and support. Ironically, this renders middle-class WLWHA more vulnerable to HIV-specific social isolation than their poorer counterparts who engage with the HIV safety net.

Recent findings from three major studies play a major role in informing HIV service delivery: continuous antiretroviral treatment is superior to episodic ART, early ART take-up reduces HIV transmission to uninfected sexual partners by 93 percent, and early ART take-up reduces serious illness and death among PLWHA by 57 percent.[35] This wave of research led the CDC to announce in 2017 that "people who take ART daily as prescribed and achieve and maintain an undetectable viral load have effectively no risk of sexually transmitting the virus to an HIV-negative partner."[36] In chapter 4, I argue that the HIV safety net plays an important, if underappreciated, role in our ability to fully exploit these discoveries and curb the epidemic through this test-and-treat revolution. I demonstrate that women's ties to the HIV safety net are vital to the effective implementation of test-and-treat in health care settings, and I highlight opportunities at the individual, institutional, and structural levels that could further maximize our substantial financial and social investments in treating and preventing HIV/AIDS. In short, investing in the HIV safety net not only encourages and supports women's transformative projects, it could also facilitate the end of the epidemic.

A successful transformative project is sustainable over time. Women often confront their greatest challenges after they have left the supportive and protective setting of framing institutions within the HIV safety net. In chapter 5, we return to the central storytellers—Beverly, Keisha, Yvette, Trisha, and Rosario—to examine the longer-term reconstruction and maintenance of their remade lives. WLWHA often produce new identities and self-narratives after undergoing change that they then operationalize. They must grapple not only with the difficult work of HIV-status disclosure but also decide how they will answer questions about past relationships, behaviors, and struggles. Sexual relationships take on new significance, and many women still grapple with the afterlife of sexual trauma and the symbolic labeling of their bodies as "contaminated" with an HIV diagnosis, despite the clear medical advances. Some have assumed leadership roles in families, organizations, and communities and must navigate these new dimensions of their social and political lives even while reconciling with the stigma and "status" that result from being HIV positive. Overall, this chapter analyzes how individuals attempting transformation renegotiate their social roles as women, mothers, intimate partners, family members, friends, political actors, and economic providers over time.

In the final chapter of *Remaking a Life,* I contemplate the implications of changing policy environments, advances in the treatment of HIV/AIDS, and other potential shifts in the epidemic for the political and social viability of the HIV safety net. With medical developments that have transformed HIV/AIDS from a terminal to chronic illness, stabilizing infection rates among certain populations, declining political mobilization, and waning public interest, many have questioned why the HIV safety net should continue to enjoy access to government resources through the Ryan White CARE Act and other policies. But the public's sense of crisis that helped define the 1980s and 1990s has subsided in part because of the gains that have been achieved. I make the case in this chapter that we must ensure that the HIV safety net continues to receive resources to sustain the successes and address ongoing challenges that allow the epidemic to stubbornly persist in some of our most vulnerable communities. Moreover, the infectious nature of the disease requires vigilance from all of us. The AIDS response therefore must be tenacious and robust, sensitive to both the inequality and the universality that drive the epidemic.

In the book's concluding chapter, I also grapple with the unfortunate irony of my analysis and its policy implications. Access to the safety net that enabled women to achieve significant and sustained life change depended on their being HIV positive. This is a sobering reality. It suggests that our societal safety net has been perversely shaped to intervene only when people are already deeply injured or assumed to pose a threat to public health, rather than playing a preventive role, insofar as the determining factor allowing women to access the social safety net was not need but a serious, transmittable, and perhaps deadly health threat.[37] The fire had to be raging before we installed the fire extinguisher.

Nevertheless, the HIV/AIDS safety net should be viewed as a model for confronting rising inequality through multidimensional and empathetic public policy. AIDS activists and advocates deserve a great deal of credit for creating a life-saving infrastructure in several major cities and helping to transform the AIDS epidemic in the United States. I conclude my analysis by underscoring its potential as a prototype for how we might assist a broader segment of the public—not just those living with HIV/AIDS—by highlighting the most important lessons from the AIDS response. We would never imagine creating a system that perversely incentivizes having HIV, and I note at the outset that none of the more than 100 women interviewed by my team over 15 years of conducting this research stated that she acquired HIV to access the HSN. The key nonetheless is to offer services to a broader array of individuals as a preventive strategy against injuries of inequality like HIV. The combination of access to healthcare, modest economic assistance, extensive social support, and an on-ramp to political and civic participation offered by the HIV safety net offers powerful lessons regarding how we can help individuals recover from some of inequality's harshest blows. Implemented in tandem with approaches that seek to reduce economic and social inequities and prevent their related injuries, effective safety nets can create opportunities that enable individuals to successfully launch transformative projects. The AIDS response demonstrates that the chance to remake our lives following tragedy and trauma should not be reserved for the most privileged among us.

CODA

Ten years after we first met her and 30 years since her initial HIV-positive diagnosis, Dawn continues remaking her life. She was recently approved through Medicare for back surgery that she hopes, if successful, will return her to the world of paid employment. Daisy is starting high school. Raising the girl as she approached her teenage years encouraged Dawn to draw on her own traumatic experiences and to use them constructively in her parenting practices. Dawn carefully manages where Daisy goes and with whom she socializes, reducing sleepovers to the homes of only a select few friends and monitoring Daisy's cell phone communication.

Dawn knows that her life as a WLWHA could have turned out much differently. Consider a story that she shares during her speaking engagements as she tells listeners what became of Jackie, the favorite stepsister who first introduced Dawn to intravenous drugs: "There are many things that you can do with your family. . . . My stepsister and I used to get high together, and we were both intravenous drug users. We shared a lot, including the HIV virus." Sadly, Jackie lost her battle with AIDS. She participated in the AIDS community with Dawn for a while, forging her own attempt at a transformation. "But, I guess it just wasn't enough for her," Dawn stated, her eyes lowering, "so she went back out there. And she didn't make it back."

When we first spoke in 2005, Dawn shared her biggest concern: the transformed lives that she and Raquel had built depended heavily on the support they offered each other. "I told Raquel time and time again, she relies on me too much. And I've asked her, 'What are you going to do if something happens to me? You need to become more independent.'"

Tragically, it would be Dawn who would hold the hand of a dying loved one. Raquel started having headaches in 2012. A CAT scan revealed stage IV cancer. "They gave her six months, and we're like, 'Yeah, right, y'all don't know Raquel,'" Dawn explained as she fought back tears. "She made it a year and a half. She fought until we told her, 'You know, you really don't have to do this for us, we got this. . . . ' We don't. But we told her that we could manage."

Losing the love of her life would be the ultimate test of Dawn's transformative project. "When she died, I was like, what will I do now? I felt lost. I understand what it means to feel lost and broken." She withdrew from much of her AIDS work, in part because raising Daisy consumes more and more of her time. Yet she still maintains a connection to that community, holding a seat on an AIDS community advisory board. She also gives back to those just starting their transformative journeys: "In my old HIV support group, [I keep in touch with] ten of us left from the original batch who started our services at that agency. So, once a year, we all just converge on the HIV support group meeting and let folks know that we've been around since the mid-80s, and don't give up. It's kind of like reunion time." Dawn has never forgotten the role that those institutional ties played, including introducing her to the love of her life and helping her anchor a new life for herself.

In the decade during which I followed her, Dawn not only maintained her strategies for negotiating challenges but also took additional steps in her transformative journey. This includes a very special one. She started the process of legally adopting Daisy: "She is my daughter. I raised her. Unfortunately, she has my and Raquel's attitude [laughs]. And she is highly sensitive to people who are ignorant about HIV/AIDS. So yeah, she's our daughter, mine and Raquel's."

1 Dying From

SEXUAL VIOLENCE, THE DRUG ECONOMY,
AND THE PERSISTENCE OF HIV/AIDS

Austin, Indiana, a rural city located about 80 miles south of Indianapolis, is home to approximately 4,200 people, 97 percent of whom are white. In January 2015, public health officials began investigating an outbreak of HIV that grew at an alarming rate, with 191 confirmed new cases by 2016.[1] Women accounted for almost half of those diagnosed.[2] The rise in new infections was traced to several factors, including an opiate abuse epidemic, poverty, and a weak local healthcare system.[3] Austin's surrounding Scott County registered the highest per capita use of OxyContin in the state.[4] High intravenous use of heroin and oxymorphone added to the crisis.

In 2015, approximately 6 percent (2,392) of the 39,513 HIV diagnoses in the United States were attributed to intravenous drug use.[5] HIV can survive for up to 28 days in a syringe, and many public health officials have recommended needle-exchange programs as a scientifically validated method of preventing the spread of HIV and hepatitis.[6] Such programs were, however, banned in Indiana, and the practice of sharing and reusing syringes was common in Austin. The *IndyStar* painted a grim picture: "Some users shoot up alongside their children or even their children's children. In the winter, as many as 20 users may huddle in a home, gathering in the one building that has heat for the day. The power of addiction is so great that even the sensation of a prick from an empty needle can bring relief."[7]

Dire community conditions were both caused and accelerated by the twin epidemics of drug addiction and HIV. In 2015, Austin's median household income of $33,000 trailed the state's median of $48,000. While the statewide poverty rate was 15.9 percent, 26 percent of Austin's residents were living in poverty.[8] Empty storefronts and boarded-up homes dotted the landscape. Austin's chief of police, Donald Spicer, included the city's "lack of opportunity, too few jobs, few resources, and few things to do" among the root causes of the city's drug epidemic. The state had slashed funding for public health in recent years and delayed expansion of its Medicaid program legislated by the Affordable Care Act. Moreover, Scott County closed its remaining HIV-testing clinic in early 2013.[9] The local health department offered HIV testing, but its unfortunate location next to the police station no doubt sent an ominous message to anyone grappling with a drug problem or fearful of Indiana's robust and punitive HIV-criminalization laws.[10] Although additional testing and HIV-related social services were available just five miles away, many residents lacked transportation or health insurance. "We saw this coming a long time ago," Dr. William Cooke, one of Austin's only physicians, told the *Chicago Tribune.* "We've been asking for help for some time."[11] After mounting pressure from public health and local law enforcement officials, then governor and now vice president Mike Pence, a staunch conservative and fierce opponent of needle-exchange programs, declared the outbreak a state of emergency and issued an executive order that authorized a targeted, 30-day emergency needle-exchange program.

The Scott County case—in which an HIV outbreak both reflected and capitalized on a community's economic, political, and social vulnerabilities—is by no means unique. The transmission of the virus occurs most frequently in the United States through sexual intercourse and, to a much lesser extent, the sharing of needles during intravenous drug use. People generally engage in these behaviors through relationships, and those relationships are embedded in social networks. Like so many social processes, as HIV travels within and across social circles, the communities in which we live and the relationships that we have can facilitate or minimize our risk of contracting the disease.[12] Two women can have identical histories of drug use and identical numbers of sexual partners, but the woman who traverses a social network with a higher HIV rate is more likely to contract the virus. Networks are unequal in their capacity to prevent an infectious disease from entering and spreading. Networks whose members are well informed about HIV, have access to regular testing, and use prevention tools such as condoms, clean needles, and antiretrovirals are more likely to experience low levels of transmission. Therefore, to understand HIV, we must look at where we live, where we work, and where we socialize as we map the social ties—short-term and long-term, weak and strong—that contribute to our health outcomes.[13]

Traveling just four hours north along Interstate 65 from Scott County to Chicago, Illinois, it is similarly apparent that to fully understand the lives of WLWHA, and highly stigmatized women more broadly, we first need to understand the environments in which they operate and the context in which they acquired HIV. By the time many women are diagnosed, they are suffering not only from the virus itself but also from the social forces and personal struggles that are simultaneously assaulting their minds, finances, and relationships. My interviews pointed to three conditions that heightened both women's HIV risk and the overall levels of distress in their lives: the aftermath of childhood sexual trauma, participation in a drug trade that is at once seductive and suffocating, and the secrecy and silence embedded in communities hit hard by HIV/AIDS. In these situations, personal, familial, institutional, community, and societal failures, missteps, and gaps powerfully converged in women's lives as accumulated injuries of inequality. Crises occurred frequently in this state, sometimes making physical death an immediate possibility. The women were suffering a kind of social death, to borrow from ethnic studies scholar Lisa Cacho, in which their value was "made unintelligible through racialized, sexualized, spatialized, and state-sanctioned violences."[14] It was often to escape this state of *dying from* that women launched transformative projects. This chapter analyzes this context of risk in more depth, but first it is important to provide some historical details about the AIDS epidemic.

AN EPIDEMIC EMERGES

In its June 5, 1981 *Morbidity and Mortality Weekly Report* (*MMWR*), the CDC reported on cases of the rare lung infection pneumocystis carinii pneumonia found in five young gay male patients.[15] While scientists believe that HIV was present years before the first cases documented in the *MMWR*, this communiqué marked the official recognition of a new disease that would come to be known as AIDS.[16] A report one month later in the same publication reported on Kaposi's sarcoma among young gay men, a rare skin cancer whose bright purple, red, or brown lesions would later be understood as one of the most identifiable symptoms of AIDS-related illness.[17] As a handful of mainstream media outlets reported on the *MMWR*s, a July 1981 *New York Times* article under the headline "Rare Cancer Seen in 41 Homosexuals" helped to solidify the initial framing of the epidemic for the general public.[18] Prior to the CDC's 1982 designation of the disease as acquired immune deficiency syndrome, terms such as *GRID* or *gay-related immune deficiency* were used early on by some media outlets and health officials, suggesting an inherent link between the new disease and homosexuality.[19]

People who inject drugs (PWID) were also afflicted with AIDS from the outset of the epidemic, although their plight was less visible.[20] Within a year of the 1981 AIDS-related *MMWR*, the CDC established injection drug use as "an identified risk factor" for AIDS. Although there was some overlap between the two groups, PWID did not receive the same level of attention as white gay men, who were framed as the earliest victims of AIDS and who quickly mobilized and leveraged their political capital to elicit answers from scientists and resources from the government. Additional challenges hampered efforts to address the increased risk for PWID, who are less likely to have consistent access to or to utilize health-care services, and whose often transient lives make it difficult to track disease progression over time. The rising death toll among PWID in the 1970s and 1980s was often attributed to any number of conditions and ongoing health concerns, in contrast to cases in which previously healthy gay men presented with AIDS-related symptoms. Lacking political clout and engaged in illegal behavior, PWID had almost no organized voice in the epidemic's early years. So while the CDC stated early in the epidemic that abstention from intravenous drug use and avoidance of needle-sharing were likely to prevent transmission, funding for harm-reduction tools such as needle-exchange programs, drug rehabilitation services, and AIDS prevention efforts faced significant resistance.[21] Much of this thinking continues, as evidenced in the Austin, Indiana, case, and will likely hamstring current efforts to confront a growing opiate epidemic in various parts of the country. This is despite clear evidence that these programs do not result in increased drug use among participants or the recruitment of first-time drug users.[22] In fact, needle- and syringe-exchange programs have been found to reduce disease incidence while providing medical testing, counseling services, referrals to drug treatment, overdose prevention, and housing and employment programs. They are also believed to reduce the number of improperly discarded syringes that can unintentionally expose children, first responders, sanitation personnel, and others to transmittable diseases.

Individuals who acquired HIV through heterosexual sex made up 25 percent of all new HIV diagnoses in 2015.[23] Most cisgender women living with HIV/AIDS contracted the disease in this way: in 2014, approximately 87 percent (7,242) of new diagnoses among women were attributed to heterosexual sex, while just 13 percent (1,045) were attributed to injection drug use. HIV is more efficiently transmitted from men to women during sexual intercourse than vice versa, due to women's longer exposure to infectious fluids and increased risk of tissue injury.[24]

As an infectious disease, HIV "can happen to anyone," as the various public service announcements of the 1980s and 1990s warned us. When HIV/AIDS gained prominence in the American collective imagination in those early years, many activists and advocates encouraged the public to view the epidemic in universal terms, reminding us that we are all biologically vulnerable to infection. The high-profile and diverse experiences of HIV-positive youngster Ryan White, tennis champion Arthur Ashe, NBA star Earvin "Magic" Johnson, and Republican National Convention speaker (and woman living with HIV) Mary Fisher helped drive this point home. This message has been an important tool in fighting the spread of the epidemic in the general population, and perhaps its greatest usefulness has been to challenge AIDS-related stigma and garner public support to fight a disease that anyone can get.

The burden of the epidemic has not, however, been borne equally or randomly across the US population. AIDS has functioned largely as a concentrated epidemic in the United States, with disproportionate infection rates among sexual minorities, black and brown communities, the poor, and transgender women. This is the inherent tension in the "it can happen to anyone" narrative: it underemphasizes the critical role of inequality in risk exposure, prevention efforts, treatment access, and the experience of living with HIV. The disease's calcifying socioeconomic, racial, and gendered dimensions call on us to interpret it as one of individual circumstances, attitudes, and behaviors that exist within and interact with environmental norms, forces, opportunities, and constraints. Stated differently, our connection to the HIV/AIDS epidemic reflects our existence as gendered and racialized bodies, each with a particular socioeconomic status and sexual identity in a society that either values or devalues those statuses by offering or withholding bodily protections. AIDS stigma was therefore generated not only because of inaccurate fears that the condition could be transmitted casually, but also because of the associations between the disease and society's most marginalized. Given the epidemic's history and the accompanying social and political stigmatization, it is perhaps not surprising that women who were already experiencing multiple intersecting traumas in their lives and neighborhoods would find themselves in the crosshairs of an HIV diagnosis. As we meet our central storytellers—Trisha, Beverly, Keisha, and Yvette—and trace their paths, we see how their personal experiences, social networks, and community context interacted in ways that heightened their risk.

PATHWAYS: COMING OF AGE WITH THE INJURY OF SEXUAL TRAUMA

Conversing with women living with HIV/AIDS for more than a decade, hearing their stories across the table, I came to dread a particular moment. When it happened, the vulnerability and pain in women's eyes shook me to my core. Several interviews into the study, I began to sense in advance that the moment would come, the life events women shared dropping clues like breadcrumbs. By the end of my fieldwork, I could anticipate, almost to the moment, when the reveal would occur.

The prevalence of early sexual trauma in the lives of WLWHA is profound and alarming. The CDC states that nearly one in five women (18.3 percent) reports having experienced rape.[25] The one-time interviews we conducted with WLWHA from diverse racial, ethnic, and economic backgrounds revealed one in four (28 percent) had been raped or molested before the age of 25, and *two-thirds* of the women with histories of drug addiction reported experiences of early sexual abuse.[26] White, black, and Latina study participants all fell victim to this experience, a highly personal injury of inequality with structural roots in gender-based violence and unequal power dynamics. And our number likely underreports the actual incidence rate, given the trauma, shame, and silence associated with this experience. As the #MeToo movement has revealed, sexual violence is endemic to our society, cutting across socioeconomic and racial lines.

Trisha McIntosh

Trisha McIntosh (white, age 55) was diagnosed with AIDS in 1996 at the age of 42. Born in Canada, she was raised by an adoptive family there. She described multiple instances of abuse at the hands of her adoptive mother's new husband and his sons. When she was about 15, she told her mother of the abuse: "She put me out of the house. She accused me of trying to steal her husband. Well, [the abuse] started when I was four years old. You don't try to steal a husband. She needed to get me psychological help, therapy, and she didn't. So, in my book, I do blame her. Children don't make those things up. They don't make them up."

Consistent with larger trends, the abuse the Chicago study women described experiencing was most often perpetrated by someone they knew. Biological relatives or close family friends were often the victimizers, but stepfathers and boyfriends of girls' mothers were the most common offenders. Echoing Trisha's experiences, Rochelle, a black 35-year-old nursing home worker, observed, "My mom was dating this man. . . . He couldn't really keep his hands off me. I was eight years old. But he really didn't start actually penetrating me until I was 14. I didn't tell my mom because in my mom's mindset, her man came before her kids. *And* I was that child that she didn't want." Drug use in the home sometimes facilitated abuse. The mother of Rosa (Latina, age 28) had a severe drug addiction and routinely brought home men from local bars who would then sexually violate Rosa. The Department of Children and Family Services stepped in, placing Rosa and her siblings in group homes when she was just nine years old. After one particularly disturbing visit to see her mother, who was jailed for the remainder of Rosa's childhood, Rosa did not see her again until she was 23.

Feminist scholars have offered numerous analyses of sexual violence to underscore girls' vulnerability.[27] Evelynn Hammonds writes, "Many young women live in . . . communities where few support systems exist to protect them and allow them to grow unmolested to adulthood."[28] Silence, dissembling, and strong investments in asserting their respectability (or their sexual prowess) become dominant strategies girls deploy to protect themselves and maintain some control over their environments after experiencing sexual violence. At a pivotal point in their development, these girls learn that their bodies are not fully within their control: they are vessels that can be readily abused, hurt, and violated. Katy (white, age 36) was 16 when she was raped during her first sexual experience: "It was a date-rape situation. I did not consent at all. So that sort of set the precedent, so from 16 to 19, sex was kind of bad." As girls, some of the women in my study also received the confusing message that their bodies could attract attention and get them access to things they wanted or needed, as Trisha explains below.

Sexual violence has racialized dimensions as well. For example, under systems of both gender and racial oppression, black women have long contended with the devaluation, objectification, and targeting of their bodies. These experiences have deep historical roots in the use of black women as sexual chattel and breeders of profit-producing slaves.[29] Media depictions, personal attitudes, and even political discourse still promulgate stereotypical assumptions about the supposed hypersexuality and wantonness of black women.[30] As a result, black girls are often perceived as less innocent, older, and more sexually experienced and available than their white counterparts, compounding their vulnerability.[31]

Abusers often threatened these girls with terrifying consequences if they dared to tell: "I've been bitter for years," Gwen (black, age 56) observed. "I was molested by my uncle and godfather for six years when I was little. I held that, because my uncle said he would kill my mother if

I told." The girls therefore learned that they would have to address their problems in isolation, and many felt they had no one to trust. June (Puerto Rican, age 48) observed that subsequent relationships were framed by one question: "Do I think I can trust somebody? Since I've been raped and molested, it's always been the issue."

When it became apparent to a teenage Trisha that her adoptive mother would offer no protection in the face of her stepfather's sexual abuse, her rebellious experimentation with drugs and alcohol intensified. When she was in her early twenties, Trisha's boyfriend was shooting drugs intravenously, and she began to use with him. Her life increasingly centered on her next high, and at 26 she moved to Los Angeles with a musician with whom she regularly freebased cocaine. They married but split up three months later when she suggested they stop using. She went back to Canada and continued her streak of drug-fueled relationships: "I kept on going, but each [guy] I picked was more abusive and more abusive and more abusive. That's the only kind of relationship I've ever had."

When Trisha's drug sources among the musicians and other men she dated began to dry up, she started to turn tricks under a series of pimps who supplied her with drugs. Trisha reflected on how her sexually abusive relationship with her stepfather groomed her for sex work: "He made me into a good prostitute. Because as I got older, I learned that I had to do [what he wanted] anyway. But he was going to buy me something if he was going to get something. So if I wanted a horse, [get me] a horse, then you can get something. So it was a gradual, almost training, to go into that business. . . . And drugs, of course, to escape."

Trisha moved around, from Canada to various cities in the United States, depending on men who sometimes protected her but more often violated her. During a relationship with one especially brutal pimp, she met up with some Chicago musicians at a local blues club in Canada she used for periodic escapes. "It was my little hideaway," she commented. "Nobody would ever look for me there." Tommy, a bass player in the band, urged her to run away. "But you just can't get away. He takes all the money. How you gonna go? And then you have no place when you get somewhere. What you gonna do?" Tommy eventually offered to find Trisha a safe place to stay if she made her way to Chicago. About two weeks later, Trisha told her pimp she was going to Vancouver to make some money turning tricks.

She packed up her things and walked away from him and the modest house she had bought with the small sum of money her adoptive mother left her after dying of cancer a few years prior: "I walked away from everything, everything. I had to. You know, it was life or death. So I got to Vancouver, and [my pimp] found me within a day." With her plan to escape foiled, she called the one person whom she felt owed her: her stepfather. "I said, 'You got to come pick me up right now.' So he came right away and got me across the border and gave me enough money to get me to Chicago."

Once Trisha made her way to the City of Big Shoulders, she promptly called Tommy the bass player. Just as he had promised, Tommy picked her up from the train station and rented a hotel room for her for the night. The next morning, he found her a room in the home of a police officer who frequented the blues club and had a wife and two kids "in a beautiful suburb," Trisha recounted. "I stayed there for about six, eight months." Unfortunately, the officer wanted something in return for his hospitality: "And then he—I probably would have stayed longer and possibly changed my life, but he starts to like me. And one night we were coming home from the [blues] club, and he pulled over and started kissing on me. And I said, 'I can't do this. Uh-um. This won't work.'"

With no place to stay, Trisha asked Tommy if she could stay with him. Although she was several months clean, Tommy's neighborhood was full of temptations. A robust drug economy was thriving: "So I went back to my old lifestyle. . . . Tommy was using, and I said, 'If I stay here with you, I'm going to be using too.' So that's what happened." Trisha then moved in with another musician until he became violent, and she ended up on the street. "I couldn't leave the drugs and the people I was around. I either lived on the street or just stayed at different people's houses or stayed in a shooting gallery or a crack house. Sometimes I stayed in stairwells. Sometimes I had to go home with men just so I'd have somewhere to get in where it was warm. I just, I had no home. I was a complete mess."

Trisha's girlhood experiences, given their troubling similarities to those of a sizable segment of the Chicago WLWHA in my study, help us understand the initial steps along the pathways from sexual violation to high-risk contexts that make contracting HIV as young adults more likely. Given their ages and the gravity of what they were experiencing, many of the women's positive coping strategies were undermined during child-hood as a result of the abuse. Filling the void was the lesson that silence—not only about sexual violations but also about difficult feelings and emo-tional struggles—was the only acceptable way to cope.[32] Borrowing a sentiment from Marlon Riggs's seminal film *Tongues Untied*, silence became a way for the young women "to grin and bear it . . . to not acknowl-edge how much their lives . . . [were] discounted each day."[33]

Tragically, the AIDS epidemic would introduce yet another domain of risk for survivors of sexual abuse: subsequent coping strategies placed women squarely in the crosshairs of HIV infection. Individuals who expe-rience adverse childhood events such as sexual abuse are more likely to abuse drugs and have multiple sex partners, and are more likely to engage in condomless sex when they become teens.[34] These behaviors become coping mechanisms when women and girls use them as a form of self-medication.[35] Women who have been sexually abused as children are also more likely to experience subsequent nonconsensual sexual contact and may find it more difficult to negotiate sexual parameters in relation-ships.[36] In Trisha's account, it is striking how often sexual contact, even outside the confines of her role as a sex worker, was undeniably transac-tional as it provided protection and a warm respite from the streets.

As we learn more about the Chicago study women, we see a connection between their personal stories of sexual trauma and the larger context, the conditions of which make them more vulnerable to acquiring HIV. Their stories corroborate much of the existing research that implicates gender inequality and gender-based violence as drivers of HIV prevalence among women. In its characterization of the global AIDS pandemic, a UNAIDS/WHO report states, "Many HIV [prevention] strategies assume an ideal-ized world in which everyone is equal and free to make empowered choices," where individuals "can opt to abstain from sex, stay faithful to one's partner or use condoms consistently."[37] Women are also more likely than men to be forced into survival-focused behaviors such as transac-tional sex for money, housing, protection, employment, and other basic needs; power-imbalanced relationships with older men; and other part-nerings in which they cannot dictate the terms of condom use, monogamy, or HIV testing.[38] Many analysts have concluded that the societal and community-based social, economic, and political statuses of women put them at a disadvantage, providing fewer opportunities to avoid or control situations and areas where HIV transmission is more likely.[39]

Sexual abuse drove many of the Chicago study women to leave their homes at a young age, only to find that the neighborhoods to which they were fleeing were under another kind of attack. Against the backdrop of a series of policies and practices that effectively weakened the economic, social, and political viability of their communities lurked a world that would seize on the young women's vulnerabilities and exploit them until they had almost nothing left: the drug trade. This world, and the networks and social ties embedded therein, deepened their traumas and marginalization, inflicting injury upon injury. Those who survived the drug gauntlet were lucky, but they also found their coping skills diminished, their relationships on life support, and death a breathlessly close possibility. In this context of sustained injury, endured by both the women and their communities, a parasitic HIV epidemic emerged and found the perfect host.

PATHWAYS: ENTERING THE SEXUALIZED DRUG ECONOMY

The sexualized drug economy functions, both economically and socially, as an intoxicating lure and escape for individuals struggling with trauma. Over 50 percent of the 84 women in the Chicago study have histories of addiction, and it bears repeating that a stunning 66 percent of this subgroup also reported histories of early sexual abuse. The issues are intertwined: the interaction between the epidemics of sexual violence and drug addiction has produced a playing field that draws in highly vulnerable women, situates them in a structure that further reduces their power, and increases their risk of contracting HIV.

The epidemiological circuitry that hobbled Scott County, Indiana, has been short-circuiting black and brown communities for decades, intensified by centuries of harsh and pernicious anti-black and anti-brown sentiment, politics, and policies in a nation that has shown little sympathy for its victims. This challenges the idea that certain groups are inherently biologically or culturally "contaminated" or "contaminating," when in fact,

HIV operates by exploiting structural vulnerabilities. Geography and class intersect with the racialized and gendered dimensions of the epidemic. An estimated 2.1 percent of heterosexuals living in high-poverty urban areas in the United States are HIV positive, a rate well above the 1 percent that designates a generalized epidemic.[40] Consequently, the CDC identifies poverty as "the single most important demographic factor associated with HIV infection among inner-city heterosexuals."[41]

Chicago's working-class and low-income neighborhoods experienced decades of racial segregation through formal and informal policies and practices and were dealt a critical economic blow in the 1970s and 1980s with the decline of manufacturing jobs, the rise of a low-wage and less stable service sector, the movement of higher-paying jobs to predominantly white suburban areas and overseas, and public policies that eroded community health resources.[42] Faced with the absence of viable economic prospects, the drug economy emerged as an alternative within poor communities, supplying both residents and outsiders who frequented the marketplace. Although the drug trade spans the globe, and narcotics can be found in some of the wealthiest corridors of society, poor communities, and especially poor communities of color, have been hit especially hard. Specifically, the targeted marketing and systematic distribution of legal and illegal drugs in poor black and brown neighborhoods has generated a barely concealed drug marketplace, with both controlled substances and alcohol becoming highly accessible and normalized as a "natural" part of the environment. From the liquor store on every corner to the dealers in the streets, the obtainability of mood-altering substances in places with mood-dampening features has set up poor communities to become major sites for the AIDS epidemic.[43]

Networks drive both the drug trade and the AIDS epidemic. As the historical and contemporary effects of residential segregation confine many people of color to low-resource neighborhoods, legal and illegal drugs traverse community networks, offering a potentially lucrative albeit highly risky financial survival strategy, a social elixir, and an opportunity to self-medicate. Addiction becomes both a contagion and an industry as friends, family members, and neighbors succumb together. Shooting galleries in which PWID purchased, used, and shared dirty works of needles and drugs proliferated in the 1980s and 1990s in abandoned and burned-out buildings.⁴⁴ The influx of crack cocaine in the 1980s ushered in a highly addictive drug that destroyed families and neighborhoods and arguably escalated the riskiness of what users were willing to do and exchange for the next high. Moreover, overwhelming blight in some areas and urban renewal and gentrification in others facilitate population movement and disrupt social networks in ways that likely encourage cross-pollination within and across networks. Community violence, another destabilizer accompanying the drug economy, is both cause and consequence of population movements. In short, the interdependence between deteriorating neighborhood conditions and the drug economy creates frighteningly perfect conditions for an infectious disease to enter vulnerable community networks and proliferate.

If money is the engine of the drug economy, sex is the fuel. The structure, culture, and codes of the drug economy position sex as a currency alongside drugs and cash. Exchanges often occur within the confines of intimate relationships: the sharing of drugs between intimate partners binds them together in addiction. Drugs can drive sex to become unambiguously transactional: trading sex for drugs or money between dealer and user, between users, or between sex worker and client.⁴⁵ Sex is often viewed as one of the spoils of a lucrative drug enterprise. Drug use can also alter sexual decision-making on the part of both women and men, clouding judgment and lowering inhibitions. As we hear from Beverly Maxwell, women play a subordinate role within this structure, rarely assuming positions of authority within the sexualized drug economy and often left paying the consequences.

Beverly Maxwell

The sexualized drug economy was growing prodigiously in urban centers just as many of the Chicago study women were entering early adulthood. The one-two punch of childhood sexual trauma and a growing drug economy robbed them of their innocence at extremely young ages. Childhood friends and first boyfriends became dealers and users in this violent yet exhilarating world, and the young women found themselves at parties, in homes, and on street corners where drugs were readily available. Early experimentation with alcohol and drugs rarely happens in a vacuum. The Chicago study women who were introduced to alcohol and drugs by family members tended to have their first experiences by early adolescence. Perhaps a parent allowed a girl to try a sip of a drink; an older sibling or cousin shared a drag of marijuana. However, most of the women were introduced to their first high by a boyfriend or friends while partying. Indeed, experimenting with drugs and alcohol at a young age is not uncommon, but the environmental context dramatically increased the ease with which youthful experimentation by the women I interviewed evolved into full-blown addiction.

This was certainly the case for 41-year-old Beverly Maxwell, who was born on Chicago's South Side. Beverly's mother Verna was left to raise seven children alone when Beverly's father, her childhood sweetheart, was killed after a confrontation with security officers in the public housing project where they lived. Beverly was only one year old at the time, but her 12-year-old brother Jerome witnessed the shooting. Traumatized, Jerome's life would "take a downfall," as Beverly described the alcohol and drug addiction he later developed after seeing "the fire coming out of the gun." The baby of the seven children (six girls and one boy), Beverly felt the void. "All I knew was something was missing, but I didn't know what until I was in school and somebody said, 'Where's your daddy?'"

When Beverly's father was killed, many lower-middle-class families, including hers, lived in the projects. Verna collected a small insurance payment, $2,500, and moved the family to a house on the far south side of Chicago. Theirs was the first black family on the block. "So, it was her and all her kids," Beverly reflected, "but she was determined to make things work and take care and she did. She did everything perfectly right." But Beverly's father's death meant her mother would have to carry a heavy load. A deeply religious and strong-willed woman, Verna started working long hours to support the family, driving a cab and cooking at a convent adjacent to the Catholic school to which she sent Beverly and her siblings: "And I remember when I was about twelve, she let me write out her checks for the month. [Afterward], she had no money. She had like $42 left. She said, 'Okay, that's good.' And I'm like, 'That's good? You just wrote out all your checks, and you have nothing.' She said, 'Yeah, but the bills are paid. We'll make it until the next paycheck comes in two weeks.'"

Watching her mother's humble struggle so close to the bottom of the economic ladder taught Beverly she would have to "start hustling" if she wanted to buy things that interested her. "I never could ask her for money after that. Any time I asked her for something, I just felt shame. I just couldn't do it. So, I started hustling." At 14, she bought her own school clothes by working under her 16-year-old sister's name to get around the minimum working age.

Like Trisha and the other women we have met, Beverly was carrying another load in her quest to "handle her own business" without burdening Verna. When she was just five years old, an electrical contractor working in her family's home molested her. Even to this day, Beverly partly blames herself: "Me being the rebel, I just had to go down to the basement and see what that man was doing in our house, 'cause that's who I was. I was one of those curious kids." Beverly never told her mother what the man had done, knowing Verna would be devastated. "I knew in my heart of hearts my mom did everything she could to protect us," Beverly commented. After Beverly's father was killed, Verna avoided dating until she remarried when Beverly was 14. When Verna went to bed at night, her new husband's friends had to leave the premises. "She was very protective of us," Beverly reflected. "So, no, I couldn't tell her because as a young person, as children, we start doing stuff to protect our parents, because we love them and we don't want to do or say anything that's gonna upset them. So, no, I never said anything."

Unfortunately, this would not be Beverly's last experience with sexual violence. She described being raped at 14 by the older brother of a boy on whom she had a huge crush. "He knew I liked his brother, he was just a dirty bastard," she commented. She tried to fill the void on her own, "because whenever a child is put in a position to be part of a sexual act, then that facilitates a process that should not have been started," she explained. Months later, Beverly, who described herself as "boy crazy" as she struggled to make sense of her sexuality, got pregnant by a 16-year-old boy who came from a well-to-do black family that owned a few local businesses. That relationship turned violent as well, as he once pinned Beverly down when she was visiting him while one of his friends tried to sexually assault her. Her boyfriend's older brother intervened to stop the attack. That fateful and tragic night ended the relationship and left an emotional scar that took Beverly years to talk about and even longer to heal. Verna pulled Beverly from her neighborhood high school and sent her to live in a local charity's residential facility and hospital for unwed mothers. She was just 14 years old.

By this time, the drug economy had grown deep roots under Beverly's feet and had infiltrated her family. Her brother Jerome was now a heavy user at 26 years old. Beverly's maternal grandmother had been an alcoholic, inspiring Verna to leave home and marry Beverly's father decades prior. Verna would then provide safe refuge to her younger siblings, who moved one by one from Mississippi to Chicago to escape their unstable home. Verna was trying to keep it all together, working long hours as a single mother and, according to Beverly, perhaps missing some of the details regarding what was happening with her daughter, who was now pregnant and a three-time survivor of sexual abuse:

> I understand that a lot of parents don't nurture their children as much because they're consumed with trying to provide for them. Work. Come home. Cook. Clean. They don't have a place to get replenished and nurtured, so they can't give me something that they don't have. Not knowing that instead of being nurtured, I'm being wounded on a daily basis.... So my mom, she did what she thought was best. She wanted to provide a home and good education for us. And in the midst of that, she had no idea what was going on.

Beverly returned to her mother's home and her local high school after giving birth to a daughter and started dating a boy whom she calls "her first real love." He was selling drugs and introduced her to selling pot in high school. After graduating in 1983 and trying her hand at electrician training at a local community college, Beverly rented her own apartment, attended beauty school, and started working as a hair stylist. She doted on her daughter, enjoying special moments with her such as putting out homemade cookies for Santa at Christmas.

Still, at 19 years old, Beverly had developed a taste for the fast life and the freedoms that living outside of her mother's home allowed:

> I had gotten addicted to the lifestyle because when I was in high school, the guy I dated sold drugs. Then I dated a guy who stole cars for a living. He had more money than the drug dealer. And then I stopped dating them, and I started hanging out with the real big drug dealers, all the big players.... I had my eighteenth birthday party at a bar, and the people didn't even know

I was underage. . . . I was way fast, you know, and I was just in the mix of things. So now once I got my own apartment, then I just really stretched out. I started selling cocaine, started fencing boosters [stolen goods]. Then I got a bigger apartment, got a new car. You know, it was just, I liked that lifestyle because it seemed glamorous at the time, hanging out with the big macs, having money to go and do things . . . going shopping once a week. . . . It was crazy, but some part of me enjoyed that.

As is true in most capitalist enterprises, the hierarchies of the drug trade shape sexual networks and accepted norms around masculinity and femininity, as dealers are able to attract women depending on their place in the pecking order. Thus, a move up the ladder potentially means access to a new set of women. Beverly had strict standards in the sexualized drug economy, applying a clear sense of ambition and expectation to her choices. She learned her lesson about dating men of limited resources after a cable company employee Beverly once dated was fired for stealing to buy her gifts. In the sexualized drug economy, dating the street corner dealers with the inconsistent income would not do: "I just had to have the most powerful man in the clique . . . the strongest . . . if you worked *for* somebody, I couldn't mess with you because I worked for me. I couldn't mess with nobody that worked for somebody else. I always had the top man. That's just the way I did things. Everybody had to be on top of their game because I was always on top of mine." Cocaine had very specific uses in Beverly's network, as a commodity to sample occasionally before a sale or as a tool with which to increase sexual arousal and one's enjoyment of a party after a couple of glasses of champagne. She was afraid at first when she saw how cocaine affected people, "but then my boyfriend convinced me to take a bump, and that's when it changed. That was our ritual. We were players, and that's what players did." Beverly certainly saw herself as part of a more exclusive wing of the sexualized drug economy: she emphasized to me that she never intravenously injected drugs or smoked crack.

Similar stories of having fun and making money in the drug-fueled 1980s could probably be told from the condos and clubs of Wall Street to the neighborhoods of Chicago. The difference was that as Beverly burrowed more and more deeply into this life, the drug economy operating within racially segregated Chicago was meting out much harsher penalties to its participants and providing much less insulation from punishment.[46]

While some politicians, media commentators, and other key influencers have rightly framed the current opioid epidemic in white communities as a public health crisis, no such framing would be extended to the drug epidemic in inner-city communities, which was almost immediately characterized as a criminal justice problem. The War on Drugs and tough-on-crime measures ushered in a highly punitive era of state surveillance in black and brown communities, including the mass incarceration of more individuals than in any other industrialized country.[47]

Beverly's friends began to get arrested and incarcerated under the heavy blanket of surveillance. She saw her friends face criminal courts without savvy attorneys just when mandatory minimum sentences for nonviolent drug offenses took effect. Neighborhood gangs and drug-dealing networks fought over territory, raising the levels of both tension and outright violence.[48] Heroin became widely available in her community, and Beverly's first time snorting it at 27 hooked her quickly. "That was a downward spiral for me 'cause everything became focused on getting it and using it and getting more and more. It became a vicious cycle."

Beverly's once cohesive network of drug-dealing associates began to fracture. She and her boyfriend broke up. With disintegrated relationships and no wealth on which to rely, Beverly had to get out and hustle for the next high. She began to "play paper," engaging in check forgery and credit card fraud. Beverly's daughter started spending more and more time under the care and protection of Beverly's sister, until Beverly decided to move with her daughter to a new apartment building. Beverly fit right in. "Everybody there hustling, and I got a hustling mentality, so I start hustling. Of course, I start dating the guy that sells all the drugs in the building. I found 'the man.'"

Fully ensconced in the underground sexualized drug economy, Beverly started to "catch cases," being arrested and brought up on various charges: "'Cause the odds of you doing wrong all the time and not getting caught just doesn't work." She faced gun charges during her time hanging out with drug dealers. She was arrested on five separate occasions for buying "spreads," wallets with credit cards and IDs stolen by pickpockets. Beverly was offering them for purchase along with the drugs she was selling. Each time, she managed to beat the charge with the help of an attorney. But her luck eventually ran out, and she was sentenced to two years in prison. She served six months, and her boyfriend picked her up in a Mercedes Benz and handed her fresh inventory. "So that kicked things right back on. Then I called up all the old connections, I get things back on, and it's just a bunch of mess all over again."

Beverly's legal troubles did not end there. She had other charges pending. The prosecutor offered probation if she could "drop clean." She couldn't pass the drug test, even after going to detox four times in four months. Her mother Verna was exasperated: "I'm tired of bringing you out here [to detox]." Beverly replied, "I'm tired of going." Beverly knew the problem, but "it still wasn't registering. How you gonna get clean if you got 100 grams of dope in your house?"

Deep crisis of the sort experienced by many of the women in my study rarely happens overnight. With its promise of easy money, emotional escape, and a good party, the drug trade attracts, and relies on, willing participants with a heightened sense of vulnerability. As their recreational use became more frequent, women found the drugs demanded more of them. If they weren't already with partners who were involved in the trade, they gravitated to those who were. They lost their homes because they couldn't pay the rent. Chemical addiction kept them captive, grabbing them by the throats whenever they thought about leaving.

Therapists who could help women heal emotional wounds were hard to come by in this era of cuts to community health centers and mental health services in inner-city neighborhoods. Jobs were scarce, but the next high was (often literally) just around the corner. Women frequently recounted to me that finding drugs in the 1980s and early 1990s took remarkably little effort: "They were everywhere." What started as an experimental or recreational tool morphed into an opportunity to self-medicate too compelling to pass up. "I was about 11," commented Charlene (Latina, age 47), whose father was a drug addict and whose mother had a gambling addiction. "That's when I tried it. But I didn't start using until I was like 16. I was very resentful. I was mad at the world; all I wanted was drugs, drugs, drugs. I didn't care about anything or anybody." As women talked about what pulled them into the sexualized drug economy and what made them stay, the very human need to feel whole permeated the discussions. They sought to control depression, anxiety, and stress. For some, anger and grief were ever-present enablers, lighting the crack pipe, thumbing the heroin needle, and pouring just one more drink. And as the women sunk deeper into street life, they were engaging—sexually or otherwise—with more and more people in this higher-risk environment.

PATHWAYS: SEX (AND SILENCE) IN THE SEGREGATED CITY

While I was conducting my fieldwork, a Chicago man in his early thirties was arrested and charged with criminal transmission of HIV, a class-2 felony. According to Cook County prosecutors, the man failed to disclose his HIV-positive status to his then girlfriend, and she later tested positive for the virus. The woman asserted she had not had sex with anyone except that man during or after that time frame. Only after the relationship ended did she discover from the man's family that his wife had died years before of AIDS-related complications. When the woman confronted the man, he admitted he knew he had HIV during their relationship and had known about it for over a decade.

The arrest drew swift criticism from members of the AIDS advocacy community, who argued that the state's laws criminalizing HIV transmission did considerably more harm than good. AIDS responders focus heavily on HIV-prevention strategies, encouraging safer sex practices and HIV treatment for those testing positive. Why would people want to get tested, they questioned, if they knew they might be prosecuted for not subsequently disclosing their status to sexual partners? HIV-criminalization laws are widely viewed by advocates, activists, and many public health officials as outdated remnants of an age with limited information about HIV, very limited options for treatment, and high mortality rates.[49] They are seen as detrimental to building good relations with communities most affected by the epidemic, where draconian approaches have been used to try to prevent disease transmission. They also have a very racialized valence, insofar as black men are disproportionately prosecuted under HIV criminalization laws nationally, and courtroom discourse often paints them as predatory, insatiable, and irresponsible.[50] Others attacked the disclosure of the man's name in the press. Now a matter of public record, the arrest essentially made his HIV status public.

Keisha Rainey

The story flickered across Keisha Rainey's Facebook newsfeed and catapulted her into stunned rage. The ethical debates surrounding the man's arrest could unfold in the background; to Keisha, this story was much more personal. There it was, a photo displaying a man she had once found attractive. The face staring back at her was that of both a stranger and the catalyst that changed her life's trajectory. In 2003, just two months shy of her seventeenth birthday, Keisha had sex for the first time, losing her virginity to the man now on her computer screen. Keisha and Jimmy met while accompanying friends on a double date. He was 22 years old, a charmer who lived near her grandmother in a neighborhood where HIV rates were among the highest in the city. Keisha believes she acquired HIV during this sexual encounter.

Keisha got sick within weeks of having sex with Jimmy. Her mother noticed and was convinced her youngest daughter was pregnant. She demanded Keisha take a home pregnancy test, having her repeat it twice after the negative result. Puzzled by Keisha's physical symptoms, her mother took her to the local clinic and commanded the doctor to order a battery of tests. Sitting across the table from me in a conference room at a local AIDS nonprofit in April 2005, Keisha's voice still flickered with emotion as she told the story: "We go to the clinic and they give me another pregnancy test. Then they test me for STDs. Found out I had chlamydia. Then all of a sudden, my mom was like, 'Well, you know what, give her an AIDS test.' And I'm sitting there looking at my mom like, a what? What do I need an AIDS test for?"

Weeks later, I go back in there and they tell me,

> "Well, come on in the room and sit down." I'm looking at this guy, and I went in by myself 'cause my mom was really angry at me. So I figured, okay, I better do all this stuff by myself. I don't know. So they call me in this room and . . . this big guy comes in and he sits in front of me. And I'm sitting there looking like, what's going on? The guy tells me, "Do you know what AIDS is?"

Keisha was stunned by the news. Searching for answers, and some accountability, her mother had contacted Jimmy a few weeks prior when she believed her daughter was pregnant. He denied being the father. When

Keisha's mother tried to reach out to him again after the diagnosis, Jimmy was nowhere to be found. The public health department was unable to locate him. Because Jimmy seemed to have disappeared from the neighborhood in which he had previously been a constant presence, Keisha came to believe he had deliberately transmitted the virus to her. But Keisha and Jimmy's presence in a neighborhood with high HIV rates meant both were navigating their early sexual experiences in a high-stakes context. Black women who are diagnosed as HIV positive often have no identified or reported risk factors and are more likely than white women to have acquired HIV through heterosexual sex rather than through illicit drug use.[51] The experience left Keisha scared and heartbroken, her adolescent naïveté and sexual curiosity delivering potentially deadly consequences.

Perhaps one of the clearest examples of how HIV operates as an injury of persistent inequality can be seen by considering the epidemic's impact on black communities. The AIDS pandemic's racialized dimensions are undeniable, especially its disproportionate impact on black people globally. Blacks were among the earliest identified PLWHA, comprising 20 percent of all cases reported in 1982 and 50 percent of all pediatric AIDS cases in 1984.[52] As early as 1986, the CDC's *MMWR* reported that blacks made up 51 percent of all AIDS cases among women.[53] In the United States, blacks accounted for an estimated 44 percent of HIV diagnoses in 2014 despite comprising only 12 percent of the population.[54] The CDC estimates that if current rates persist, half of all gay and bisexual black men in America will acquire HIV during their lifetimes.[55]

When I have conversations about my research with black women from various walks of life, many offer a theory to explain the disproportionately high HIV infection rates among them. They see a clear link between the epidemic among black men who have sex with men (MSM) and black women, charging the former group with being the direct cause of infections among the latter. Media obsession in the late 1990s and early 2000s with so-called men on the down low (DL) promoted this narrative. "DL men," primarily but not exclusively identified as black, are thought to classify themselves as heterosexual and may even be involved in long-term heterosexual relationships. Yet unbeknownst to their female partners, these men also secretly engage in sexual relationships with other men. Several high-profile television and print news stories, talk shows, and fictional and non-fictional accounts revealed the secret lives of men who identify themselves as "living on the down low."[56]

The DL cultural obsession of this period blasted a powerful undercurrent in the discourse on HIV in black communities.[57] I interviewed a woman who described the anger, suspicion, and sense of betrayal she felt toward black gay men:

> It just angers me because many of them have children . . . [so] at one point in your life . . . you've had relationships with women. And I think to myself, are you gay or are you not gay? It angers me a little. Not a little, a lot. It angers me a lot . . . I don't feel that reaction with gay white males because I've never dated white men. I feel that reaction with gay black males . . . because I think they're giving it [HIV] to us. I think they don't know what side of the fence they're on, and I think they should make up their minds and stay on it. And if they want to be on the fence, then at least have the guts enough to tell the women that, you know, "I sleep with men." There are some women who will still see them, but I think they just don't have the guts to say that.

Many black women share this frustration, offering knowing nods of agreement when this topic comes up in beauty shops and cocktail circles I've traversed, recounting their own dismay with black men who "refuse to stop pretending and just come out of the closet."

However, a closer look at the cultural signficance of this discussion in and for black communities suggests that the DL debacle almost undoubtedly undercut life-saving and scientifically accurate discussions of the drivers of the AIDS epidemic among blacks. The research linking practices around sexual self-identification to HIV rates is complex. Historically and presently, gay and bisexual men are the population most affected by HIV. In 2017, they accounted for 66 percent (25,748) of all HIV diagnoses.[58] Several studies have indicated that black MSM are less likely than white MSM to identify as gay and are less likely to disclose their sexual identity or behavior to associates.[59] A 2008 study found that men living with HIV/AIDS who have sex with men and women (MSMW) and who are less connected to a homosexual identification are more likely to engage in unprotected sex with female partners without disclosing their HIV status, and black and Latino MSMW are more likely to report unprotected sex with a female partner without HIV status disclosure than are white men.[60] However, researchers also find little evidence that having a non-gay identity increases HIV risk-taking behavior with male sexual partners among black MSM, and may in fact be associated with lower sexual risk-taking. This suggests that unprotected sex between black women and black MSMW who fail to disclose their sexual histories likely accounts for *some* portion of HIV rates among women. But the magnitude of this relationship is widely overstated in light of other research pointing to even stronger drivers of HIV rates among black women.

Given this reality, the public discourse on the issue proved highly problematic, outweighing many of the stated protective intentions of those involved in promoting the discussion. The DL conversation revealed that individuals sometimes maintain silence and secrecy to protect "normalcy" and to preserve social resources such as status, legitimacy, and belonging as they interact in a range of environments. Black LGBTQ individuals risk losing positive connections to a racial community that shares their experiences with racism, and they risk being overlooked or discriminated against as racial minorities in predominately white LGBTQ spaces.[61] Silence becomes a form of protection. However, the public's simultaneous fear of and obsession with black sexuality and black masculinity overshadowed a more nuanced discussion of the relationship between homophobia, racism, and HIV/AIDS and instead fueled a spectacle. Further, the down low discourse is framed around shame and blame, its racialized overtones suggesting something much more sinister than simply being in the closet, a strategy that men and women of *many* racial backgrounds adopt to avoid homophobia and stigma.

Black men, frequently portrayed in public discourse as absent figures or the root causes of the perpetual penury of black women, were foregrounded and depicted as black women's very present, irresponsible, and deceitful contaminators at the height of the DL fascination. Black gay and bisexual men saw their status calcified as a group undeserving of empathy and resources within black communities.[62] Struggling against an escalating AIDS epidemic, they were largely relegated to the status of lures of otherwise straight men and therefore seen as indirect hazards to the health of black women.

Perhaps one of the deadliest enduring consequences of this conversation is that it sent a message to black women that as long as they can be sure their intimate partners are not on the DL, they are largely protected from HIV risk. This has left an indelible imprint on how black women understand their own sexual health. Another lasting byproduct of the DL spectacle is that it pits black women against black men in the AIDS conversation, hindering the creation of a unified strategy to target HIV in black communities. Crafting HIV prevention messages for black women has proven to be an uphill climb for AIDS activists and advocates, given that much of their audience has been primed to engage the question of HIV solely from the perspective of how DL men are putting them at risk.

In fact, a complex web of challenges—structural, political, cultural, and interpersonal—led to the epidemic's startling and devastating consequences in black communities and set the stage for Keisha's experience. To be clear, racism has been a pernicious catalyst in the AIDS epidemic.[63] From a policy standpoint, the weak public health response to the needs of black and brown communities undermined the capacity to build a strong HIV prevention and treatment infrastructure from the early years of the epidemic, and debates over whether communities of color are receiving a level of support commensurate with the size of the epidemic in these populations continue. More than 90 percent of new HIV infections in the US are transmitted by persons who do not know they have the virus or are not receiving treatment.[64] This underscores the importance of early diagnosis and linkage to medical care to reduce the number of new HIV infections. Among racial groups, though, blacks are the least likely to receive medical treatment after diagnosis, resulting in greater risk of transmission within the population.[65] Simultaneously, demands for abstinence-only school curricula and limited sex education have left communities with inadequate information about sexual health.

Several studies point to higher rates of sexually transmitted infections (STIs) in black and brown communities due to a number of factors, including a dearth of testing and treatment opportunities.[66] Certain STIs can increase the risk of HIV infection by causing lesions on the skin, through which HIV can enter the body. Historian of science Evelynn Hammonds examined racial disparities in syphilis rates during the twentieth century to argue that negative moral judgments of black sexuality have likely contributed to longstanding and persistent disconnects from treatment and medical care for STIs among blacks.[67]

The incarceration boom that was ostensibly designed to eradicate the sexualized drug economy has ironically also contributed to the proliferation of HIV and other sexually transmitted infections by linking prisons with neighborhoods. The HIV infection rate in prisons is three times higher than in the general population.[68] However, according to a growing consensus among scholars, most HIV-positive prisoners do not acquire HIV while in prison.[69] Most acquire it in their home communities prior to incarceration, often through their participation in, or social proximity to, the sexualized drug economy.[70] One of the most significant mechanisms underlying the relationship between mass incarceration and HIV rates may be more indirect: cycling in and out of correctional facilities undermines the stability of relationships because "the partner entering prison is now at risk of forming new (sometimes coercive) sexual connections with a pool of individuals [who may participate in] high-risk behaviors. . . . The partner who remains behind . . . forfeits the social and sexual companionship of the incarcerated partner and may pursue other partnerships to satisfy those needs."[71] Further, while many prisoners living with HIV/AIDS are able to access healthcare while incarcerated, once they are released that care often becomes inconsistent or nonexistent.[72] This makes it more likely that these individuals will transmit the virus to others post-release as a result of rising and unchecked viral loads.[73] Our criminal justice policies therefore have long-term health consequences not only for prisoners, but also for the communities to which they are returning and the social networks they are (re)entering.[74]

Political and cultural dynamics within black communities play a major role as well. Political scientist Cathy Cohen is widely credited for her analysis of the laggard response in addressing HIV in black communities in the 1980s and 1990s.[75] She argues that religious doctrine as well as a politics of racial respectability among black church leaders and politicians, black media, and others drove the silence and reluctance to acknowlege HIV/AIDS as a political and community issue. This strategy has deep historical roots within black communities that must counter a white-controlled racial order that promulgates racist discourses and logics of black inferiority, black pathology, and black immorality to justify barriers to political, economic, and social advancement. As historian Evelyn Brooks Higginbotham posits in her seminal work on black middle- and working-class women who politically organized in the late nineteenth and early twentieth centuries, respectability politics

> demanded that every individual in the black community assume responsibility for behavioral self-regulation and self-improvement along moral, educational, and economic lines. The goal was to distance oneself as far as possible from images perpetuated by racist stereotypes. . . . It was particularly public behavior that they perceived to wield the power either to refute or confirm stereotypical representations and discriminatory practices. . . . There could be no laxity as far as sexual conduct, cleanliness, temperance, hard work, and politeness were concerned. There could be no transgression of society's norms.[76]

The AIDS epidemic therefore represents a crisis of respectability for those who maintain this ideology. Cohen convincingly argues that this fueled reluctance among community leaders to rally behind those most likely to be exposed to the virus—gay men, PWID, impoverished women, and sex workers. That fierce commitment to respectability and fear of being linked to yet another stigmatizing identity drove currents that even today run through the black community and will reappear throughout this book. Cohen argues that this fear, coupled with a slow response to rising HIV infection rates among blacks by the federal government, many white-dominated HIV advocacy organizations, and the general public, allowed the epidemic to gain a foothold black communities are still struggling to loosen.

In addition to noting the structural drivers of HIV/AIDS, it is worth underscoring that unequal gender dynamics continue to play important roles in the epidemic among women: Keisha and Jimmy's five-year age gap and her legal status as a minor when they had sex highlights how those power modalities can operate when younger girls partner with older men. This is highly reminiscent of Sanyu Mojola's analysis in *Love, Money, and HIV: Becoming a Modern African Woman in the Age of AIDS*, which reminds us of the importance of the transition to adulthood as a pivotal and highly vulnerable moment for HIV transmission among women.[77] What echoes in both Keisha's and Beverly's stories is Mojola's discussion of how young Kenyan women, as "consuming women" who desire access to the material goods promoted in a global economy, partner with older men who can provide those goods at the cost of heightening their risk of contracting HIV. Lastly, it must be noted that the sex ratio in many black communities contributes to dense social–sexual networks within an economically and racially segregated context, as "the shortage of men places women at a disadvantage in negotiating and maintaining mutually monogamous relationships."[78]

This complex sexual playing field, with its political, economic, and social landmines, leaves teenagers like Keisha with limited tools to take control of their sexual health and manage unseen vulnerabilities. Ten years after AIDS activist Rae Lewis-Thornton's landmark appearance on the cover of *ESSENCE* magazine in 1994 next to the headline "I'm young, I'm educated, I'm drug-free, and I'm dying of AIDS," Keisha contracted the virus, demonstrating in sharp relief black women's long history of struggle against the epidemic.

Nonetheless, a gendered analysis that acknowledges only women's oppression can fail to recognize men's fears and vulnerabilities as well.[79] As men navigate and are called upon to reinforce norms of masculinity in these environments, they, too, struggle under risky conditions. They create relationships within and across networks that are sometimes transactional, sometimes emotional, and often both as they seek love, comfort, safety, resources, pleasure, and power in the quest for survival and mobility. We can only speculate about what and when Jimmy knew about his HIV status, and why he chose silence as a coping strategy. But as AIDS scholars Lisa Bowleg and Anita Raj observe, the reality is that black men and women "live, work, socialize, worship, and form romantic and sexual relationships in the same communities, and as epidemiological data document, share sexual risk within their communities."[80] Keisha and Jimmy were doing what many people their age do: trying to make a romantic connection. However, they were doing so in an environment of higher risk because of the ways in which the epidemic had infiltrated their world and generated a complex landscape with a number of hazards. Silence, blame, and avoidance of difficult subjects can easily become the tools by which individuals navigate the terrain and further fuel an epidemic.

PATHWAYS CONVERGE: THE DIAGNOSIS

By the time they were diagnosed with HIV, many of the Chicago women who depended on the sexualized drug economy were in deep crisis. They were *dying from* massive, sustained, and untreated injuries inflicted by sexual, physical, and emotional violence, addiction, and sometimes homelessness. HIV was just one of many contributors to their physiological and psychological distress. They were eating poorly if at all, not sleeping, self-medicating, and engaging with healthcare professionals only through emergency-room visits. Their economic resources were tied almost exclusively to the sexualized drug economy. They had damaged relationships with family members, and some were not on speaking terms with their parents, siblings, and adult children who had had enough. They lacked security, feeling their bodies and possessions were under constant threat. When they received the news of their life-threatening illness and needed all the support and strength they could muster, most of these women were in fact at their weakest points. In our interviews, several women shared that they had thought about or attempted suicide, devastated by the additional layer of stigma the diagnosis applied, like salt poured into gaping wounds.

After four unsuccessful attempts to pass court-mandated drug tests, Beverly finally admitted that she had a serious problem and asked the court for help: "I turned myself in May 10th of 1994. May 11th was my clean day." As part of her deal with prosecutors, she would complete a month-long stay in jail while waiting for a bed to become available in a rehab facility. While in jail, Beverly visited the clinic to address a yeast infection and decided to take a test offered by a handsome and friendly HIV counselor named Thomas: "I saw him there, we chatted when I was [in the clinic]. I figured, I'm gonna get the test because I wanted to holla at the brotha, a fine black man, you know."

Thomas gave Beverly a piece of paper containing a number linked to her test results, per the protocols of anonymous testing. During the weeks in which she was awaiting her results, she was transferred to the drug rehab facility. Thomas found her there and delivered the news that the test had come back positive:

> I forgot I took the test because I didn't think I was at risk because of whatever reason. I didn't have enough knowledge to see my risk at the time, even though I sold drugs, I dealt with men that sold drugs, and I used drugs. But I wasn't an intravenous drug user. . . . I didn't stand on the corner and prostitute. I wasn't a gay man. But I had sugar daddies. I had multiple sex

partners. But I knew the exact number of men I slept with. So it still didn't seem to fit. I didn't seem to fit in this category. Can't be so.

A second confirmatory test came back ten days before Beverly's thirtieth birthday. What happened next is revelatory. Still at the drug rehab center, Beverly called her mother Verna, sobbing into the phone to the woman who carried the family on her back:

I'm crying so hard. And she's like, "What's wrong, honey?"
"Mom, I'm dying, I'm dying."
"Huh, you're gonna die? What do you mean you're gonna die?"
"I got the virus."
"What? What do you mean you got the virus? What virus? You talking about having what Magic Johnson got?"
"Yeah, the virus and I'm gonna die."
"Honey, honey, calm down, you're not gonna die. You're not gonna die. Listen, listen, listen. Just listen [soothing voice]. On Monday we're taking your sister, who has just gotten her test. She's going into surgery on Monday, and it does not look good. They're gonna remove the breast."
I had a sister who got diagnosed with breast cancer one month before my diagnosis. So on this particular Friday . . . it was a Friday, I'll never forget and then my mother said:
"Just hold on, just hold on, hold on. Stop crying. Just listen, just listen [soothing voice]. Your sister's going to surgery on Monday and, baby, it don't look good at all. So we will deal with her, then we gonna deal with you. But right now, you ain't gonna die. I need you to stop crying, and I need you to hold on. Now could you just do that for me? Just . . . just let us deal with her, then we gonna deal with you. Because hers is much worse and they gonna take the breast off on Monday and it doesn't look good."
So the way she said it was like, "Listen, we got another crisis before yours. But you hold on to yours, and we gonna handle it. Stop crying, you're gonna be all right. Don't worry. Don't worry about it, you're gonna be . . . it's gonna be all right."
And that's the way we did it. "Deal with her. Then we'll deal with you."

Verna's response illustrates mothering in the crossfire. Mothers living in highly disadvantaged contexts often find themselves confronting multiple simultaneous life-threatening and life-draining issues. Lacking even the everyday financial wherewithal, let alone wealth, to help address these problems, one of the most powerful tools at their disposal is their ability to navigate the devastating currents that whiplash them, to triage the crises. Verna engaged her tools: weighing the severity of multiple crises, making strategic decisions about which to confront first, and assuring both of her children that she could be counted on for support. Critical for Verna was her immediate understanding of HIV/AIDS as a virus, "like Magic Johnson's," something that was not cause for immediate panic, the basketball legend's vitality and visibility serving as her guidepost.

Recalling her numerous emergency room admittances starting in the 1980s, Trisha remembers health providers telling her about the importance of getting tested for HIV. Sex workers face higher HIV infection rates in part because of inconsistent condom use, high numbers of partners, and for some, drug use and mental health issues. Their circumstances also may discourage or prevent them from accessing HIV prevention resources as they grapple with stigma, lack of access to healthcare and other social services, and poverty.[81] But Trisha refused to take the test. Untreated gonorrhea had destroyed her ability to have children. She had liver and kidney problems and had suffered several strokes, likely cumulative damage from the effects of drugs. She had frequent mouth sores, one of the most common symptoms of HIV. At one point she had lost so much weight she could barely wear a bra as her chest wasted away to childlike proportions. She was still battling hepatitis C when we had our first interview in 2010. As she recalled, lying in that hospital bed in 1996 with pneumocystis carinii pneumonia and being told "the infectious disease doctor is coming to see you tomorrow," Trisha knew what it meant, and a flood of emotions came over her:

> Saying to myself, "I really did it this time." I wanted to kick myself in the butt. I said, "You have gone too far. Now what? Now you're going to die." And you realize, you don't want to die. So I went through my little changes of really looking back on what I did to myself. And now the position I was in. And then I remember, I dealt with it for a few days and then I asked the doctor, "Well, how long do I have to live?" And he said, "Five years maybe." I said, "Okay. I'm going to make the best out of these five years."

The diagnosis was not a surprise; Trisha learned about the dangers of sharing needles, ironically, from a person with whom she shared needles. She watched friends waste away and die, recalling the menagerie of medications she had seen on one friend's bedroom dresser. But dying companions and street acquaintances never discussed what ailed them.

The diagnosis did not, however, spark immediate transformation. Instead, Trisha fell deeper into the abyss. "Once I got healthy enough, I went right back to those streets and I was using, like, 'I'm gonna enjoy these five years.'"

It was in fact quite common for women, upon receiving an HIV diagnosis, to return to risky behaviors. Most interpreted the news as a death sentence and believed their demise was imminent. This is not surprising, because protease inhibitor–based antiretroviral therapy was not widely available until 1996 (prior to that, AZT, a controversial drug widely considered toxic and only moderately effective, was used to treat patients). Even with the introduction of newer HIV medications, access to them has been uneven across populations.[82] But Trisha is describing another kind of barrier: she was in no mental or physical state to wage a battle against HIV. For her, the easiest and most comfortable course of action was to ignore the health risk and resume her previous coping and survival strategies. When Trisha returned to life on the streets, she made a point of not telling anyone about her diagnosis. "No, I might have gotten myself killed," she commented—accused of infecting her compatriots or customers. HIV therefore simply took its place at the end of a long list of traumas Trisha knew not to discuss.

Yvette Simmons

Many women's stories bear strong similarities to those of Trisha, Beverly, and Keisha. But the AIDS epidemic is complex and nuanced in part because there are multiple pathways and contexts that lead to HIV transmission and shape women's experiences once diagnosed. Some of the Chicago women were diagnosed in the early 1980s after receiving blood transfusions. Others reported that they acquired HIV from their husbands, some of whom were former or current PWID or had engaged in unprotected sex before or during the marriage. A number of the women were diagnosed during prenatal visits to their doctors and were immediately offered medication to prevent perinatal (mother to child) transmission. In fact, when diagnosed, many women were leading stable lives at some distance from the sexualized drug economy and other higher-risk contexts.

For example, Yvette Simmons grew up in a close-knit and stable working-class household in Maryland. The reserved youngest daughter of five children met a boy in high school who became her high school sweetheart. She found herself pregnant at 19 but broke up with her baby's father within a year of the birth of their son Steven:

> Steven's father was so funny. Oh, my goodness, I think he pursued me from the time I got into that high school until I graduated. But I didn't want to have anything to do with knuckleheads. I had a plan. I think because my mom had five kids and struggled, I didn't want to be anything like that. So I planned on having a full-time job and this nice house and no kids. . . . It didn't seem like he would be very responsible. I said, "You know what, he's just going to cause me problems. And I just need to figure out what I'm going to do and take care of myself and my child."

Her ex-boyfriend continued to be a part of Steven's life, but they would not be together. When Steven turned four, Yvette enrolled in college at 24 years old. Recounting what happened next still makes her emotional:

> I hope I don't cry. It was my very first semester. And there was a blood drive and fair in the student center. I love stuff like that, so I went and got my blood drawn. HIV did come to mind. I don't know why I thought about this, because I wasn't promiscuous, I wasn't an IV drug user, I'm not gay. And so I thought if everything comes out right, "I'll be set. I'm in college, I'll have a great job."

The thought of HIV crossed Yvette's mind because of stories she had heard about people learning they had HIV when they donated blood. Like Beverly, though, she quickly dismissed it after rationalizing that she didn't fit the category of someone with HIV. The Red Cross called her back two weeks later: "And so I went, and the woman who told me [I have HIV] was pregnant. And I'm crying and I'm thinking, 'Oh, my tears are going to get on your baby! Are you going to get it?' It was really bad. It was really bad."

Given that Yvette had been tested when she was pregnant with Steven and was HIV negative at that time, she and the healthcare worker deduced she must have seroconverted more recently: "I knew it couldn't have been more than two or three guys, so I narrowed it down like that. But I still don't know for sure. I was kind of a naïve, gullible person. I'm probably a little naïve and gullible now. I often thought by not asking a guy to use condoms, that would prove to him how trustworthy I was and how clean a person I was. And so I never did."

Yvette's assumptions about the norms and signals around sex were not unusual, as many women in this study shared the belief that having unprotected sex demonstrated cleanliness, trust, and connection. Elisa Sobo captures the complexity of women's sexual agency in her book *Choosing Unsafe Sex*, pointing out that the expectations and understandings undergirding heterosexual unions in fact encourage unprotected sex.[83] Through cultural messages and social norms, women like Yvette are socialized to be more vulnerable to "wishful thinking engendered by hopes for their relationships [as well as] desires to preserve status and self-esteem."[84] Such risk denial is inextricably linked to the need to believe that their own unions meet expectations, that they are wise enough to assess their sexual risk, and that the men in their lives are monogamous. These persistent mental frames can make an HIV diagnosis all the more startling.

DYING FROM: THE CONTINUED RACE TO THE BOTTOM

Keisha's post-diagnosis struggle played out in perhaps one of the most challenging of venues: high school. Jimmy was still out of the picture, effectively disappearing from Keisha's life until she would hear of his arrest. As she began learning more about HIV and how to best manage it, she and her parents had to decide how Keisha would continue her education. For her parents, dropping out was not an option. "My mom is like, 'Live your life, keep going.' That's easy for people to say who don't have it. Everybody thinks you can just take the pills and be fine, but emotionally it's a lot harder. You don't have a normal life." Keisha was clear that she did not want to remain at her current school. She was terrified of being ostracized not only within the walls of the school but in the nearby neighborhood where she and her family lived.

Keisha convinced her parents to allow her to transfer to a school where there were fewer friends and acquaintances, a school with a very small percentage of black students that would overlap with her overwhelmingly black social network. They chose a public high school with a large Latinx and Asian student population. There, Keisha hoped to keep a low profile as she grappled with her newly discovered health status:

> [After my diagnosis] I was basically traumatized for a while. Went to school, did my work, that was it. My dad was very supportive [and would ask], "How do you like the new school?" Then [long pause] . . . my status got out there. A girl was there [long pause] . . . and I guess we were cool. Then we got into an argument about something, and she went around telling everybody she wanted to fight me, but when she fought me, she said she wanted to put some gloves on because she didn't want to spread any blood. And that got back to me. Well, I just . . . that wasn't the time to mess with me, you know. I was already really angry. I remember what . . . well, I remember exactly what I did. One of my friends told me, "The girl is upstairs, you know, and you can go get her." I went upstairs, took the lock off my locker, met her on the second floor. And I said to her, "Why did you say what you said about me?" She tells me, "Come on, you know, I don't want to fight you." I'm like, "I ain't talking about that, I just want to know about you talking about putting on gloves and everything." She said something smart and I don't know what happened after that, 'cause I just . . . I just went at her. Afterwards, I went to jail because a police officer pressed charges against me because I fought the police officer [breaking up the fight], which I didn't even remember I did. I was so angry that day, I . . . I don't know, I really don't even . . . I don't even remember what happened from the time I fought her. The next thing I know, I remember . . . I asked her why she did it, then I went from that to . . . I was sitting down with handcuffs on. That's all I remember. That was the first time I had anything, altercations, anything. I was the quietest person. I never say nothing to nobody. But that . . .

Keisha believes the girl learned about her HIV status through a mutual friend in whom Keisha had confided:

> This was the time where it was fresh. My diagnosis was fresh. I was getting different opinions from different doctors. So me and my family . . . well, me and my dad really weren't automatically saying okay, we're positive. I was getting an opinion here, an opinion here, an opinion here. All of the opinions were coming out HIV positive, but we just weren't accepting that. And one day the doctors did actually tell me that [I needed to accept that I was definitely HIV positive]. And then I went to school that day, and I felt . . . all the emotions came over me. People kept asking me what was wrong, and I talked to my best friend, I told her what happened. And it basically went like that.

The school administrators allowed Keisha to remain enrolled despite the fight. She returned after a suspension and focused on completing the requirements for her diploma. She graduated, but not without navigating difficult social terrain as a teenager living with HIV: "I didn't go to prom. I would come in the lunchroom, and the faces are automatically looking. I could see people just looking at me all crazy. So after a while, I started sitting by myself because I didn't want to . . . I didn't want no one asking me questions. Didn't want any of that. Some of the teachers were asking me, 'Was it true?' I just was like, 'Yeah, it's true.'"

After completing high school, Keisha headed to a local community college. She met a handsome guy named Marcus who approached her on the street. It was exhilarating; after her isolation in high school, now she finally had a guy showing serious interest in her. Seven years her senior, Marcus persuaded her months into the relationship to move out of her family home. As I got to know her over more than a decade, I saw how deeply attracted Keisha was to the idea of traditional family life; she was drawn to men who boasted that they could provide that, even if there was no evidence they could actually deliver. Marcus was the first to make such claims, and he backed it up by suggesting she move in with him at a point in her life when Keisha seriously doubted she could have "a happily ever after" given her status. She jumped at the chance.

Keisha lied and told her mother she was headed for Job Corps to get out of the house: "I wrote my mother a letter one day out of the blue and just told her I wanted to be independent." Her mother was perhaps distracted with struggles of her own. Her marriage to Keisha's father was ending, crumbling under the weight of what was becoming his growing drug addiction. And tensions between Keisha and her mother were escalating. "I don't think I would have left my mom's house if I weren't HIV positive. I would have been able to live with her." What was it about her HIV status that made living under her mother's roof untenable? "She kept telling people," Keisha explained:

One day, before Marcus, I invited this boy to my house. And she thought we were having sex, but we weren't. The guy was fully clothed, I was fully clothed, nothing was going on. But I was scared to death [when she came home], so I hid him under my bed. I was scared to death because I knew my mom was gonna go crazy. So she sent me to the store. Oh my God, this guy is in my house! I didn't know what he was gonna do. So eventually, when I came home, my mom said, "Oh, we're about to change the furniture in your room around." I already knew she knew that he was in there. . . . [He came out of my room] and was saying, "Well, I love her . . ." and he wants to spend the rest of his life with me. And she's like, "Well, did you know she is HIV positive?" And I'm standing like, oh, God. No. And that guy left and never came back. And after that, I was pissed at her. Because I could have had a relationship with him. And like I said, if I wasn't positive, none of that stuff would have happened.

It is unclear what Keisha's mother hoped to gain by disclosing her daughter's HIV status to would-be suitors. Arguably, she was trying to ensure the young men had critical information that could have implications for the health and safety of both her daughter and the young men. She frequently said to Keisha, "Well, you've got to tell people that you're positive, or they'll kill you." Perhaps she feared Keisha could be subject to intimate-partner violence or held criminally liable for not disclosing her HIV status to sexual partners. Or perhaps she was simply at a loss about how best to parent a daughter through sexual maturity, a daughter who was navigating her late teen years and early adulthood with a life-threatening diagnosis that is sexually transmittable. To Keisha, however, her mother's sharing of this information seemed like a deliberate attempt to embarrass and punish a daughter she saw as sexually irresponsible.

Keisha disclosed her HIV status to Marcus, and to her great relief he stuck around. They used condoms occasionally, but not consistently. He told her he was HIV positive as well, but to this day Keisha doesn't know if that was true or just something he told her so she would not press him to use condoms.

Once Keisha moved in, the living situation with Marcus deteriorated at breakneck speed. He had exhibited some controlling behavior when they first began seeing one another, and it escalated once Keisha was living with him, isolated from her family in a south suburb of Chicago known for high levels of poverty and unemployment. Marcus would stay out late into the night and then come home demanding sex. He had final say on where she went and convinced her she needed to drop out of community college. She tried to make it work, clinging to her ideals of domesticity by regularly cooking him dinner on a hot plate while he barely kept the heat and gas bills paid. Within a month, Keisha knew she had to get out of the situation. "It wasn't what I thought it was gonna be. What he portrayed it as . . . it was like, 'Come move with me. We can live this life.' He made it sound like it was gonna be all roses. And then when I get there . . . " He used the fact that he was significantly older than Keisha to his advantage: "He told me what I could do and when I can do it, how I can do it. He had too much authority over me. And me being so young, he figured I didn't know nothing. With him, I found myself withering away. Basically dying. I even stopped taking my medicine."

I met Keisha just two years after her diagnosis. She was 19, six months pregnant with Marcus's child, and had been living in a homeless shelter since leaving him. For Keisha, stigma was a lens through which she interpreted her life and the possibilities before her, and she made very consequential decisions using that narrowing lens. Twenty-six-year-old Marcus had convinced her to leave her mother's home and move into his, where physical isolation from the rest of the world became a way of life until she effectively escaped. He had promised to love her regardless of her HIV status when she believed no one else would.

I once heard a woman living with HIV say that stigma is like cold air: you don't see it, but you feel it. Due to anticipated, internalized, and experienced stigma, an HIV-positive diagnosis ignites a crisis of respectability. In addition to the physical challenges and other crises they faced, many WLWHA experienced periods in which they were essentially *dying from* the burden of this social marker. The possibility of social death—the loss of familial connections, identity, intimacy, and social standing—was a clear and present danger.[85] A blood-borne disease, HIV was the symbolic evidence of moral failure; now the shame was pulsing through their bloodstreams. Without a cure, this status would follow them for the rest of their lives and potentially degrade any claim the women might have to love, respect, and peace.

Almost from the moment of her diagnosis, Yvette began attempting to restore and affirm her respectability. She already felt pressure to marry after becoming an unwed mother at 19 in order to be "an upstanding member of society and fix my social standing." Her HIV status pushed those impulses into overdrive. She completed her bachelor's degree in social work and earned several credits toward a master's degree. She started dating a man she met at an HIV support group and married him after a six-month courtship. Keisha and Yvette were not the only women I interviewed who made hasty relationship decisions based on the fear of being alone and unwanted; more than one-third of the Chicago women described making similar choices. Yvette's marriage lasted only eleven months as it became clear they had little in common except for their HIV status. "I was desperate to get married," she explained. "I was desperate to find this enchanted, happily-ever-after relationship, and I wanted it badly . . . to feel like an upstanding member of society. . . . I guess I thought my happily ever after was a man." Notably, this represented a shift from Yvette's high school ambitions of an independent life with a great job and a house.

When we met in 2007, Yvette had yet to disclose her HIV status to her family, with the exception of her oldest sister, Sherry, whom she had told in case something happened to her. She was concerned about the prejudice and ignorance she might face if she revealed her status to others. "I'm so afraid of telling people, because it would really hurt my feelings if someone went into the bathroom after me with Lysol and bleach. Or after me using a plate or a fork, they would just put it in the trash."

Yvette was also, however, deeply concerned about another kind of "death," the loss of the esteem her family felt for her. "Because I was an irresponsible teenager, getting pregnant younger. And I didn't have a successful marriage, and I feel like that was kind of irresponsible. I don't want to be seen as being irresponsible once again [because I have HIV]." Yvette was over a decade into a lucrative career working for the government. Although others in her family had attended college, she was the first in her family to graduate. She had bravely made the move to Chicago from the east coast; she had a sister whose first airplane ride did not take place until her mid-forties, when she visited Yvette. Her sisters and nieces viewed her as a success story and role model, the one who "made it." What would it mean if their most successful family member had "the virus"? "I'm a role model to my nieces, and I want to tell them because I don't want them to make the same mistakes I did. But, again, I don't want to be treated negatively either." Yvette described living a double life: "It's become such a part of me, because I've had it for so long. I don't know, it's kind of normal now."

Despite her outward appearance of success, signs of Yvette's struggle were evident in our first interview. A deep sense of shame undergirded

many of her comments. When her marriage and other subsequent relationships failed, Yvette slumped into a depression and gained 35 pounds.
She described herself as overweight and without prompting from me vol-
unteered that she thought it was because she was afraid of relationships.
She had been "keeping the weight on, trying to keep men at a distance."
This came up again in a subsequent interview, and her elaboration was
striking: "The weight also limits me in that the men who come to me, I
don't have as wide of a choice. So I'm less likely to pick a bad man." Not
only did Yvette not trust men to do the right thing, she also did not trust
herself to choose the right man, still heaping punishment on herself for
picking the man from whom she acquired HIV. Yvette's now-adult son
Steven was living with her when we met. She was friendly with coworkers
and had a few close girlfriends. But given her secret, Yvette was very much
alone, hiding in plain sight.

HIV/AIDS AND THE PROBLEM OF "THE OTHER"

HIV/AIDS, unlike many other diseases, has a particular cultural significance that obliges people living with it to grapple with some of the weight-
iest and most contentious issues threaded through our social fabric: sex,
sexuality, money, race, gender, drugs, and the unequal access to resources
that allows some social groups to insulate themselves from injuries of inequality while others are highly vulnerable. This is an infection that many
believed, and continue to believe, is a kind of punishment, a moral adjudi-
cation. From the residents of Austin, Indiana to the Chicago women in my
research, it might be tempting to assign sympathy or blame to these individuals and the various people in their lives, designating heroes and vil-
lains in the story of AIDS.

This temptation exists because HIV/AIDS is not only a medical epidemic but also a social and cultural Rorschach test that pushes our views
about difference, ethics, morality, and complex inequalities to center
stage. The need to rhetorically classify people living with HIV/AIDS and
groups most affected by the epidemic has long guided the political and
cultural debate.[86] The mode through which an individual reports acquiring the virus and the measures she or he takes to avoid transmitting it to

others are viewed as "respectability proxies" that allow our moral measuring sticks to tag some as "innocent victims of the epidemic" and others as "those who should have known better," or even worse, as those who "earned their fate."[87]

HIV/AIDS is also emblematic of "the Other."[88] Cultural theorist Stuart Hall observes that "the Other" has become essential to how we make sense of our own lives and ascribe meaning. The frame provides the opportunity for us to view our own choices through the lens of "the Other" and to pronounce that we are not alike. We often see "the Other" as a weak individual with moral deficits, and this is compounded by, and even rooted in, racial animus, homophobia, sexism, and anti-poor sentiment.[89] In the assessments of some, "the Other" does not deserve a second chance or even compassion. Those commodities are reserved for those who are like us and remind us of ourselves.

Insofar as the presumed guilt or innocence of "the Other" remains fully operational in discussions of HIV, the women I interviewed must contend with its deep and bruising stigma. Many therefore confront what feminist scholar Michele Tracy Berger terms "intersectional stigma," marginalization based on both HIV and other disadvantaged statuses.[90] For example, long-standing and embedded stereotypical notions about the supposed lasciviousness and irresponsible behaviors of black and brown women interconnect with beliefs about the immorality of women living with HIV/AIDS. This "sexualized racism," as Patricia Hill Collins describes it, frames these women's sexual options and decision-making.[91] Low-income women, especially those experienced with drug addiction, are branded with yet another discrediting social marker when they are diagnosed HIV positive. Even for middle-class women, an HIV diagnosis challenges the idea that they are "respectable" women who have "done things right." As respectability is often socially reinforced as a requirement for women's social and economic success, even their prospects for upward mobility can be called into question with an HIV diagnosis. These cultural-historical traps drive the assaults on women's self- and societal worth and fuel the silences that ignore threats to their health.

Until we abandon this thinking, these hard-and-fast distinctions between the "deserving" and "undeserving" will continue to play an influential role in determining the allocation of attention and resources, potentially deepening the very inequities that contribute to the disparate infection rates among certain populations. I contend that rather than sympathizing with some while blaming (or distancing from, or shaming) others, we should think about the AIDS epidemic through a dual lens of empathy and humble curiosity. Many of us have never lived the harrowing experiences Trisha, Beverly, Keisha, and Yvette describe, but perhaps we can empathize with what it's like to make questionable decisions in the quest for love or financial security. We might see ourselves as far removed from the sexualized drug economies of Scott County and Chicago, but we know what it's like to want to remove the sting of devastating pain, of trauma, as expediently as possible. Perhaps we can relate to what it's like to seek pleasure, safety, and connection while navigating life's vicissitudes. And perhaps we did everything "right," closely following societal conventions, only to face crisis when we least expected it.

Apropos of humble curiosity, some might approach this discussion by assuming that because the women in my research are marginalized, they lack the education or judgment to have anything useful to teach us. By listening to what these women have to say, however, we can be humble students who realize just how much we can learn about inequality, public policy, societal epidemics, healing from trauma, and life transformation by drawing from their perspectives.

We might also be tempted to frame the women's experiences solely through the lens of victimhood, viewing them as women who were robbed of all agency. That, however, would be inaccurate. Trisha, Beverly, Keisha, and Yvette offered their own reflections on how they exercised agency, on mistakes they made along the way, and on their willingness to own some of the circumstances that led them to this point. All of them pursued joy and pleasure, valid and legitimate dimensions of human behavior, through intimate relationships and, in some cases, drug use. Sex and the earliest stages of drug use represented freedom and power, the expression of some level of control over their bodies. To fully understand AIDS, we must understand how these complicated truths of human behavior fit into the epidemic. This lens is also useful for comprehending the early turn of events that eventually spiraled into *dying from* for some women: when women became mired in shame rather than affirmed through accountability, they often continued down destructive paths.[92]

As inaccurate as it would be to deny that these women possessed agency, it would be quite problematic to ignore the conditions that severely constrained their choices and opportunities. They exercised *restricted* agency. Their very natural pursuit of validation, happiness, and love existed within a context of heightened structural risk. They weighed numerous risks—economic, emotional, physical, social—with HIV circulating as just one of several potential dangers. Each woman's choices and decision-making were inextricably linked to her personal dreams, fears, and traumas; enacted and negotiated through interpersonal connections and violations; and embedded in environmental vulnerabilities, temptations, and opportunities (or lack thereof). Given these complex issues, recognizing the interplay between a woman's self and her environment is a much more useful way to understand not only HIV/AIDS but inequality in general. It also requires us to think about accountability—at the individual, community, and societal levels—as the women's stories reveal the gaps and exposures that led to their acquiring HIV. Too many of the women in this research had experienced multiple traumas before the actual incident that gave them the virus, including childhood sexual abuse, the rigors of the sexualized drug economy, and coming of age in communities characterized by gaping vulnerabilities and strategic silences.

This represents the common thread between the people of Scott County, Indiana, and the Chicago women living with HIV who were a part of my research. HIV/AIDS is a global pandemic shaped by social inequality.[93] Marginalization on the basis of race, class, gender, and sexuality plays a significant role in determining who faces the highest risk of HIV infection, who is most likely to receive life-saving treatment, and how the epidemic disproportionately affects certain communities. And the results of this inequality are costly. Experts estimate that the cost of lifetime HIV care for those who acquired the virus during the Scott County outbreak is close to $59 million if treatment costs remain the same.[94]

Later we will examine what happened when the Chicago women attempted to halt the downward momentum of their lives. Despite the obstacles, hope managed to find cracks in the concrete of despair for a significant number of these women. The most successful found ways to hold themselves accountable rather than shamed and blameworthy, and through that process they found ways to hold to account those with considerably greater power. They sought out support structures to combat their invisibility and to help them navigate their new status. Some of the most economically, physically, and emotionally distressed women sought new outlets for survival outside of the sexualized drug economy. Many discovered they could save themselves and remake their lives by replacing one set of networks with another, networks that offered life instead of death, promise and opportunity instead of degradation and violence. What greeted the women was the HIV safety net, a billion-dollar infrastructure of public policy, institutions, networks, and a culture that would prove highly effective at presenting an alternative to *dying from*. In the next chapter, we consider how this life force, the HIV safety net, emerged out of the shadows of an epidemic to transform *dying from* to *living with*.

2 The Safety Net that AIDS Activism Built

The caretakers of the earliest AIDS patients—those lovers, friends, family members, doctors, and nurses who were not afraid to hold the hands of the dying—likely did not realize then that they were laying the groundwork for what has become one of the most effective policy innovations of the last 50 years. They recruited important, albeit sometimes reluctant, allies to the fight: sympathetic lawmakers and government bureaucrats who injected words of caution and pragmatism while ensuring that needed resources would be available; medical providers and scientific researchers who acknowledged the importance of taking up a cause with implications that extended beyond their examining rooms and laboratories; and social service providers who could help implement the vision on the front lines. From the grass roots to the rarified air of the political elite, there is a grand experiment under way; it is only decades old but has nevertheless proven to be highly successful in helping to transform lives. Its mission is simple: move people from death to life. Debates within the community about what that goal means and how we get there persist. Should the AIDS response focus on a purely clinical definition of what it means to live and die: getting life-saving drugs into bodies? Or is a more holistic interpretation called for, one that works to improve overall health, social, economic, and political outcomes for populations most affected by HIV/AIDS and that pushes against the inequities that fuel the epidemic?

The story of AIDS activists who opened the eyes of the world to a devastating epidemic is now well known, chronicled in books and film.[1] Their political demonstrations and marches became defining moments of 1980s and 1990s America, fundamentally altering how investigators conduct medical research and doctors practice medicine to make the patient a partner rather than solely an object. People with HIV spoke up: demanding more rights for patients, access to healthcare and life-saving drugs, and research to understand what was happening to their bodies.

AIDS activists and advocates were involved in another critical effort at that time, a lesser-known, often overlooked part of the AIDS response. As these individuals fought for treatment and dignity—locking arms; learning as much as they could about the disease that was inexplicably ravaging their communities; confronting the ignorance, silence, apathy, and antipathy that threatened their lives and the lives of people they cared about— AIDS activists and advocates were simultaneously building one of the most effective health and social support safety nets of the twentieth century. With healthcare services, modest economic assistance, extensive social support, and political and civic engagement as its pillars, this now billion-dollar infrastructure stands as an underappreciated yet highly effective model for assisting marginalized populations, demonstrating how effective public policies, robust institutional networks, and multicultural coalitions can address injuries of inequality.

CONFRONTING THE POLITICS OF DISGUST: THE EARLY YEARS OF THE HIV/AIDS SAFETY NET

The AIDS epidemic was framed from the outset by what political scientist Ange-Marie Hancock terms the "politics of disgust," an emotion-laden response to policy demands based on longstanding beliefs and stereotypes about the population at the center of the debate.[2] When AIDS emerged in the United States, the majority of reported cases involved gay men and intravenous drug users, fueling a disease narrative that emphasized individual behavior and stigmatized identities. Many warned that AIDS was "the modern plague," divine punishment for personal failings related to homosexuality, promiscuity, and drug use.[3] These views have manifested at times as a religiously inflected politics of disgust and have fueled the controversy over policy responses to the epidemic.[4] Therefore, challenging dominant narratives that portray people living with HIV/AIDS as immoral, powerless, socially dysfunctional, irresponsible, and unable to contribute to society because of their alleged deviance has been an integral part of confronting HIV/AIDS.

Gay (mostly white) men began to formally organize to confront the emerging threat shortly after the CDC released its 1981 *Morbidity and Mortality Weekly Report* and media outlets began to cover this new disease. The epidemic represented, in the words of historian Julio Capó Jr., "one of the greatest assaults on queer communities already vulnerable to state violence, negligence, erasure, and marginalization."[5] As sociologist Steven Epstein points out, gay men both suffered from and contributed to the notion that AIDS was "a gay disease."[6] Recognizing the need for greater coordination in the effort to address "the gay cancer" or the "gay-related immune deficiency or GRID," on January 4, 1982, playwright Larry Kramer and five others officially established the Gay Men's Health Crisis (GMHC) in New York City. The group formed after a community gathering at Kramer's apartment that occurred soon after the first cases of AIDS were reported. As perhaps the earliest nonprofit and community-based AIDS services provider in the United States, GMHC became a critical source of information, community organizing, and advocacy for the gay community as public health officials struggled to manage the crisis.

GMHC also formally organized what sympathetic friends, lovers, and family members began doing informally: lending daily living assistance to those suffering from AIDS. As the mysterious disease progressed, patients were increasingly unable to care for themselves as diminished immune systems subjected them to opportunistic infections. In the absence of viable treatment options, providing emotional support and caregiving to help those afflicted by AIDS made it possible to confront the disease immediately, to do *something*.

The services offered by GMHC created a foundational model for AIDS care as members pieced together the offerings as needs emerged.[7] A telephone hotline provided information to worried callers and a buddy service helped patients make doctor's appointments. The organization connected clients to housing assistance when their families cast them aside because of AIDS stigma. It connected PLWHA to lawyers who provided free or low-cost legal services to help people develop end-of-life plans or seek legal advice following discriminatory experiences. It referred people to funeral homes willing to take the bodies of those who succumbed to AIDS and ensured that hospitalized patients were visited. It brought groceries and meals when people could no longer cook for themselves or work. Facing high levels of stigmatization from some family members, health providers, and the general public, PLWHA could access assistance at GMHC offices away from the harsh glare of public judgment. Many of the organizers had worked in social services. As service provision became more extensive and sophisticated, GMHC eventually sought federal, state, and local government funding to support its efforts, essentially formalizing the relationship between the budding HIV safety net and the state.

As it evolved from its grassroots beginnings, GMHC, according to Philip Kayal's early history of the organization, became "well-housed, professionally staffed, and remarkably well appointed."[8] It utilized what would become a central organizing principle in AIDS services: care based on case management—the provision of comprehensive, wrap-around services organized by a key point person, the case manager. Support groups were also a critical aspect of care, encouraging people to share their stories and view themselves as peer advocates. GMHC identified early on the need to address overlapping physical and mental health issues, and case managers were expected to understand the science of the disease and the emerging treatment options, making their approach to care truly holistic.[9] When New York's statewide AIDS Institute opened, it modeled itself on GMHC, tapping former executive director Mel Rosen to run the organization.[10]

While GMHC established itself at the center of what would become the HIV safety net, pressing issues within the epidemic would challenge its approach. GMHC received criticism for its somewhat stilted, institutionalized feel and more moderate stance toward political activism in support of AIDS and gay rights, opting to seek legitimacy in the eyes of federal, state, and local government funders.[11] Among those voicing this critique was Larry Kramer himself, whose view of GMHC's direction began to diverge sharply from that of many within the organization.

The AIDS Coalition to Unleash Power (ACT UP) emerged in 1987 to drive a decidedly more activist agenda: pushing for treatments rather than focusing on services; positioning itself in opposition to, rather than as a partner of, the state; and serving as a voice of the community, not a bureaucracy serving the community.[12] President Ronald Reagan's downplaying of the epidemic and failure to publicly mention AIDS until 1986, as well as his political allies' cold-hearted attacks against gay men and others most affected by the epidemic, positioned the federal government as an early foe of the AIDS movement, notwithstanding the efforts of some at the National Institutes of Health (NIH), CDC, and other agencies to understand and contain the epidemic. ACT UP founding member Peter Staley, addressing the government's lackluster response, characterized PLWHA as "threatened with extinction," requiring them "to stand up, and to fight back."[13] With some overlap between those involved in GMHC and ACT UP, the latter aggressively fought the Food and Drug Administration (FDA) for fast-tracked drug trials, pushed for more federal dollars for AIDS research, demanded seats at the table at NIH and other key decision-making bodies, and advocated for change in other state practices. ACT UP waged a highly publicized fight against the institutionalized practices of the research, clinical, and pharmaceutical industries, accusing all three of not moving fast enough to fight the epidemic and bringing problematic assumptions and beliefs to bear on the fight. These efforts not only led to changes by government officials, the medical community, and corporate leaders in their approaches to HIV/AIDS, but to other diseases as well, by reframing how we think about the individuals at the center of an illness and by altering the strategies and procedures for medical research, pharmaceutical testing and distribution, and doctor-patient relationships. Epstein writes:

> Perhaps the most striking feature on the landscape of AIDS politics is the development of an "AIDS movement" that is more than just a "disease constituency" pressuring the government for more funding, but is in fact an alternative basis of expertise. The members of this movement are not the first laypeople to put forward claims to speak credibly on biomedical matters. But this is indeed the first social movement in the US to accomplish the large-scale conversion of disease "victims" into activist-experts. In this sense, the AIDS movement stands alone, even as it begins to serve as a model for others.[14]

AIDS activists stormed the stage at the Second National AIDS Forum in Denver, Colorado in 1983 and demanded to be called "people with AIDS" rather than "AIDS victims." They pressed for PLWHA to be represented at the table for policy decisions and demanded to be treated with dignity. In what came to be known as the Denver Principles, these tenets informed the founding charter of the National Association of People with AIDS (NAPWA). The growing AIDS community adopted another value that would become fundamental to the HIV safety net's evolution: strong partnerships and overlap between providers and recipients of services. With an explosion of peer-led AIDS organizations, AIDS "victims" could become AIDS survivors, and AIDS survivors could become AIDS activists and service providers within this organizational structure.

Gay men used their networks and resources to grow and expand both their AIDS activism and services. Due to the fairly recent mobilization of gay activists after the 1969 Stonewall riots, an infrastructure supporting gay political rights was already in place that could readily adopt AIDS as the next significant threat to the community and use similar tools and strategies of protest, including those borrowed from the civil rights movement that took place throughout much of the twentieth century.[15] Gay rights activists took a page from black freedom struggles, creating a social movement that challenged structures of domination and had an organizational core that served as an instrument for social change. This self-actuated collective action was critically necessary in the wake of structures, policies, and a dominant culture that largely overlooked or punished those most disproportionately affected by the growing AIDS epidemic.

As in the civil rights movement, LGBTQ individuals deployed the cultural resources and organizational structures of their communities in order to wage a war against AIDS and the apathy and antipathy that fueled it. Major cities around the country housed organizations, newspapers, bars and clubs, bathhouses, bookstores, and other spaces in which gay men could congregate, share information, and create strategies for fighting AIDS. A small health infrastructure for gay men was also in place, with specialty clinics and providers who could address STIs and other health concerns in a non-stigmatizing environment. As a sizeable HIV/AIDS infrastructure emerged in New York City, there was a parallel emergence of similar systems of support in other cities with large gay communities, including San Francisco, Los Angeles, and later, Chicago. The San Francisco AIDS Foundation (SFAF) was established in the same year as GMHC. They were joined by organizations such as the Shanti Project (also in San Francisco) and Howard Brown Health in Chicago, which had been offering health services to vulnerable populations confronting terminal, life-threatening, or disabling illnesses and conditions since the 1970s.

The SFAF, GMHC, and other organizations also initiated specific efforts to address the emerging epidemic among people who inject drugs, including having information and resources available to PWID through their AIDS hotlines. SFAF's BleachMan campaign played a major role in pushing forward the approval of needle exchange in the area. Although some gay men injected drugs, the majority of PWIDs affected by HIV/ AIDS were not gay, creating an early link between the LGBTQ community and others affected by the epidemic. These shifts introduced more class diversity into the nascent HIV safety net as the client services departments of organizations such as SFAF and GMHC shifted from serving mostly middle-class (mostly white) gay men to serving a growing number of low-income clients, many of whom were people of color.

The fight against AIDS was also waged on the cultural front. AIDS activists fought homophobia to answer the politics of disgust that added fuel to the epidemic. They worked vigorously to educate the public, offering detailed, eloquent, and sympathetic media portrayals to "reveal to the larger heterosexual world the emotional toll that AIDS has taken in gay communities while breaking down stereotypes about gay life."[16] Other affected populations did not wage the same full-frontal attacks on the cultural representation of HIV/AIDS, for reasons that will be discussed throughout the book. But gay men of various racial backgrounds leaned heavily on popular culture to gain public sympathy and change the narrative through films, books, and plays such as *And the Band Played On* and *Angels in America,* as well as in the work of black gay cultural icons such as Marlon Riggs, Essex Hemphill, and Joseph Beam.

To be sure, the growing economic, cultural, and political clout white gay men possessed gave them the resources needed to create and sustain a nascent patchwork of political and service organizations. Phill Wilson, a black gay man who worked in several AIDS organizations prior to becoming the founder and executive director of the Black AIDS Institute in 1999, explains:

The front of the spear *looked* like the rich and powerful sons [of the elites]. So you could look and say, "Oh that could be my son . . . " And then the other thing is—separate from perception—the resources that they brought to the table. Because for a huge percentage of those men, their lives were intact when AIDS hit. They weren't dealing with all of the other marginalized issues. Larry Kramer was a rich successful playwright when AIDS hit. Peter Staley was a bond trader, so they had resources, they had [powerful networks]. So that made a difference.

These early AIDS activists leveraged their simultaneous positions of status—as white men—and marginalization—as sexual minorities—to make a forceful claim against being "scripted out of narratives of American national belonging."[17] A population that had been hidden, maligned, and poorly understood was able to tell its stories, build institutions, and gather political support by revealing some of the "junctures and disjunctures in our beliefs about sexuality and sexual practices as well as the anxieties in American life about sex and morality."[18] These efforts on the political and cultural front in turn expanded how we might understand the core concept underlying the *dying from* to *living with* ethos: threatened with extinction, these individuals stood up and fought back. These early efforts laid the groundwork for the embryonic HIV safety net and positioned it to make a robust claim that could be institutionalized and expanded not only for national resources but for dignity in the face of marginalization.

A SUPPORT SYSTEM FOR WHOM? THE FIGHT TO EXPAND THE HIV SAFETY NET

> There are (s)heroes all over the place in the history of women and HIV.
>
> —Terry McGovern, Founder, HIV Law Project

In its earliest incarnation, the network that constituted the nascent HIV safety net had a defining characteristic: it focused almost exclusively on the needs of white gay men. Their experiences were presumed to represent the default HIV/AIDS experience, and this frame often neglected the struggles of other groups who walked alternative paths and had different needs because of their race, gender, class, or sexuality. This did not mean that early AIDS work was exclusively conducted by and for white gay men. Several lesbians, transgender women and men, and black gay and bisexual men were involved in early AIDS mobilization through their work in the LGBTQ rights movement. In addition, women from a variety of backgrounds joined in the protests, raised significant dollars, and worked alongside men in the hospitals, food programs, hospice facilities, and other institutions providing services for PLWHA. Even GMHC eventually made that abbreviation its official name to signal a more inclusive mission, serving a small group of women from its earliest years but growing into a series of programs staffed by and serving women.

Yet the urgency of the AIDS epidemic demanded that women not simply serve alongside men and follow their lead. While the 1980s and 1990s brought national visibility to the lives and deaths of white gay men, many others who were suffering and dying during that same period were effectively invisible. As more and more women came forward to reveal that they too were HIV positive, they confronted the burgeoning HIV safety net. Their labor changed how support services are delivered, bolstered the voices of women in AIDS policy-making, built new communication channels to reach women living with the disease, revised the narrative about women in the epidemic, and even challenged how we understand the disease itself. However, those gains would not come without a fight.

"AIDS Looks Different in Women":
Inside the Early Struggle to Count Women

Cultivating a growing passion for women's rights and poverty law, Terry McGovern, a white female New York attorney, accepted a job at the Legal Aid Society after graduating from Georgetown Law School in 1986. She then moved to MFY Legal Services, which began in 1961 as Mobilization for Youth, a large community-based antipoverty program, and became MFY Legal Services in 1968. MFY was just one example of the many ways in which AIDS services would have surprising links back to the antipoverty programs of the 1960s. In the mid-1980s, MFY was perfectly poised to enter the fray of the growing fight against the discrimination that was becoming rampant in the early days of AIDS. But due to confusion and misinformation, even some on the MFY staff were reluctant to take on these cases, fearing for their families' safety. Terry remembered how some coated their desks with Lysol following intake visits from clients with HIV.

It became apparent to Terry that a series of battles had to be fought for low-income PLWHA. Several of MFY's cases involved gay men fighting for the right to remain in the public housing units where some had spent decades building homes, as leases bearing the names of now-dead lovers offered no legal standing against eviction. While GMHC and other organizations were fighting to protect rent-controlled private units so that the lovers of deceased AIDS patients could remain in their homes, MFY was doing the work in the public housing market.

Terry began noticing another troubling trend: a growing number of women with HIV seeking assistance. Many had histories of trauma resembling those of the Chicago study women. Terry and an attorney working pro bono with MFY began digging into the cases and quickly learned that there was no legal infrastructure to protect women living with the disease. Like the men, the women coming to MFY were desperately ill and highly stigmatized. But they lacked one critical element: an AIDS diagnosis. Gay rights organizations had successfully mounted a powerful civil rights lobby in Congress in the late 1980s to protect PLWHA under the Americans with Disabilities Act. A momentous legal development for the community, this qualified people with an AIDS diagnosis for Medicaid, Social Security disability assistance, and housing programs. "They fought really hard to get that," Terry acknowledged.

Because AIDS is a syndrome, though, physicians diagnose the disease based on certain known symptoms. It so happened that the symptoms that the CDC used initially to define AIDS for diagnosing physicians were those disproportionately found in male AIDS patients. HIV-positive women often lacked the bright red skin legions of Kaposi's sarcoma that affected mostly men but were instead presenting with gynecological cancers, advanced pelvic inflammatory disease, and recurring yeast infections. Unfortunately, those symptoms fell outside of the CDC's case definition of an AIDS-related illness. Terry explains:

> So I was seeing this really weird phenomenon where these women were coming in, and they had fallen into a complete state of everything going wrong. They couldn't qualify for Medicaid and disability. If you take a case

because somebody's been denied Social Security disability, you appeal, you get their medical records. That was the context in which I saw all these cases. T-cells are basically a marker for how healthy your immune system is. And in the early days, it was a marker of how long you were gonna live. And these women [out of a normal range of 500–1600] had like six T-cells, ten T-cells, and all over their records, there would be all these gynecological conditions, bacterial pneumonia, tuberculosis, all kinds of stuff. But their records would say "Doesn't have AIDS." And then I would go to hearings with them and basically the administrative judge would kind of accuse them of overstating their illness. So you couldn't win the cases. And often women would die before I got the rejection.

The issues were hopelessly tangled. Conditions that were not part of the original AIDS case definition, such as tuberculosis and bacterial pneumonia, were illnesses disproportionately affecting poor people with HIV. They often struggled to maintain jobs because of their illness and other barriers. Their applications for Social Security, Medicaid, and other programs were denied because they had not been officially diagnosed with AIDS. Moreover, lacking income while suffering from a debilitating illness, they struggled to find stable housing. Taken together, these issues put poor, single, HIV-positive mothers at considerable risk of losing their children to the foster care system. "Nobody had thought about women," Terry lamented. "Nobody had thought about children. It was very sad and really outrageous."

Terry approached the nascent AIDS services network in New York looking for answers. At that time, GMHC had few female clients, so Terry attended an ACT UP/NY meeting and stood in the back, absorbing the conversation. ACT UP had also noted that the CDC's definition of AIDS seemed to exclude women. The problem, they charged, was that early studies of AIDS had focused disproportionately on white gay men, and the resources dedicated to studying HIV among women were woefully inadequate. "So we realized," Terry explained, ". . . that this whole system around relief for people with AIDS was really problematic for women." Many had in fact paid into the Social Security system through employment taxes, and now they were unable to access those disability dollars. To borrow from scholar Alexis Shotwell's characterization, disease classification was operating as a political formation with material effects.[19]

Terry left the MFY after the organization was prevented from filing class action lawsuits by its politically appointed board of directors at the

Legal Services Corporation. She recruited a young attorney from MFY, Martha Jones, who would become a renowned historian years later. Terry founded the HIV Law Project in 1989 with funding from several small New York foundations. Gathering a number of her clients' medical records, she filed a class action lawsuit against the Department of Health and Human Services in 1990, charging that the government's AIDS definition overlooked disease symptoms in women and arguing that it was inappropriate for the Social Security Administration (SSA) to use that definition to determine eligibility for disability benefits. Recorded as S.P. v. Sullivan, the case was so sensitive that Terry had to use the plaintiffs' initials in court documents to conceal their identities.[20] To demonstrate her claim's scientific credibility, Terry and other advocates encouraged doctors to publish their observations about female patients. These physicians were having their own struggle getting their colleagues to recognize the significance of the epidemic among women, given the systematic underemphasis on women's health research beyond the subfield of obstetrics.[21]

Terry soon realized, however, that the cause needed willing and knowledgeable spokeswomen to raise public awareness and pressure government officials. Around this time Terry was hearing from formerly incarcerated clients about the "Muslim lady in Bedford Hills." Katrina Haslip, a black woman from Niagara Falls, New York, was a venerable jailhouse lawyer who had gleaned much information during her work assignment as an inmate in the library of New York's Bedford Hills Correctional Facility for Women. Katrina had become a valuable resource for her fellow inmates, pointing them to law books and other resources as they fought their cases. For her part she developed another area of specialization: she had been reading everything that she could find about HIV, the illness with which she was diagnosed in 1988. After her own experience with the sexualized drug economy, Katrina returned to Islam, the faith of her childhood upbringing, and was known to greet her fellow prisoners wearing a hijab. At the time, the New York State Department of Health was reporting that almost 20 percent of the incoming women in Bedford Hills were HIV positive.[22] They were experiencing severe stigma from inmates and guards alike, as facilities around the country were placing inmates living with HIV/AIDS in substandard isolation units managed by medical staff, many of whom knew very little about the disease.[23] Inmates at Bedford

Hills had formed the AIDS Counseling and Education (ACE) Program in 1988 with the approval of prison administrators, and the women organized a collective that offered peer education, counseling, support, and health advocacy pertaining to HIV/AIDS. Katrina became a leader, writing:

> These women believed that none of their peers should be discriminated against, isolated, or treated cruelly merely because they were ill. . . . These were the women who understood my silence and yet felt my need to be heard. . . . I had never noticed in my peers this ability to care so deeply. For I, too, had labeled them as prisoners, cold and uncaring. Yet they had managed to build a community of women: black, white, Hispanic, learned, illiterate, robbers, murderers, forgers, rich, poor, Christian, Muslim, Jewish, bisexual, gay, heterosexual—all putting aside their differences and egos for a collective cause, to help themselves. I could not believe my eyes. Right before me lay a model of how we, as a whole, needed to combat all the issues AIDS brought, and we were building it from behind a wall, from prison. We were the community that no one thought would help itself.[24]

Terry wrote to Katrina in Bedford Hills, and the two formed a friendship. One of Katrina's frequently stated observations made a strong impression on Terry: "AIDS looks different in women." When Katrina was released in the fall of 1990, she was hired as an AIDS advocate and helped motivate the women involved in Terry's class action suit to speak out. The Women's Caucus of ACT UP was also organized for the fight, launching highly visible demonstrations at HHS offices in Washington, DC, proclaiming that "Women Don't Get AIDS, They Just Die from It." Activist women of color living with HIV/AIDS—including Phyllis Sharpe, a plaintiff in Terry's class-action lawsuit, and former sex worker and writer Iris De La Cruz—offered moving testimonies as demonstrators spiritedly chanted, "How many women have to die before you say they qualify?"[25] Katrina attended the ACT UP demonstration in DC, violating the terms of her parole to lend her voice to the struggle. As ACT UP activists like Maxine Wolfe, Linda Meredith, and others mounted a national direct action campaign to challenge the CDC and NIH to change the case definition of AIDS and to increase the amount of research on HIV among women, respectively, Katrina became a regular and vocal presence at various gatherings.

Waiting for the case against the federal government to wind its way through the courts proved agonizing. Terry and her team routinely filed motions in family court to preserve clients' rights to visit with children who had been removed from their homes due to their mother's physical deterioration, homelessness, or issues that pre-dated but were often related to their HIV status. As the HIV Law Project attorneys fought to maintain that bright spot, their clients died one by one. Local health departments encouraged the group to press on, as they too witnessed the explosion of women with serious HIV-related illnesses and desperately needed greater access to resources earmarked for people with AIDS.

Katrina's health declined precipitously over the course of the fight. She did not qualify for a home health attendant or other resources through the Division of AIDS Services because she too lacked an AIDS diagnosis. As she repeatedly fell at home due to weakness, Terry "literally had to send clients to help her get up from the floor of her house to take her to the hospital."

Finally, the CDC announced that it would expand the case definition of AIDS starting in January 1993 to include those with CD4 (T-cell) counts below 200, pulmonary tuberculosis, recurrent pneumonia, or invasive cervical cancer. "Katrina's dying in the hospital, and I went to tell her," Terry recalled. "She was really angry, because it didn't have to be that way. She didn't have to struggle the way she did." Katrina died on December 2, 1992, exactly one month before the CDC's new AIDS case definition would take effect. She never received services or disability benefits reserved for people with that designation.

Partly as a result of the changes in the case definition of AIDS, the CDC saw a spike in AIDS surveillance statistics among women.[26] This change effectively forced the SSA to expand AIDS-related disability criteria, allowing more women and low-income individuals to qualify for Medicaid and Social Security. But this development was about more than government benefits, Terry explained. "That was one aspect of it. It was also about whether you were spotting people who might have AIDS and counting them. It was about who was vulnerable and how that got defined, and what we did about it." It was also about science, as the discovery of effective treatments depended on a full consideration of the evidence in both men and women that could be utilized to accurately reflect the realities of the disease.

The HIV Law Project faced its share of opposition. From Terry's vantage point, the resistance appeared to come from several directions. First, there seemed to be "a total lack of understanding of what goes on for women, poor women, and people living in public housing with HIV. . . . You had different sectors of society affected by HIV. So all the things that exist in society—racism, sexism—all were front and center in the response to HIV/AIDS." Second, even some AIDS organizations seemed less than eager about the HIV Law Project; Terry sensed fear on the part of some that the pie was only so big and the resources for which they had fought so hard would be redirected to other populations.

Terry also eventually recognized structural barriers to the creation of evidence, including the evidence that she needed to assist her clients. Under the vigilant watch of activists, policy officials, and a general public urgently needing answers at the height of the epidemic, the scientific research community had to grapple with the reality that many women with HIV were not previously healthy patients who had suddenly fallen ill. Women as well as men of color who were diagnosed with HIV were often poorer than their white male counterparts and suffered from preexisting health issues that could make it challenging to isolate the specific effects of HIV. As she explained in her frank, no-nonsense style, Terry could not help but perceive frustration from some government officials who were under intense pressure: "I think it was like: We have this beautiful epidemiological study of what has happened for people who have a healthy immune system if they become HIV positive, and we see these diseases that we don't see otherwise. Now you're introducing this whole mess of people who have all these other health conditions, who maybe used drugs, and maybe have vaginas. How are we going to measure this disease now? That's very messy for science and for policy."

Yet the changing of the case definition of AIDS and the other victories won by the HIV Law Project produced watershed moments. The understanding that the disease presents differently in women had economic as well as health implications. It was an important scientific discovery and a critical moment for the access to the safety net that it granted to women. As one fellow advocate described admiringly, "Terry fought long and hard, and you know, she won. And it was advocacy like nobody's business to make certain that women were included. People were dying, people were sick, and the system wasn't together yet. So you had to fight really hard." Terry, however, gives credit to someone else, as I learned when Terry pulled a photograph from the wall of her office at Columbia University, where she is now on the faculty. It was an image of Katrina Haslip, a black woman defiantly holding a bullhorn at a protest in front of a federal government building. "All of the safety net stuff that exists, really, we had to fight and claw our way [to earn]," Terry reflected. "And frankly, it was always led by HIV-positive women of color, against incredible odds and obstacles." When the HIV Law Project created an initiative to train women to participate in AIDS advocacy, they named it the Katrina Haslip Technical Assistance Program.

Services: Women-Focused, Family-Centered

Many women were introduced to AIDS work through the devastation of their own diagnoses. In the mid-1980s, Patricia Nalls, a happily married Guyanese national of East Indian descent, was working as a community organizer for a global anti-hunger nonprofit. As nonprofit professionals, she and her husband had just bought a new home in Washington, DC, and were awaiting their third child. When their daughter was born in 1984, the baby's health problems started immediately and stumped physicians. "They did all kinds of tests on her," Pat explained. "It was the liver. It was the heart. It was cystic fibrosis. It was just a zillion things." After two years of focusing on their ailing daughter, Pat's husband Lenny began to lose weight and battled a recurring cough that doctors diagnosed as a symptom of allergies. Finally, during a trip to the emergency room after he became too weak to move, doctors asked Lenny more questions about his health history, suspecting that a treatable bleeding ulcer was the real cause of his health problems. When he disclosed that he was eleven years clean as a recovering drug addict, doctors conducted an HIV test. The test confirmed that Lenny had AIDS.

Lenny died within months of his diagnosis. In another almost insurmountable blow, Pat and Lenny's three-year-old daughter died of AIDS-related complications just six months later. The couple's other two children (a daughter and a son) were HIV negative, but Pat herself was down to just 80 pounds, learning shortly after Lenny's diagnosis in 1986 that she too was HIV positive: "As a mom, you put your children first. I took my baby all over the country to seek care. I even took her to the Mayo Clinic. But we don't tend to care for ourselves. . . . I was no different than most moms. When she passed on, I was doing everything in my power for her, while I was very sick and was told I had no T-cells. They also told me to prepare for death. I bought my [burial] plot."

It was 1986, and by this time AZT was becoming more widely available. The drug could keep death at bay, but now new emotions flooded in with the overwhelming grief: isolation and survivor's guilt. "My husband begged doctors to give him AZT, but they told him they couldn't because it was not yet approved for use." Pat was the only woman she knew with AIDS, and she told no one about her diagnosis: "I literally remember being in the closet. They used to deliver this little machine to my home to do this medication treatment, Pentamidine, to prevent pneumonia. And you had to suck and breathe through the machine. And I would literally go into a closet, lock the door, and do the treatment, because I was so terrified that my kids would get scared that their mommy was gonna die if they saw me."

By this time, the mobilized gay community had established its nascent AIDS infrastructure. Terrified and needing support, Pat ventured out and began to attend AIDS support group meetings. She met others with her diagnosis, but no women: "I thought I was the only woman with AIDS because I had never seen another woman, so I just didn't know what to do, where to turn." While the men seated around her were pleasant, she felt worlds apart from them:

> The guys were wonderful, but their lives . . . I would start talking about, "I'm in a panic, I'm gonna die, and I have two children. I don't know who's going to keep my kids." Those are the types of things I was focused on. And I went from two incomes to a fixed income [after Lenny died]. I had a mortgage to pay. I didn't know how I was going to get through any of this stuff. What I found is they just kinda dismissed it and moved on to another conversation. So the guys were talking more about [living well before they died]. They're enjoying trips to Europe, and enjoying their fine china for dinner, and you know, I can barely stay two minutes past the meeting time because I had to get home because I had to pay a babysitter to keep the kids. And they would have dinner before or after groups, I couldn't do anything. I had to race there, race back as fast as I could. I did socialize a little bit with the

guys when I could, like, if they had a gathering or had dinner or something. But I just felt like I wasn't getting anything from the group, so I eventually stopped going.

Pat was determined to move from what had become her physical and emotional state of *dying from* to a new reality of *living with* AIDS. Because she encountered no institutions focusing on women's experiences, she created her own, providing women with a gateway into the HIV safety net. In 1990, she asked her doctor if she could post a flyer in the waiting room looking for other women with HIV/AIDS. She installed a second phone line, terrified that her family would pick up the phone and learn of her status: "Lo and behold, the phone started ringing, and folks started calling. None of us wanted to show our faces, so we would just talk on the phone. . . . We were all talking the same language about the same fears and concerns."

Meetings over the phone turned into in-person gatherings at Pat's home for those willing to forgo a bit of their anonymity in exchange for a supportive collective and Pat's home-cooked meals. At first, the women shared information about how to stave off the nausea and other symptoms caused by medications, or how to put together a will and custody plan for post-mortem care of their children: "We shared our very limited resources because we were all sick. We were all on fixed incomes, so we shared extra food, transportation. . . . And so, it really became a network of women just honestly trying to help each other, even when we were a support group with no money. Just a safe space to share, weep, and prepare for death." They went to HIV testing locations and provided the group's phone number to clinic staff. "We said, 'We just want to do this. You don't have to pay anything. When a woman tests positive . . . tell her she can call this number and one of us will be there to greet her, to hold her hand, to support her through the devastation of the diagnosis, to let her know we're here for her and her children, and to take her to the doctor.' And so we began just by doing that."

Pat learned what would become one of the earliest lessons to emerge around AIDS services for women: WLWHA often needed more than medical services; they needed a holistic approach to care. As Dr. Frances Ashe-Goins, a black female federal government official who worked on HIV for much of her career, explained, "In my experience in the early years of the epidemic, many of the men with HIV/AIDS were single. However, the women with HIV/AIDS had children, husbands, and were caregivers for family members. They came with different issues of care." Moreover, many of them lacked economic resources. Pat and her group would therefore extend emotional and disease management support into material and logistical support; they were all intertwined. "When you start a group," she explained, "it's very difficult to just do a support group and say, 'Bye, I'll see you next time,' and people are needing stuff. So you had to quickly figure out, where are the resources? Where do I send her? How do I help her? And that's when we quickly realized there was really nothing for [women]."

What would officially be established as the Women's Collective in 1995 in Washington, DC, began to confront some of the disadvantages that women in the growing AIDS service community faced. The agency received a small grant to provide case management and, as Pat described it, built an infrastructure "from the ground up to serve women, knowing their needs." For example, service providers were distributing food to the homes of PLWHA in single-serving containers for the presumed single gay male client, rather than family meals for women who often had multiple mouths to feed. "I swear I know women died from starvation," Pat lamented. "They took their [single-serving] meal, and they fed their children, and they weren't eating." Transportation vouchers to help patients make doctor's appointments failed to acknowledge that women might need additional bus passes for their children, and the lack of transportation often meant missing appointments.

As Pat and others continued their work, another truth surfaced: the epidemic's impact on children. In Philadelphia, Alicia Beatty, the daughter of one of the city's most prominent black pastors, was recruited to the AIDS fight by formidable reproductive rights advocate Dorothy Mann, executive director of the city's Family Planning Council for over 30 years. In 1990, Mann asked Beatty to lead a program focused on the needs of women and children in the growing epidemic, with a specific focus on helping families navigate systems of care. As the first director of what would become known as the Circle of Care, Beatty recruited pediatricians, infectious disease doctors, nurses, attorneys, social workers, and others into a citywide network focused on wrap-around care for women and children affected by AIDS.

The Circle of Care organized comprehensive services that would become one of the precursors to a national model of HIV/AIDS care that could confront what providers were seeing on the ground. Carole Treston is the executive director of the Association of Nurses in AIDS Care (ANAC) and the former executive director of the AIDS Alliance for Women, Infants, Children, Youth and Families. When she was starting out in the late 1980s and early 1990s as a nurse in north Philadelphia at St. Christopher's Hospital for Children, the intensive care unit was seeing a spike in the number of gravely ill children. Carole and her colleagues began tracking cases that matched the emerging AIDS profile, which was evolving as doctors and researchers puzzled over whether children could be victims of a disease originally described as GRID (gay-related immune deficiency). In the first week of case-finding the team identified 31 children who were either currently in the hospital, were recently discharged, or had recently died from what they realized was AIDS-related illness. Within a month the number had climbed to 70. Within two or three months, there were 100 children suffering from AIDS. "All of them," Carole, a white woman who was in her thirties at the time explained, "had either a sick mom, a deceased mom, or a lost mom with the grandmother taking care of the child." By the late 1980s, with a small grant and a staff of five, St. Christopher's opened a pediatric AIDS clinic.

The sexualized drug economy had hit North Philadelphia hard. It was the height of the crack epidemic, leaving many residents in poor health. As Carole and her team came to know the women who visited the clinic regularly with their children, many of these caretakers revealed histories of their own childhood sexual abuse and ongoing struggles with intimate partner violence. Mental health issues were pervasive. As we have seen, while the epidemic among women is not monolithic, across the country it has always disproportionately and aggressively ensnared those already caught in webs of trauma.

Mothers were coming to the clinic at St. Christopher's emaciated and wasting away. "It was awful," Carole pensively recalled. "I barely think about it because it was really awful. . . . You would see somebody, and then a month later, they'd start to look a lot thinner, and then a month later they were wasting, and then a month later they weren't there anymore." It was one of only two pediatric AIDS clinics in town and white, black, and

Latina mothers were crowding the waiting room. The healthcare staff frequently had to call 911 to get emergency care for mothers at death's door: "The grandmas were really the unsung heroes of the day," Carole reflected. "They were poor women themselves. They were now caring for not only that one daughter's child, but maybe two or three others because these were multigenerational issues, and they had no benefits at all other than maybe medical assistance."

Carole and the other healthcare providers asked the mothers and grandmothers to bring their babies in for regular HIV antibody testing until the children were fifteen to eighteen months old. "So imagine," Carole explained,

> what it was like for these moms coming in every month, sick themselves, trying to get the answer. Did they pass it on to their baby? Often, a mom only found out she was HIV positive when the baby tested positive. There was no prenatal testing; there was no testing at delivery. The only time anybody got into care was when they had AIDS. So either the baby got sick with an AIDS-related illness first, and that's how the whole family found out, or mom was sick, and eventually, maybe her kids would get tested. The parents, the grandparents, the guardians were flocking to us because finally they had some answers, even though they weren't the answers that they wanted. . . . But the mothers were falling apart in the waiting room. It was devastating. It was awful, awful.

Carole began attending Circle of Care meetings with other local health professionals who were following the epidemic and crafting protocols for care. She vividly described spending hours studying the science, knowing, just as gay men had come to realize, that fluency in the scientific language of AIDS was critical if one wanted credibility among the activists, policymakers, and scientific elites. "Part of your job," Phill Wilson of the Black AIDS Institute explained, "is to learn the precision of the language and the [scientific] methodology. Because the ways we talk about these things are not accidents." Activists, advocates, and service providers who were focusing on women, people of color, and those who inhabit multiple marginalized statuses understood that the AIDS infrastructure was becoming institutionalized, and it would be critically important to gain insider status and legitimacy to have a voice in what was shaping up to be a massive effort to combat the epidemic.

Without sophisticated prenatal HIV-testing tools or established treatment protocols, offering social services was *the* primary strategy through which early AIDS clinics like St. Christopher's provided assistance. "We tried to manage the opportunistic infections," Carole explained, "but there was no treatment." Hospitals and community organizations targeting AIDS, homelessness, drug addiction, and mental health therefore partnered to create one-stop shopping in the two Philadelphia pediatric hospitals that brought together physicians, nurses, psychologists, drug and alcohol counselors, and peer advocates or "buddies" who coupled emotional support with transportation and other logistical assistance. They also added social workers to the team, and they helped patients access subsidized medical assistance and, eventually, Social Security benefits. Patients could even meet with attorneys from local AIDS legal services organizations to fill out guardianship papers for their children's care and access emergency financial assistance through funds raised by the Circle of Care.

Funding for this growing network of providers was made possible largely through the lobbying of Dorothy Mann, who regularly pressed Pennsylvania Senator Arlen Specter. She invited Specter's staffers to visit hospitals like St. Christopher's to see patients firsthand. Specter, a Republican with stints in the Democratic Party bookending his career, chaired the Labor Appropriations Committee and emerged as a chief champion of what became known as the Pediatric AIDS Demonstration Projects. Thirteen sites were established across the country to develop care and treatment models for children and women with HIV/AIDS. Dr. Ivy Turnbull, now deputy executive director of the AIDS Alliance, worked at the Brooklyn Pediatric AIDS Network in 1992. "We provided one-stop shopping," she explained. "It was a coordinated, comprehensive, culturally and linguistically competent model of care. . . . Because you cannot take care of the baby without taking care of the mother. You cannot take care of the mother without taking care of the rest of the children in the family, [HIV] positive or negative."

It was grueling work, with intense emotional highs and lows. The multidisciplinary teams of care professionals learned the ins and outs of their patients' lives, with several people troubleshooting to help address challenges facing mothers and their children. Ivy explained:

> Because we had children, one of the most difficult things was losing a lot of babies. With the horrors of the epidemic, we initially spent a lot of time

helping folks prepare to die . . . because we knew what was going to happen. So we were very much involved with their families, because we knew that one day . . . And so that preparation was very much at the heart of what we did. And sometimes we used to have case conferences about it and, depending on how many T-cells Jackson had or Mary's opportunistic infection, we would know, "It's time." And we all understood what "It's time" meant. What we didn't expect . . . was that they would live. We saved a lot of kids. So as these kids got older, and the moms were alive, we realized that we had not taught them how to live.

Thus Ivy Turnbull and her colleagues were facing an undeniable reality as the infrastructure for women and children grew: to be effective one had to grapple seriously with one of the epidemic's root causes, poverty and its intersections with race and gender. Marsha Martin is an African American social worker who has focused on HIV/AIDS issues in several government agencies, including the departments of Health and Human Services, Housing and Urban Development, and Veterans Affairs. She began her career in the early 1980s, though, working in a mobile medical outreach unit for the homeless in midtown Manhattan. While AIDS was devastating some of the most affluent segments of the gay community, it was simultaneously ravaging the most destitute corners of New York City streets. Times Square had become a settlement area for substance users and former patients of shuttered psychiatric hospitals. Marsha was tapped to direct the Office of Homelessness and Single-Room Occupancy (SRO) Housing under then mayor David Dinkins, where she helped develop the first housing programs for PLWHA.

On weekdays, Marsha was overseeing a program in which *half* of the city's SRO housing was occupied by PLWHA. On weekends, she witnessed previously healthy men who were her fellow worshipers at Riverside Church deteriorate rapidly: "There was this wonderful man that went to our church. His name is/was Jack, white gay man. I'll never forget it. In two years, he had 44 friends die. And Jack was in his mid-twenties. This is the impact the early epidemic had on people. And I say, this is the epidemic that built [services] we didn't have. I call it 'the house that Jack built.'"

Advocates and service providers involved in combatting homelessness, drug addiction, and mental illness in urban centers across the country were in agreement with the LGBTQ community and women's health advocates about the need for comprehensive services for their rising numbers of clients with HIV/AIDS. Not all of their clients fit the emerging public face of the epidemic of a white gay male, but their needs seemed just as great if not greater because of their severe economic and social disadvantages. Hale House Center, a Harlem home for children who were born addicted to drugs that was founded in 1969 by Clara McBride Hale, or "Mother Hale," began taking in HIV-positive babies or babies who were orphaned by the AIDS-related deaths of parents in the 1980s. "The child welfare agencies were absolutely overwhelmed—a lot of mothers didn't make it," Marsha recounted. "You had so-called boarder babies being born in hospitals, nobody touching them, nobody cuddling them, nobody doing anything with them, because nobody knew what to do. But you have this black woman, Mother Hale, who opened up her home to these children where nobody else did."[27]

In 1989, stunned by the number of black men, women, and children dying alone in Harlem Hospital and by the lack of a coordinated response to AIDS in black faith communities, immunologist and minister Pernessa Seele founded the Balm in Gilead. Reasoning that the black church played an enormous role in the lives of black people and served multiple roles as a community social service agency, a site for political organizing, and a spiritual sanctuary, Seele saw the church as an important institution from which to mount a full-scale attack on AIDS. Other small programs emerged as a result of her leadership, mostly in progressive churches such as the Upper Room AIDS Ministry in Harlem, which provided case management, food, respite care, and AIDS outreach.

Thus, while many "mainstream" AIDS service organizations were adding programs for women, several women recognized a greater need. Some wanted a more expansive approach to AIDS work that grappled with injuries of inequality being inflicted at the intersections of race, class, and gender. They were frustrated by the smaller fractions of organizational budgets, "second-thought" programming, and lower institutional priority that seemed to befall any group outside of the assumed white gay male experience of HIV/AIDS. Many women's experiences as mothers shaped their vision of a more expansive and family-centered safety net. They started their own grassroots AIDS service organizations across the country where, as one founder told me, "the primary reason for opening our doors every morning is to serve women." Organizations such as the

Chicago Women's AIDS Project in 1988, Iris House in 1992 in New York City, and Christie's Place in 1996 in San Diego were founded to offer services and encourage women to take control of their health.

Many of these organizations were funded by the Ford Foundation, which made an early commitment to supporting grassroots organizations that were addressing the epidemic among women and people of color. This was spearheaded by a highly dedicated program officer: Terry McGovern, who was now working for the foundation. "I was just really burnt out," she commented about her 1999 departure from the HIV Law Project. "I think just the cumulative impact of all of that loss and having to fight so many battles ... I really tried to give a boost to the women's organizations through Ford and actually give them the capacity to fight. That was really quite a privilege." Embracing a holistic approach to care, emphasizing the impact of HIV/AIDS on both themselves and their children, and acknowledging how poverty and racial inequality were not only drivers of the epidemic but realities that had to be considered in the engineering of services, women activists and advocates were remaking AIDS service provision.

"We Have to Know Who Else Is Out There":
Establishing Channels of Communication

When the AIDS epidemic hit, existing social networks among gay and bisexual men in major US cities offered important preexisting communication channels that enabled them to share information and build community. For WLWHA, these channels had to be built from scratch. I met Rebecca Denison while attending meetings of the Women's Research Institute (WRI), a collective of WLWHA, advocates, researchers, and policy specialists who gather annually to reflect on a chosen area of AIDS research and strategize about how to better connect the emerging science to the needs of women. Rebecca was a passionate and thoughtful contributor to the discussion, her words infused with a long history "in the epidemic." Rebecca was diagnosed on June 16, 1990, having taken the test as a show of support while accompanying a friend to testing. She had been with her husband for five years and only had a few relationships prior to that. While she had unprotected sex and "understood there were risks, I was in complete denial," she explained to me over breakfast in Oakland, California. While in her twenties, she had asked about HIV testing, but her doctor led her to believe that she had nothing to worry about, likely because she was a middle-class white woman with relatively few partners.

Rebecca became very sick, however, just a few months after she had started seeing her prior boyfriend in March of 1983. Doctors couldn't pinpoint the cause of her illness. Rebecca now believes that was acute viral syndrome, an illness that can appear approximately one to four weeks after HIV transmission. Nevertheless, when the HIV counselor informed her seven years later that her test was positive, she was stunned:

> And I wanna be clear when I say these things because I think it's very easy when people say, "I didn't see this or I didn't do that." It's as if people are trying to say "I'm innocent" or even that other people deserved it. I want to be very clear that I'm not trying to say that. But what I am trying to say is, sometimes I wonder how the epidemic would have been different if the virus had first been seen in the children of white senators. . . . If we noticed it in pediatrics first and associated it with sex related to conception rather than sex related to gay men, would we have responded as a nation or as a world differently to that? Or if the epidemic first hit Americans with power and privilege, perhaps the resources would have been allocated sooner to identify a cause and treatments. But because it was first identified in some of the most marginalized people in the world, I think . . . [it made] it easier for people to say, "I'm not that. I'm not them. So it's not my problem."

As Rebecca struggled to make sense of the news, she vividly recalled encountering an ACT UP demonstration in the streets of her Bay Area community. "AIDS is a disaster, women die faster!" the protestors shouted, handing Rebecca a leaflet that warned, "Men die 18 months after a diagnosis, and women die 6 months after a diagnosis." Still in shock, she took what had been ACT UP's message about the lack of services for women as a prognosis and began planning the last six months of her life. She spoke to her husband, who was traveling in a rural area of Central America. She informed him that she had been diagnosed with HIV and that he needed to come home immediately. As she waited for him to make the days-long trek, Rebecca wondered how they would pay for healthcare services given that she had just resigned from her job to return to school. Her husband had no health insurance. Perhaps the AIDS network could be helpful, she thought, having observed San Franciscans quickly establish their own wing of the HIV safety net through the San Francisco AIDS Foundation and other organizations.

Like Terry McGovern in New York and Pat Nalls in Washington, DC, however, Rebecca was shocked to discover that so few resources existed for women. She joined her local ACT UP chapter, then the group sent her to Washington, DC for the first national conference on women and HIV/AIDS:

> At the conference, a woman named Michelle Wilson organized a support group for positive women. And we all just sat in this room and I thought, "Oh my God. We all have it." And that was one of the most powerful moments of my life, to just sit in the room with others for the first time and be with people who were very different—we were from all over the country and all different backgrounds—but we. . . [had] that one thing in common. And around that same time, I received in the mail my first copy of "The Positive Woman," which was Michelle's newsletter, and I was like, "Oh my God, I'm not alone." And it just meant so much to me. We needed something like this . . . to share information about what was in the Bay Area.

ACT UP's Golden Gate chapter strongly encouraged Rebecca to start a new organization focused on women. They suggested the name WORLD (Women Organized to Respond to Life-Threatening Diseases), which Rebecca thought was pretentious, "Like really, I'm going to call it WORLD." But ACT UP members, increasingly schooled in the art of organizing, argued that it would be savvy to give the organization a more discreet name to protect members' confidentiality: "You'll have a name that doesn't make family or friends think anything of it if an envelope or phone message comes in. WORLD can be a bank, it can be an environmental organization, it could be anything."

From the start, WORLD members agreed that the organization's leadership should reflect those most impacted by the epidemic, decreeing that WLWHA and women of color had to comprise at least 50 percent of its board of directors, and that all programs would be initiated by and for WLWHA.

ACT UP learned that the US surgeon general, Dr. Antonia Novello, would be visiting Stanford University. Flexing their growing political clout, ACT UP members contacted Novello's office and said that WORLD was requesting a meeting with the surgeon general. To everyone's astonishment, the meeting was granted. Rebecca would become a reluctant spokesperson:

And I'm like, what are you doing? We don't exist. And then I went to another AIDS conference, and I'm sitting in the back being all meek. And one of the panel presenters says, "By the way, there's a new organization called WORLD. Their delegation is going to be meeting with the surgeon general at Stanford this weekend. If you'd like to be part of the delegation, please meet with Rebecca after this presentation. Rebecca's sitting right there—Rebecca wave your hand!" I'm like, what the hell?! So that's how a delegation of HIV-positive women from WORLD met with Antonia Novello, the surgeon general.

Among other programs, WORLD members organized retreats, a speakers' bureau, peer advocacy, outreach to incarcerated WLWHA, and HIV University, which became a national model that educated women about treatments and other issues. One of WORLD's first services was a newsletter that shared women's stories and offered information and resources. As a white middle-class woman, Rebecca resolved from the start to recruit a diverse set of voices. She contacted AIDS service organizations that engaged with women of color, introduced herself, and asked them to inform their clients about WORLD. Rebecca's husband, who tested HIV negative, created the newsletter's masthead. "Here's your newsletter," he encouraged; "Go write it."

On May 1, 1991, just months after Rebecca's HIV diagnosis, WORLD released the first issue of its newsletter. Women gathered in Rebecca's living room, stuffing envelopes addressed to clinics, community organizations, and anyone else who had discreetly requested a copy. The newsletter offered women's stories and the latest news on policy, prevention, and emerging treatment options. By the time the last issue came out in 2003, Rebecca, exhausted, had produced 142 monthly issues. It reached 12,000 readers in over 85 countries, publishing the stories of over 300 women living with HIV/AIDS.

Taking Control of the Narrative: How Women Fought to Define Themselves in the AIDS Epidemic

Alongside new HIV/AIDS service organizations, communication channels, and major legal victories, women in the epidemic knew that they needed a more organized and forceful policy voice. They needed to be in the rooms where decisions were being made about not only the scientific research being conducted but also the epidemic's emerging health and social policy infrastructure. Even the question of how the epidemic was being defined at the intersection of race and gender became an important topic of policy debate. Being counted was critical: it properly focused attention on the epidemic's devastating impacts in communities that needed scientific research and prevention and treatment dollars. Phill Wilson of the Black AIDS Institute had this to say:

> [Black AIDS activists and advocates said to] the CDC, you need to unpack your data. Because they were delivering the data, but they weren't breaking the data down demographically [until the mid-1980s]. And then we saw immediately that black and Latino people were disproportionally impacted. Back then . . . 25 percent of the cases were black. And even the earliest data showed that black women relative to white women were off the charts. There's never been a time when the majority of the cases among women weren't black. So this kind of "changing face of the epidemic," the language that people adopted, was all bullshit. The epidemic never changed its face.

It was clear that the AIDS community needed more voices to raise issues facing women, especially women of color. In 1989, black feminist activist Dázon Dixon Diallo established SisterLove in Atlanta, the first organization in the Southeast to focus on WLWHA or those at higher risk of contracting the disease. A campus activist at Spelman College, Diallo was motivated to start SisterLove after becoming frustrated with the dearth of organizations working at the intersection of HIV, sexual health, and reproductive justice. She and I sat in an aging converted Victorian mansion on the southwest side of Atlanta, that now housed several grass-roots reproductive justice organizations. We talked about her decades-long advocacy experiences:

> People ask, "Well, how did you get involved in this work?" And I say, "Rock Hudson." And that's always my short answer, but it's the truth. I can remember as plain as day, in the summer of 1985. You rotated jobs at the Feminist Women's Health Center, where I was working; and that week, I was working phones. Rock Hudson announced his AIDS diagnosis. AID Atlanta, which up until that point was only serving men who had sex with men or gay men, used to be the host for the National AIDS Hotline. Their phones just started ringing from women who were either sick [and] didn't know why, or were just freaked out by this news and wanted to know more about AIDS. But

AID Atlanta couldn't answer some of the women's questions, so they started fielding them over to us at the Feminist Women's Health Center. Well, we didn't have any information about HIV/AIDS, because we're reproductive health and weren't paying attention to that. And so the phone just started ringing off the hook, and I literally said, "Well, we need some help."

Dázon helped AID Atlanta build its HIV services for women. When the program dwindled after staff shake-ups, Dázon moved the work back to the Feminist Women's Health Center. It struggled to gain footing there as well, taking funding hits ostensibly due to the organization's other work related to abortion rights. But Dázon wondered if she was also witnessing reluctance on the part of the reproductive rights community to take on AIDS: "HIV just never was a priority anyway, because of the population, because it wasn't an income generator, because it still was 'AIDS,' and it had a whole lot of stigma attached to it."

Nevertheless, Dázon was able over the years to grow SisterLove into an important player in the AIDS policy arena. A compelling and persuasive speaker with a master's degree in public health, her voice as a health advocate for women resonated from community groups to Washington policy circles; she was a grassroots organizer with significant policy bona fides. For Dázon, *how* we talk about women and HIV/AIDS, or the framing, is critically important to how we think about HIV/AIDS prevention and treatment policy:

> Changing the narrative has become one of the core elements of how we do this work in HIV. It has been extremely important to say that women are not just vectors of the disease because we can get pregnant [and transmit the virus to babies]. And we're not all just victims of the disease because we're all on the receiving end of the fluids most of the time. But to say that we can be agents on our own. *That we can be self-determining around our own prevention and our own protection,* and that is the conversation that we have pushed in terms of changing the narrative. [emphasis added]

Fighting for women's whole selves to be seen and heard as beings with political, economic, social, and even sexual lives and investments would be risky. Black feminist scholars describe a politics of silence in which black women have historically reacted to repressive discourses on race and sex with "silence, secrecy, and a partially self-chosen invisibility."[28] Women, especially women of color, were in a paradoxical position from the start: they wanted to help shape their destinies in the evolving HIV/AIDS discussion, but their visibility could make them targets of a politics of disgust that had a long and brutal history of training its sights on black and brown women. The narratives circulating around women living with HIV/AIDS had already taken on a racialized tinge in the 1980s and 1990s. Early news stories appeared to depict white women as innocent victims of HIV transmission via blood transfusion while presenting black women and Latinas as the guilty, irresponsible, and drug-addicted mothers of "boarder babies." The former group was positively reflected in the courage of white women like Mary Fischer, who spoke at the Republican National Convention, and Elizabeth Glaser, the celebrity wife of actor Paul Glaser and a vocal advocate of the pediatric AIDS community. The latter group was an obvious close cousin of the crass "welfare queen" stereotype (a lazy, unwed mother who dines on steak and drives a Cadillac), the stigmatizing public identity assigned to poor black and brown women by Ronald Reagan in the 1980s.[29]

Although women of color were disproportionately affected by the epidemic, there would be no public equivalent of an Elizabeth Glaser (or a Magic Johnson for that matter), highly visible PLWHA who dispelled stereotypes and gained access to the corridors of power. The stigma that women of color experienced therefore was acute, racialized, and gendered, zeroing in on how they might have acquired HIV and what it signaled about their morality as women and their fitness as mothers.[30] The devastating political vulnerability of black and brown women caught at the intersection of the political construction of the welfare queen, the new stereotype of the reproductively irresponsible "crack mother," and the emergence of HIV cannot be overstated.[31] Women of color living with HIV were tattooed with pernicious assumptions about their alleged sexual deviance, racial inferiority, female irresponsibility, and economic undeservedness, as they saw themselves reduced to one-dimensional caricatures. As Marsha Martin observed:

> Who were perceived to be the women living with HIV? Drug users and prostitutes—now which one do you want to be? Were you going to stand up and say, "Oh hi, I'm living with HIV, and I'm a sex worker? I'm a drug addict? I have a lot of baby daddies?" So it became, "I'm not that! I don't want to be that!" So all of that is going on for these women. And immediately the questions are, "How'd you get it? Who did you get it from? Don't you know?"

These narratives of pathology did in fact appear to shape both policy creation and implementation, setting up a pernicious interplay between the social construction of these women and their material conditions as WLWHA. The skepticism toward her clients at the HIV Law Project that Terry McGovern perceived among the Social Security administrative judges recalls the treatment of women who were denied welfare benefits.[32] Legislators in some states began introducing mandatory HIV-testing policies in the late 1980s and early 1990s for pregnant women. These programs were purportedly designed to protect babies, but they often imposed punitive tactics on mothers and offered almost no support services for those who tested positive. David Holtgrave, a leading HIV researcher who previously served as the director of the Division of HIV/AIDS Prevention—Intervention Research and Support at the CDC, illuminated the debate over HIV testing in the early 1990s:

> We had as treatment AZT, which was of some use, but of course not nearly as good as the antiretrovirals that we have now. So, at that time, there were still differences of opinion in the field about HIV testing. Some people increasingly were saying it's important to be tested to know your serostatus, so there can be a pathway to getting into treatment. At the same time, other people were very concerned about testing, in that if the treatments weren't especially effective, and if people were concerned about stigma that would arise by testing HIV positive, what that might mean in terms of your insurance, discrimination, and stigma. Now in 2017, there's still far too much HIV-related stigma and discrimination, but there was even more . . . in the early 1990s.

As women participated in these national policy debates, perhaps what most upset Pat Nalls and the growing Washington-based Women's Collective was a policy issue closer to home: watching the child welfare system absorb the children of friends when mothers were hospitalized or deceased.[33] The women tried to offer each other assistance, with children of Women's Collective participants often staying in Pat's home even though she was ill herself and worn down from managing others' children in addition to her own. But the women found their stigmatized treatment within the child welfare system infuriating. "Oh my God, you had a battle to fight [with child protective services] to prove you did nothing wrong," Pat explained, echoing Terry McGovern's observations about what was happening in New York. "You got sick, and when you add HIV to that scenario, 'You couldn't have been a good woman, so you don't deserve to have your babies back.' So the battle was so hard."

These narratives were so threatening that they forced many women into silence. As an HIV-positive mother in the early years of AIDS, Pat worried about the implications of revealing her status: "We were so petri-fied of how this would interfere with our children's lives. Are they going to get kicked out of school? Are their friends going to stop playing with them? Are their teachers going to treat them differently? We were so obsessed with that, that even things we wanted to do [politically], we wouldn't do because we were so afraid of how it would impact our chil-dren." This reluctance shaped how many WLWHA engaged with AIDS activism, occasionally leading to clashes with other members of the com-munity, especially, as Pat describes, several women in the ACT UP move-ment who did not understand the issues for women of color:

> I remember some of us from the Women's Collective were at an AIDS con-ference and trying to be very discreet about our HIV status, the few of us that were there. And I remember there was this really active ACT UP group. But then they told us that they wanted us to go on the Washington Mall and "act out," or whatever they were doing. And it could get violent. And I remember we were all looking at each other, "Oh my God, I'm gonna die, no we can't do that." Some of us said, "Yes," and then we changed our minds. Those ACT UP women, they just looked at us like we were horrible for not doing that. We were horrible, horrible women for not going on the Mall. They started telling us all of these things like, "How dare you? How come you're here? Why don't you want to do this? You're not part of the cause!" and we're like, "No, we're scared, we're just scared." Well, we got this pres-sure from these women, and they were mostly white lesbians. . . making you feel like, "So what's up with these women of color? . . . Why aren't they com-ing out there?" that type of thing. . . . I remember that day in that room and we were . . . all of us left kinda feeling so lost. So there were so many pres-sures and so much judgment coming at us, often from other women.

Scholar Cathy Cohen asked how queer activists might build political coalitions with women, particularly women of color, who may fit into the heterosexual category but whose sexual choices are not perceived as normal, moral, or worthy of state support.[34] Although ACT UP and its Women's Caucus had successfully engaged with and effectively leveraged

Katrina Haslip and the clients at the HIV Law Project in important public demonstrations, Pat's comments reveal that this was not the preferred mode of engagement for all women affected by the epidemic. The prospect of participating in a visible and potentially contentious demonstration on the Washington Mall felt to Pat like she was being asked to charge into a blazing building without fireproof gear. Her words reveal the complex dimensions of both AIDS activism and the struggle women of color living with HIV/AIDS experienced fighting for air at the intersections of gender, race, class, and sexuality.[35]

With the initial framing of AIDS as a "gay disease," an existing infrastructure within the LGBTQ community lent considerable support to activists as they summoned the courage to openly acknowledge their HIV status and literally "put their bodies on the line" to advance the cause. With the exception of lesbian, bisexual, and some transgender women, WLWHA were, by and large, not embedded in this community in the early years of the AIDS response. Many of their friends and families did not even know that they were HIV positive, let alone have the preparation and political desire to support them if they too stood out in front. Women who were not also a part of the LGBTQ community, especially women of color whose racial communities were slow to confront the reality of AIDS, did not always feel the same assurances of backing and protection. They were reluctant to reveal publicly yet another stigmatizing social marker. As AIDS advocates on the front lines of the fight in organizations like ACT UP touted "silence = death" as their slogan, women of color living with HIV grappled with the reality that making noise could be just as deadly.

Women within the AIDS movement therefore from the beginning recognized an uncomfortable truth. On the one hand, the silence regarding the high numbers of women, black and brown people, transgender individuals, and poor people who were acquiring HIV was both deafening and deadly. On the other hand, white gay men, serving as the face of the disease, aggressively fought for, and most notably *seized*, a level of public attention that laid a foundation for significant resources and political clout with which to confront the epidemic for years to come. Their willingness to be visible benefited communities beyond their own. SisterLove founder Dázon Dixon Diallo's observation would be echoed by many advocates whom I interviewed:

It's not the most comfortable acknowledgment for some people. But I unapologetically acknowledge that we have to be grateful to some degree that HIV/AIDS showed up the way that it did: in a Western country in white men. Regardless of the fact that these were gay men, I think that ... that partially helped because it's still a marginalized group of people. But they are in the margins *of the most privileged people.* And so, if we start with that fact, that, but for the sake that white men were dying—*young* white men were dying—it galvanized. They were able to use that white privilege, and that male privilege, *and* that sense of otherness that they shared ... to change everything.

Although WLWHA and their allies may have relied less on highly visible and controversial tactics of political protest, they nevertheless participated meaningfully in the emergence of the HIV safety net. Female AIDS activists and advocates took an alternative strategic approach to political activism and influence. They knew that other women were struggling in the shadows, their invisibility and fear of disclosure silencing their struggles and needs. Therefore, many activists and advocates chose to become deeply engaged in advocacy from within, battling within the institutional walls of hospitals, local departments of public health, churches, and other entities to ensure that the needs of women and people of color were being addressed. They challenged newly created AIDS organizations to expand and reimagine their services. And they asserted their voices and began, as we will see, to participate in highly meaningful policy discussions. C. Virginia Fields, president of the National Black Leadership Commission on AIDS, summed it up this way: "Policy drives budgets. At least you have a chance of fighting for more resources if you have policies that hold people accountable."

INSTITUTIONALIZING THE HIV SAFETY NET:
THE RYAN WHITE CARE ACT

Without widely available and effective treatment options, AIDS continued to aggressively claim lives and devastate communities throughout the 1980s and early 1990s. The HIV safety net was rapidly evolving from a patchwork to a sophisticated network. However, it would take a massive

infusion of public resources for that network to become fully institutionalized as a national infrastructure.

Senator Ted Kennedy of Massachusetts was an early ally of AIDS activists and introduced legislation to encourage public and nonprofit institutions to continue their early work in HIV services. Many saw the same
looming reality. With the growing numbers of people contracting HIV,
large segments of the public would be unable to afford medications and
medical care, creating an even more serious public health emergency.
Furthermore, as thousands of PLWHA watched their health, finances and,
in some cases, support systems deteriorate, something had to be done to
address their basic needs. These issues could undermine the efficacy of any
new medical advancements discovered to stop the epidemic.

When Kennedy's bill was first proposed, many AIDS activists and advocates noticed the lack of attention to the needs of women. One voice at the
forefront was that of Elizabeth Glaser. She contracted HIV in 1981 through
a blood transfusion that she received while giving birth to her daughter
Ariel. She unknowingly passed the virus to Ariel through breast milk and
later gave birth to Jake, who contracted the virus in utero. Glaser was
stunned by the lack of research on children and HIV: the few drugs available to treat the virus had not been tested or approved for children. After
losing Ariel to AIDS-related complications in 1988, she co-created a foundation dedicated to addressing the dearth of pediatric AIDS research.
Glaser headed to Washington, where she met with President and Mrs.
Reagan, representatives at the NIH, and members of Congress. She became
a frequent visitor to Washington, and the Pediatric AIDS Foundation
became a major granting agency for research. When Glaser lost her battle
with AIDS in 1994, the foundation was renamed the Elizabeth Glaser
Pediatric AIDS Foundation, and it continues its work in the United States
and abroad.

With her considerable political clout, Glaser successfully lobbied with
others to have the Pediatric AIDS Demonstration Projects folded into the
bill. Shortly thereafter, on August 18, 1990, the Ryan White Comprehensive
AIDS Resources Emergency (CARE) Act was signed into law by
Republican President George H. W. Bush. Bush was viewed by many
within the AIDS community as having a mixed record: he cut funding for
AIDS research at the NIH and oversaw the institution of a travel ban that

prevented people with HIV/AIDS from entering the country. This prevented the United States from hosting the International AIDS Society Conference until 2012, after the ban was lifted in 2010. The signing of the CARE Act stands, nevertheless as a game-changing moment in the history of the AIDS epidemic.

The notion that AIDS services should be coordinated and comprehensive was a signature aspect of the law and the backbone of the national HIV safety net. Its funds provide critical relief for communities battling the rising costs of medical treatment and care among their HIV/AIDS patients. The CARE Act provided $220.5 million in federal funds for community-based care and treatment services in its first year, and the program was funded at $2.32 billion in fiscal year 2016. Managed by the US Health Resources and Services Administration (HRSA), it is the nation's largest HIV-specific federal grant program and currently provides funds to over 2,500 organizations across the country. Just one month prior to the passage of the Ryan White CARE Act, Congress enacted the ADA, prohibiting discrimination against individuals with disabilities, including PLWHA. Capping off a truly important year in the history of the HIV safety net, in November 1990 Congress passed the AIDS Housing Opportunity Act, creating the Housing Opportunities for People with AIDS (HOPWA) program to provide housing assistance to PLWHA.

From the beginning, supporters of the Ryan White CARE Act carefully threaded the needle between the realities of the epidemic and public perception to generate political commitment. The act was named in honor of Ryan White, a young white hemophiliac who contracted HIV through contaminated blood products and was expelled from his Indiana middle school in 1985 because of the disease. Even though the CDC had demonstrated by 1983 that HIV could not be transmitted through casual contact or by food, water, air, or environmental surfaces, millions around the country saw on their nightly news broadcasts the vitriol from community members that White and his family faced. White went on to become a prominent AIDS activist and educator, testifying before the US President's Commission on AIDS in 1988, just two years before his death and the passage of the CARE Act. His mother, Jeanne White-Ginder, was a formidable AIDS activist in her own right. White's identity as a young, white, heterosexual male, and his acquisition of HIV not through sex or drug use but through a blood transfusion, represented exactly the kind of image that activists, advocates, and service providers would need to circumvent the politics of disgust and garner wider support.

Indeed, the HIV safety net, with the CARE Act as its centerpiece in the United States, stands as a somewhat unusual safety net *because* it received, and continues to receive, bipartisan support at the federal level. Dr. Jennifer Kates, one of the country's foremost experts on healthcare policy, described the bill thus: "The CARE Act is a story about the AIDS activist community demanding healthcare to have their lives saved. They felt that the government needed to do more. There was a recognition on the part of many political leaders that this was the right thing to do. And that was combined with the federal government's recognition that there was a lot of financial pressure on states to support people living with HIV." Caring for the growing numbers of PLWHA was becoming a costly proposition for states that were paying for AZT and health services. At the time, AZT cost approximately $10,000 per year, per patient, making it the most expensive drug released in history. In light of the prospect that every senator and congressional representative could potentially bring cost-relieving federal dollars back to their states to address the epidemic, the bill had 66 cosponsors—45 Democrats and 19 Republicans—and the Ryan White CARE Act passed with strong bipartisan support.[36]

The CARE Act is composed of six parts, each with stakeholders representing wings of the AIDS community. As one advocate put it, "We go into a room and battle our policy positions because the money comes in different ways." Each section of the law has a unique funding allocation. Part A of the act provides an emergency relief grant program for HIV healthcare services administered in metropolitan areas with high numbers of HIV/AIDS cases. These stakeholders tend to be providers in the major cities most visibly affected by the epidemic, such as San Francisco, New York, and Chicago; although some advocates have questioned whether funding should be redistributed given that over half of new HIV cases were in southern states in 2017. The AIDS Drug Assistance Program (ADAP) falls under Part B, providing FDA-approved medications to low-income people living with HIV who have limited or no health coverage from private insurance, Medicaid, or Medicare.[37] HIV/AIDS program directors across the 50 states, united through the National Alliance of State and Territorial AIDS Directors

(NASTAD), are vigorous protectors of this aspect of the law. The ADAP was rolled out in 1987 and paved the way for the Ryan White CARE Act. Because ADAP funding is capped at a certain level with every reauthorization, when demand for treatment increases and states begin to experience patient wait-lists, NASTAD leads the fight for increased funding. Part C funds provide comprehensive primary healthcare services in outpatient settings for PLWHA, and this portion of the policy draws its most vocal supporters from the directors of community health centers. Part D provides grant funding to deliver family-centered, comprehensive care to women, infants, children, and youth living with HIV. Part E of the program gives the Secretary of HHS the authority to use up to 5 percent of supplemental funds appropriated under Parts A and B to address needs during public health emergencies, such as aiding people requiring HIV/AIDS care and treatment in disaster areas. Part F supports the development of innovative models of HIV care and treatment, including AIDS Education and Training Centers to train healthcare providers, and other programs.

The Ryan White Part D program would come to symbolize the government's commitment to women and children in the epidemic. They were viewed as a protected class, especially among more conservative members of Congress and the larger public, who resisted pleas from gay communities for support but who were willing to assist women and especially children, who were viewed as innocent victims of the epidemic. But despite Part D's political valence and growing evidence of the efficacy of the wrap-around care model of the Pediatric AIDS Demonstration Projects, funding for this part of the law was uncertain. In fact, the lack of a highly vocal advocacy group in Washington representing women and children meant that no resources were originally dedicated to Part D of the CARE Act.

The small but growing community of activists and advocates who focused on women and children mobilized. Linda H. Scruggs is an African American AIDS activist who was diagnosed during a routine prenatal visit when she was thirteen weeks pregnant. "I was there when we were negotiating the Ryan White program," she recalled. "The CARE Act was not built for women. That was a fight, to include women and children." David Harvey, a trained social worker with ties to policy circles and a background in disability legal rights, was hired to open a Washington, DC, office of the National Pediatric HIV Resource Center. He would go on to serve as the first executive director of the AIDS Alliance for Women, Infants, Children, Youth, and Families, which was established in 1994. Although initially led by a white gay male, the AIDS Alliance essentially served as one of the first and most influential advocacy groups specifically focusing on women in the epidemic, encouraging WLWHA from all over the country to lobby their congressional representatives, as Linda did, to allocate money to Part D. "And then by joining forces with the rest of the HIV community," Harvey reflected, "we were able to grow the money over the years so that we had a direct funding mechanism that really zeroed in on the needs of women and kids. It was a very significant policy development to get that program in place."

The success of the Ryan White program did not quell existing tensions between the various constituencies of the HIV safety net. As women's voices gained strength, they increasingly trained their sights on the implementation of the CARE Act. One powerful mechanism that emerged from the policy involved HIV Health Services Planning Councils. The Ryan White Planning Councils, as they would come to be known, are volunteer, federally required bodies that work to organize, prioritize, and allocate the CARE Act's Title I/Part A funds within cities, states, and other localities in order to develop and operate effective and cost-efficient systems of care for PLWHA. The planning councils establish priorities and develop comprehensive plans for how HIV health services should be organized and delivered in their respective communities.

From the beginning key officials pushed to ensure that the people sitting around the table in these discussions mirrored the demographics of the epidemic. As David Holtgrave, formerly of the CDC, explained,

> There was increasing understanding that the most effective thing to do was to talk to people, to talk to communities you wanted to reach, and to ask, "Whose opinion matters to you? Who do you trust? Whose voice is important to the community?" Then taking those voices and being able to . . . work with the peer opinion leaders as the messengers to the community, so that you could make sure that the messages were culturally appropriate and related to what people were interested in in the community.

The bedrock of the planning councils, consistent with the long history going back to the Denver Principles, is that PLWHA make up a portion of the membership, enabling the HIV safety net in each locality receiving Part A funds to be shaped by those most affected by, and knowledgeable about, the epidemic. This is an extraordinary mechanism for a safety net to utilize.

Once again, women and people of color had to work strategically *within* the largely white male–dominated AIDS services network while pushing to ensure that their perspectives were included and the unique needs of their communities addressed. The structure of Ryan White encourages both collaboration and friction between the groups. Debates over how to allocate funding play out in conference rooms of AIDS organizations and city public health offices all over the country. Marsha Martin described the dynamic in the early years in this way:

> Since the planning council is the local vehicle for prioritization of the dissemination of [Ryan White] funds, whoever is sitting at the table is who is going to get the funds. It's not legally that way, but it's sort of like, if nobody is at the table that understands that prenatal transmission is a huge problem and can't speak on it, then no one's gonna put money aside . . . [and] say, "Oh well, we should make sure there's some resources for babies." So you needed an intelligent, informed planning body to make sure that your responses . . . [are] consistent with the community need.

The dynamics of privilege and disadvantage were sometimes palpable at these meetings. At the HIV Law Project's Katrina Haslip Technical Assistance Project, "We'd actually practice" to prepare for the meetings, Terry McGovern explained:

> Women would go and participate in a planning council meeting, and they'd come back to the group and say, "I felt totally humiliated. I was not treated like an expert." Even me, as a white [middle-class] female lawyer, half the time people would say, "What you're talking about is anecdotal. It's not science." So we very actively processed all of that, and worked on their skills. . . . They could actually really help others if they would assume kind of a leadership role, and overcome this kind of huge racism, sexism stigma. They could actually save a lot of people.

Thus, in a trend reminiscent of the strategies that gay men adopted to establish themselves as experts in HIV/AIDS conversations, it soon became a national effort to ensure that women had a voice in the growing leadership of the HIV safety net.[38] Terry continued, "We were very stealthy about targeting and getting women appointed to [planning councils and advisory boards], because otherwise, nothing would have changed. So there was a very strategic kind of process, all around the country. We had to work really hard to make sure that women's needs were addressed."

Chicago study women Dawn Stevens and Trisha McIntosh have each served on the Chicago planning council. Dázon was chairing the Metro Atlanta planning council when I interviewed her in 2016. Several members of WORLD participated in planning councils in their cities as well. Pat Nalls served on a Ryan White planning council in Washington, DC, and reflected on her experience in the early years: "I found my voice there and realized how the system worked. And I became a very, very, very strong advocate for women. . . . I started saying to my women's support group, 'Come on, we're gonna all go there. And we're going to show them we're here.' So we started going as a group. Folks were shocked to see there were that many women with HIV in the city at that time."

These interventions created what Michele Tracy Berger has called a workable sisterhood, as women across the country learned how to advocate on behalf of themselves and others.[39] As Terry observed: "At the Katrina Haslip Project, we did this very intentional program where we would teach women about Social Security, what the CDC does, why family court law looked like it did—turn the lights on about all this stuff—and all of this sharing of information about how problematic these policies were really had a transformative effect."

Women also began forming their own partnerships with government officials to move their agendas forward. Trained in nursing and public health, Frances Ashe-Goins regularly convened women activists, advocates, and service providers in her role as deputy director of the Office of Women's Health in HHS from 1996 to 2014.[40] This office went on to create National Women and Girls HIV/AIDS Awareness Day. "When we brought people together," she commented, "women with HIV learned that they were not alone. They learned that there were advocates for them, on the *inside* of government." They had opportunities to interact with officials from the CDC, HRSA, NIH, the Substance Abuse and Mental Health Services Administration, and other federal entities to share their experiences and advocate for their needs. Ashe-Goins continued: "We had federal agency partners that would indicate that they had programs that

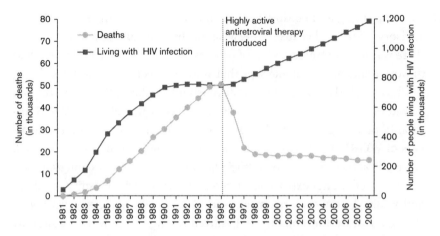

Figure 2. Estimated number of persons living with HIV infection (diagnosed and undiagnosed) and estimated AIDS deaths among adults and adolescents in the United States, 1981–2008. Source: www.drugabuse.gov/publications/research-reports/hivaids/how-does-drug-abuse-affect-hiv-epidemic.

could address issues sensitive to women, or they would indicate their willingness to work together to develop a program to do this to help the women. It was a great collaboration to meet the needs of women and their families."

The investments in the HIV safety net, coupled with the widespread distribution of highly active antiretroviral therapy, created a sea change in the fight against HIV/AIDS in the late 1990s. The clearest success is the reduction in perinatal HIV transmissions by more than 90 percent through universal "opt-out" testing of pregnant women, and through family-centered services funded by Part D of the Ryan White CARE Act. The graph above illustrates the estimated declines in AIDS-related deaths overall starting in 1995 with the introduction of ART.

The strong results that the AIDS community was able to deliver further solidified its bipartisan support. Although federal and state politicians have certainly at times aggressively sought to shape aspects of AIDS policy to match their ideological leanings, the AIDS community has leaned on the evidence, convincingly making the case for the importance of sustaining the HIV safety net. For example, a 2015 study of over 8,000 PLWHA in the US found that 72.8 percent received care at Ryan White–funded facilities, with the greatest utilization taking place among young people ages 18 to 29, women, blacks, Hispanics, the uninsured, and those with less than a high school education and income at or below the poverty level.[41] Ryan White–funded facilities were more likely to provide case management, mental health, drug counseling, and other services than providers funded by other sources. Notably, while the percentage of patients prescribed ART was similar at both types of facilities (adjusting for patient characteristics), poor patients attending Ryan White–funded facilities were more likely to be virally suppressed. In short, medical services alone do not appear to produce the kinds of outcomes that we are seeing: Ryan White programs that provide support services are critical to helping PLWHA remain in care and adhere to treatment.

COMPLICATED ALLIANCES: EXPANDING THE HIV SAFETY NET THROUGH BLACK POLITICAL POWER

Eight years after the 1990 passage of the Ryan White CARE Act, 33 black AIDS advocates and activists gathered at CDC headquarters to meet with officials about the epidemic's impact on black communities. They had been invited by Dr. Helene Gayle, then head of the CDC's National Center for HIV, STD and TB Prevention, who sent word of very troubling data to be published in an upcoming MWWR about the epidemic's trends among blacks. Gayle would be called away on other business and could not attend the meeting, but participants who listened to the presentation given by CDC staff were shocked by statistics estimating that African Americans accounted for 49 percent of all AIDS-related deaths in the United States.[42] It was known that the epidemic was having a disproportionate impact on black communities, but the numbers were still astonishing.

The tension in the room was palpable. As Marsha Martin, who attended the meeting as chief of staff to then HHS Secretary Donna Shalala, described, "They presented the data and everybody was sort of aghast. And then the [CDC people] started talking about strategies. And honestly, it was at the point when they started talking about developing new brochures [that] the people in the room became incensed and said, 'Are you kidding? You're talking to us about brochures and our house is on fire!'"

Debra Fraser-Howze, founding executive director of the National Black Leadership Commission on AIDS (NBLCA), was one of the participants in what came to be known as the Palm Sunday Meeting at the CDC, because it took place a week before Easter 1998. "We shut it down!" she told me proudly as we talked 20 years later. Once a New York City teen mother on welfare, Fraser-Howze later earned a master's degree and used her political savvy and deep connections to black civic, political, and religious leaders to build NBLCA. "We wouldn't let them go on with the presentation." The meeting participants demanded to see top CDC officials immediately and were told that the officials overseeing the HIV program were out of the building at other meetings. Fraser-Howze recalled, "We told them there would be no more discussion with us, 'because now you're going to see the community in a way that you don't want to see us. Because we're sick of you, CDC! . . . Leave us alone, and let us figure out what to do.' And they did. And we came up with a plan."

The CDC meeting attendees got to work, drafting a strategic plan for addressing HIV/AIDS in black communities and agreeing to call for President Bill Clinton to declare a state of emergency in response to the AIDS crisis among blacks. The plan was to then draft legislation seeking to expand AIDS services in black communities and improve the technical capacity of black HIV/AIDS providers so that they could meet demand and better compete for Ryan White dollars. Despite the access to funding that black AIDS organizations received under the CARE Act, the resource disparities between black-led and white-led AIDS organizations started early and only grew, driven largely by the inequities in wealth and political clout among the populations they served.

The meeting attendees dispatched Dr. Beny Primm to Washington, DC. Primm, a respected leader in HIV medicine who had worked on mental health and addiction issues under several presidents, met with congressional leaders, including Louis Stokes, the first black congressman elected in the state of Ohio, and Maxine Waters of California, then head of the Congressional Black Caucus (CBC). The CBC organized a listening session and invited HHS Secretary Shalala. Black activists and advocates lined up at the microphones to air their concerns. "Everybody put their dollar on the table," longtime AIDS activist Cornelius Baker described, recalling speech after speech admonishing the Clinton administration and asking what would be done. As a government insider, Marsha Martin remembered the gathering as if it were yesterday: "We all sat there and listened to the community be angry and furious, starting with Maxine Waters [who offered vocal criticism]. And we were in a small hot room . . . about 200 people. And then we were back at HHS coming up with a plan of what we were gonna do, calling the members of Congress on the right and the left. Everybody understanding that this was an absolute imperative." As Helene Gayle explained, "When the CBC called for the state of emergency, people recognized the urgency of it . . . the CDC leads with the data and felt a real responsibility to communities as a public health agency. I think there was a lot of support."

Despite strong lobbying from Representatives Waters, Stokes, and a cadre of black AIDS advocates and activists, President Clinton declined to declare a public health emergency, unwilling to trigger the accompanying mandated federal resources per the Public Health Service Act because it did not fall within the specified guidelines. After pressure from Waters and others, Clinton publicly described HIV and AIDS as a severe and ongoing health crisis in racial and ethnic minority communities, but stopped short of declaring a federal emergency focused on just one racial group. The bill desired by the Palm Sunday meeting participants then met several challenges as forces both inside and outside the AIDS community questioned whether new legislation should focus only on the black AIDS epidemic, whether newly allocated funds should go only to black-led AIDS organizations as opposed to any organization that served minority clients, and the size of the funding allocation itself. Many black AIDS activists grew increasingly concerned that this broader approach, while inclusive of all racial minorities and poised to provide some assistance to black communities, would not sufficiently attack the disparities in the organizations and the outcomes of the epidemic in the most disproportionately affected group.

After an intense policy-making process, on October 28, 1998, the CBC announced the creation of the Minority AIDS Initiative (MAI). President Clinton, Secretary Shalala, Congressman Stokes, Congresswoman Donna Christensen, and Congresswoman Waters were all on hand to mark the occasion. The MAI would receive an initial appropriation of $156 million in fiscal year 1999 to improve the nation's effectiveness in preventing and treating HIV/AIDS in African American, Hispanic, and other minority communities.[43] In fiscal year 2015, the initiative received $425 million. It funds several AIDS organizations and programs run by local and state governments and community healthcare providers. Congresswoman Waters remains an ardent supporter, consistently circulating requests to leaders of the House Appropriations Committee in support of funding the initiative and advocating for its growth.

When the bill passed in 1998, the MAI looked very different from what the Palm Sunday meeting participants had originally imagined in that conference room at the CDC. Many, like Helene Gayle, credit the MAI with raising awareness of the epidemic in communities of color, building a stronger safety net and strengthening organizational capacity in minority communities, and developing a new cadre of AIDS leaders through its grantees. Others see the MAI as a policy of unrealized potential, much more diffuse in terms of its focus and who benefits from it. "What we got was really watered down from what we were demanding," Debra Fraser-Howze commented, "where everybody took a piece of the pie." The AIDS community, it seemed to her and many other black advocates and activists, was willing to take on racial disparities in the epidemic, but it would do so while maintaining many of the power dynamics embedded in the growing safety net. "The other thing was," Fraser-Howze continued, "while we were fighting for the policy, whenever we would go into the black community and talk about this funding, they would get up and scream at us and tell us that we didn't do enough." Blacks occupied a number of key positions in the Clinton administration, including Gayle at the CDC, Surgeon General David Satcher, and key officials working on AIDS policy in both HHS and the White House. Yet their efforts did not translate into resources on the level many had hoped, caught in the dynamic tension between their responsibility to craft HIV/AIDS policies for all Americans and their recognition of the disparate impact of HIV on black men and women. When the MAI bill passed, Mario Cooper, a prominent black gay rights activist who died in 2015 of AIDS-related complications, was quoted in the *Washington Post* as saying, "For those who have been out there toiling . . . it's a shot in the arm. But it's really only chump change for what is going to be needed for this horrible disease."[44]

SPACEMAKING: TRANSGENDER WOMEN
IN THE HIV SAFETY NET

Tiommi Luckett took her inspiration from the transwomen activists who preceded her, those who had been active participants in LGBTQ struggles and contributors to the AIDS movement from the early years of the epidemic.[45] Marsha P. Johnson, the gender-nonconforming activist credited as a leading force behind the 1969 Stonewall riots, was also involved in ACT UP.

Diagnosed as HIV positive in September 2012, Tiommi was fortunate to receive treatment and within six months had an undetectable viral load. A few years later, a nurse in her doctor's office asked if she would be interested in speaking at an event in Washington, DC, on Medicaid expansion in her home state of Arkansas. "I said yes to the question," she explained when I interviewed her at the 2018 International AIDS Conference in Amsterdam. "But I had no idea what was in store for me." A couple of months after her visit to Washington, Tiommi was asked to speak in other venues on behalf of transgender rights. From there, she attended the "HIV Is Not a Crime" Training Academy, a gathering of activists, legislators, lawyers, people living with HIV and other experts to discuss and plan ways to reform and modernize laws that criminalize HIV. There Tiommi learned just how much her HIV status jeopardized her freedom. She recalled that when she was diagnosed, a healthcare worker asked her to sign a document before providing her with services; it acknowledged that if she did not disclose her HIV status to a sexual partner, she could be charged with a felony, punishable by 30 years in prison under Arkansas law. If she didn't disclose her status to a medical provider, she could be charged with a misdemeanor, even with an undetectable viral load that rendered her virus untransmittable. As she looked around at those gathered for the training academy, she realized just how dire the consequences were for PLWHA, especially transwomen, whose vulnerability was already heightened. Unable to find jobs due to employment discrimination, some transgender individuals engage in sex work as one of the few economic strategies available to them. Tiommi described her own experience:

> Before my documentation was changed, everything said male. I had a male's name, but I presented as female. No one wanted to hire me. . . . So when I got my documentation changed, I was able to get in, but that was my story.

That's not the story of every trans person out there. It's not so easy to get a job, and so sex work becomes the work that they have to engage in. And with a positive diagnosis, if you do sex work, even if there are no HIV criminalization statutes in that state, you can still receive sentence enhancements for solicitation. Because you're positive.

While many within the AIDS community point out that sex work is a choice for some and should be afforded certain human rights protections, they are also quick to assert that it should not be the *only* choice for those who have no other means to subsist.[46] Transgender women, especially those who participate in sex work, live under threat of sexual and physical violence, and high levels of stigma can often lead to drug addiction, depression, and other mental health challenges.[47]

Tiommi's work in the HIV and transgender communities continued to grow. She served as a blogger and advisory board member for various AIDS and transgender organizations and held a seat on the Arkansas Ryan White HIV planning council. She did it "to get my words out there," she reflected. "People relate. Women relate to what I am saying. It started to break down the differences in our lived experiences, and it brought me closer to a community of people that I trust." As is the case for so many women, Tiommi's connections to the HIV safety net provided a social, political, and economic lifeline. "Before my HIV diagnosis, I was an addict, a sex worker, someone with a history of incarceration. I tried to be the life of the party because I felt like I wasn't loved and because I was different. I always put up a façade that I was happy. Then I said, 'You know what? It's time for me to live for me. I can't live for how people want me to be.'"

The indication that things were changing in a meaningful way at the policy level was brought home to Tiommi when she and other transgender activists were invited to the White House in 2016. The group arrived at the gathering with two things: a policy agenda and data. The organization Positively Trans had organized a survey. "We knew that they were gonna tell us: 'There's not enough data,'" Tiommi explained. "Well guess what, we have it for you. We've done the work for you. We did a needs assessment." The meeting was attended by leaders of the transgender advocacy community; transgender women and men working in the Obama administration; scholars; members of the AIDS community; and other federal officials. They sat around a rectangular table, "and we were able to *see* each other," Tiommi emphasized with pride.

Hearing Tiommi describe the White House meeting reminded me of David Harvey's reflections when AIDS activists were invited to the White House during the Clinton presidency more than 20 years earlier. These invitations are deeply symbolic signals of inclusion and indicators that the highest echelons of American power are willing to listen, even if every policy dream is not ultimately realized. David Harvey reflected thus:

> I will never forget the first time the HIV community went to a meeting in the White House after Clinton was elected. I was there, together with some other very vocal, strong-willed people. I'll never forget walking through those gates and walking into the White House, into the Roosevelt Room, for a meeting with one of the president's advisors. You could hear a pin drop; everyone's silent. And everybody was just kinda in awe. It was the first time we'd ever been in there, and it was really . . . oh, it was really something! And then some of us started speaking up. Of course, I think that the item then was healthcare reform, because the Clintons set right out to do healthcare reform, and we wanted to make sure that people with HIV were protected. So, we had a lot of access in the Clinton administration. They created an AIDS czar position. That was a focal point of a lot of work. We did a lot of work with the agencies, and Congress. We had a lot of influence.

Now the transgender community would finally have its opportunity to articulate its needs in this hallowed setting. Tiommi recounted how the activists seated around the table spoke about their fundamental right to self-definition, health, and safety. They advocated for access to trans-affirming healthcare (including hormones), economic opportunity, HIV decriminalization, and a commitment from the administration to help battle trans and HIV stigma. They called on HRSA, CDC, the Office for National AIDS Policy, and other federal agencies to end the routine practice of categorizing transwomen as men who have sex with men.[48] "To be identified as a man by the government, no matter how we look," Tiommi explained. "That [misgendering] is what leads to us being killed. We never know how safe we are. . . . But then we have to actually claim to be a man in order to receive services."

The activists gathered also called out some of the troubling dynamics that were happening within the AIDS community. HIV/AIDS program funders, they argued, needed to reconsider some of the criteria for higher-paying jobs and grants that were in place. In practice, they served as barriers to entry for the transgender community. "One thing we [reinforced in subsequent meetings]," Tiommi continued, "was that a lot of transwomen living with HIV will not have the credentials on paper, but they will actually have the experience to do the work. So what came from that meeting was that they removed the stipulation that in order to receive funding, you had to have a bachelor's degree. That's important, to allow us the space that we need to do the work ourselves, as it pertains to our community."

Throughout the discussion at this historic meeting, transwomen of color, and especially black transwomen, were front and center. They would not be silenced by a politics of racial respectability, nor by racial bias that threatened to put their needs last. Tiommi declared:

> We went there, and we made ourselves visible. That was not an easy meeting to sit through. Tempers flared, egos were checked, because in that meeting there was still an element of anti-blackness. And we called it out for what it was. You will not silence black transwomen and allow white transmen to talk. We're not doing that. Like I said, it was a lot to deal with. We got through it, and we were invited back. And so a second meeting happened later that year, in September, where they discussed what they had come up with from our meeting. So they heard us.

As a result of these ongoing conversations, several funders developed opportunities specifically for the transgender community in order to redistribute some of the resources going for AIDS work. "We were no longer grouped with the MSM community," Tiommi explained, "or having the funding divvied up 75 percent to MSMs and 25 percent to the trans community." Further, when President Obama announced the updated version of the National HIV/AIDS Strategy, the needs and contributions of the transgender community were explicitly stated. "So we got the federal government to acknowledge us as the community that we are. Now, we are a movement within a movement," Tiommi said proudly. While the pace of change is arguably too slow for many, especially as the post-Obama era political winds threaten to halt and even reverse the momentum, transwomen are challenging the HIV safety net to expand the boundaries even further to ensure that they too have access to its transformative effects.

COMPETITION AND CONVERGENCE: BUILDING A TRULY
INTERSECTIONAL HIV COMMUNITY

Today, the billion-dollar HIV/AIDS infrastructure stands as an underappreciated yet highly effective model for assisting marginalized populations, demonstrating how centering their voices, leveraging institutional
networks, and generating coalitions across race, class, sexuality, and gender can help address injuries of inequality. The safety net created by the
AIDS community represents an intersectional politics in action at the
level of both policy and institutions, making women's transformations
from *dying from* to *living with* possible. This is done in several ways.

First, in building the HIV safety net, the AIDS community created a
space in which to confront the pervasive politics of disgust directed toward
groups most affected by the epidemic while reshaping the public narrative
in ways that have produced, and are produced by, victories won through
political power brokering and the empowerment of PLWHA. It draws on
affected communities that have experienced trauma and stigma in many
forms—from the devastation of diagnosis to lifetimes of marginalization—
to tell important stories and glean valuable and diverse lessons that
advance its goals. It then simultaneously and effectively draws on its stock-
piles of privilege, as the community adroitly leverages celebrity, wealth, and
cultural capital to advance its agenda and counteract destructive public
narratives. This balance of privilege and marginalization offers an array of
potential strategies through which to mobilize and contributes to the AIDS
community's effectiveness at speaking truth to power and defining its own
story.

Second, the HIV safety net relies on a deep commitment to encouraging
those most affected by its policies and programs—PLWHA and those at
higher risk of acquiring HIV—to play active roles in the decision-making
and agenda-setting of organizations within the system. AIDS services are
therefore heavily influenced by the voices of the population they serve, as
experiential knowledge augments scientific evidence to shape programs and
services. This safety net was built *by* the community, *for* the community.

Third, women, gay and bisexual men of color, transgender individuals,
low-income people, and others have consistently challenged the AIDS
community to "expand the tent" and define *community* in the most

inclusive terms. These groups have demanded an intersectional approach to the AIDS response, implicitly and sometimes explicitly adopting a black feminist framework articulated by scholars such as Kimberlé Crenshaw and circulating in texts such as the iconic Combahee River Collective statement. "The most general statement of our politics at the present time," the essay contends, "would be that we are actively committed to struggling against racial, sexual, heterosexual, and class oppression and see as our particular task the development of *integrated* analysis and practice based upon the fact that the major systems of oppression are interlocking. The synthesis of these oppressions creates the conditions of our lives."[49] By increasing access to culturally sensitive services, sharing decision-making power, and lending attention to the unique needs of all of the populations deeply affected by AIDS—not just white gay men—those operating in this tradition continually push the AIDS community to stay true to the mission of moving people from *death* to *life,* in the broadest sense of those terms. They also expanded what it means to be an AIDS activist-expert, bringing to bear their own experiential knowledge and engagement with science and policy to make the fight against AIDS even more inclusive. Arguably, this priority has been the greatest source of conflict within the AIDS response community; it is also, however, one of its deepest sources of strength. The labor and demands of the diverse communities affected by the epidemic have driven advances in the science of HIV/AIDS, improvements in services, and decisive victories in policy advocacy.

To be sure, it is not the case that women, and especially women of color, stand simply as beneficiaries of the political activism of gay male AIDS activists. Rather, the support is multi-directional, and the contributions of many different groups have expanded what is possible for all. Gay and bisexual white men used their economic and cultural capital and white male privilege to lay the foundation for the HIV/AIDS agenda and to politically protect it throughout the decades. Gay and bisexual men of color leverage their liminal status between the LGBTQ and black communities to shine a light on both racism within the LGBTQ community and homophobia within communities of color to improve services. Women push different levers of power because of their status as mothers and the framing of their babies as "deserving" of support. Some have also exercised their racial and/or class privilege to advance the political claims of WLWHA and to enter certain political spaces, while others who are highly marginalized bring their sharp survival skills to bear as they fight back against exclusion and injustice. And it took Ryan White and Magic Johnson to be important symbolic markers of the movement for the general public. Part of the success of the AIDS movement therefore is the way in which it has adroitly leveraged the politics of privilege and the bitter consequences of oppression for political advancement. The composition of this coalition paved the way for gains that perhaps would not have come about without these disparate groups working together.

Despite, or perhaps *because* of, tensions between the various constituencies most affected by HIV/AIDS, the HIV safety net has been built through the activism of a passionate community and its ability to strategically deploy its political, economic, and social capital. Through subsequent reauthorizations of the Ryan White CARE Act, the community has had numerous chances to reflect and evolve, ensuring that what began as a mobilization against a politics of disgust has become a politics of transformation. "None of us wins everything," David Harvey commented. "And then we go forward to Congress with a unified front and advocate for what we want. It is a very powerful alliance. And in one way, shape, or form, that process happens in each of the policy reauthorizations."

The infrastructure that was built in response to AIDS also relies on synergistic relationships among the HIV/AIDS research, clinical, human service, and activist communities, as the safety net was built from the ground up rather than from the top down. These networks constantly challenge each other to notice blind spots, and each contributes to the safety net that is in effect today. These relationships were hard fought, especially in the early stages, when activists and HIV-positive individuals found themselves on the margins of professionalized AIDS knowledge production and, as Deborah Gould captures in her "emotional history" of ACT UP, the targets of "aggressive indifference, extreme negligence, and punitive policies regarding AIDS."[50] Nevertheless, through those struggles, AIDS activists and advocates, with the support of policymakers and other elites, have been able to create and sustain an effective infrastructure for confronting a raging epidemic.

．　　．　　．　　．　　．

The HIV safety net is not a perfect system; no system is. From the struggle to address the epidemic in the American South to the lingering challenge of ensuring that women, poor people, transgender people, and people of color (especially black MSM) have the same access to care, political clout, and career opportunities as their white gay male counterparts, tensions remain. The HIV safety net operates like any other playing field of power. Public attention, social recognition, scientific focus, research dollars, programmatic funding, political access, career opportunities, access to services, decision-making authority, research publication authorships, and the legitimacy to "represent" the epidemic all serve as currency. The AIDS response has become not just a humanitarian effort but a business, with inequalities that mirror everyday life. The marginalized sometimes marginalize others, despite good intentions. "This was a boys' game, and it's still a boys' game," Linda Scruggs commented. "And I think there . . . [have] been very few of us women who are HIV positive, and especially HIV positive [and] of color, who really have learned to play that game." As I listened to the Chicago study women, I was struck by the way in which a successful policy intervention that was built and animated through multicultural grassroots activism produced a remarkably durable safety net and a launching pad for personal and political transformation. In the next chapter we will examine how some Chicago study women found their way into this infrastructure and were able to launch transformative projects.

3 Living With

I arrived precisely at noon on a brisk March day in 2005 and anxiously glanced around for Josie (black, age 35), one of the earliest participants in my research study. I had interviewed her a month prior, and she suggested that I observe one of the monthly support group meetings that she leads for women living with HIV/AIDS. She completed peer facilitator training through a local AIDS organization and described how she educated herself about both the science of the disease and the psychological impact of stigma. Fittingly, when Josie decided to disclose to her employer that she is HIV positive, she brought literature to educate him about the disease and about her legal rights under the Americans with Disabilities Act.

As I hurriedly checked the directory posted in the lobby of the eight-story gray office building on Chicago's north side, I heard Josie calling my name. We hugged and she escorted me into a large conference room on the first floor. "I want to introduce you to somebody," she explained as we approached a middle-aged white woman with reddish brown hair wearing a crisp pumpkin-colored blazer. Trisha McIntosh held out her hand and explained that she too was a peer facilitator in the city's HIV support groups for women. "I want to be in your study," Trisha proclaimed, at which point I explained that for this small pilot phase, we were focusing on black women, given their disproportionate numbers in the epidemic. Little did I know then that Trisha would in fact participate in the study when we expanded it five years later, and I introduced the Canadian native's story in chapter 1.

Due to scheduling confusion, it turned out not to be Josie's turn to facilitate the support group meeting, which she believed had given her the authority to invite me as her guest.[1] She would not receive the $25 stipend for leading the meeting offered by the AIDS service organization on the second floor, but there would be other opportunities to lead. I stepped out while Josie asked the six women assembled if I could sit in during their session. They graciously agreed, offering me a seat at the conference table. They passed around the fruit, water, sandwiches, and cupcakes that various members had contributed for lunch. As we waited to begin, Josie leaned over to describe to me just how important groups like these were to her: "It's our responsibility to help other women going through this. We've gotta help those that are just finding out [that they have HIV] and don't know that you can still have a life. We gotta reach out to them." As we settled into our Ryan White–funded support group meeting, I was witnessing one of the policy innovations described in chapter 2 come to life.

At about 12:15 p.m. the meeting started. Tammy, a white woman perhaps in her forties with frizzy blond hair and a tattoo on the inside of her right forearm, welcomed everyone and commanded, "Okay, let's check in." Betina, a fortyish black woman with a gummy smile and thin black hair gathered into a hair clip, gave her name and, to open the proceedings, announced that she had been diagnosed 20 years prior and was "feeling fine." Betina reminded everyone of the ground rules: "Don't interrupt and let everyone have their say. Don't break confidentiality. No one is better than anyone else."

One by one the women around the table gave their names, shared when they were diagnosed with HIV, and relayed how they were feeling and what issues concerned them. Joanie, a white woman in her forties or fifties with a worn face and very thin frame, described feeling particularly good because she had just found housing. Tammy then described her frustration at still being unable to obtain Social Security disability assistance but was happy to be out of her nursing home residence for a few hours. Trisha and Josie offered Tammy advice about how to appeal the Social Security denial, informing her that there was an AIDS advocate in the building who might be able to help.

During her turn, Josie described feeling "blessed" and reported that she had been in the hospital a few weeks earlier with sinusitis and a 102-degree fever. She had a spinal tap and they "checked my brain for parasites," she commented. "Yeah, we gotta watch out for the parasites," Trisha nodded and flashed a sly smile.

What I would come to realize was that all of the participants were survivors of the sexualized drug economy. As each woman spoke, the others nodded in agreement, offering advice, congratulations, and affirmations that each was doing the best she could. Those on the receiving end thanked the group and explained that they "just needed to keep reminding themselves." It was as if each woman was trying to drown out a lifetime's worth of destructive messages, with those seated around them providing a Greek chorus of affirming voices, a positive feedback loop that perhaps none of them had ever experienced.

Trisha, seated commandingly at the head of the table, projected a very different presence from the woman who had entered rehab five years earlier on death's door. She spoke in a gravelly voice with hints of slightly slurred speech, the lingering evidence of the years of distress. Her knowledge of the resources in the area and her wealth of strategies that could help the women in the group overcome emotional turbulence was extensive. Although she was light years away from her life in the sexualized drug economy, her time there granted her experiential capital that was extremely valuable to the women seated around her. My host, Josie, whose addiction to drugs began *after* she was diagnosed with HIV, held court at the opposite end of the table, equally impressive with her command of information. When Josie briefly went quiet during the conversation, Betina asked, "So what do you think, Josie?" soliciting her counsel. Josie spoke calmly but passionately, often invoking God and spirituality. Trisha and Josie basked in the respect the others paid to them as leaders, a subtle competitive tension holding the space between them.

Margaret, a black woman with shoulder-length Jheri-curled hair, described struggling recently with the experience of seeing her sister lying on her deathbed, sick with cancer. Margaret said that she was determined to stay positive and sober: "I believe in God, and I know that He's got me, but I need someone down here. I feel like it's just me and I ain't got nobody. It's like at two and three in the morning when I'm alone and I'm struggling the most." Trisha interrupted Margaret to tell her that she was sorry she had not called. "I wasn't trying to accuse anyone," Margaret shrugged, "It was just how I felt." "I know, but I feel bad," Trisha responded, carrying the responsibility of offering support. Josie interjected, encouraging Margaret to stay faithful and to call her. "I work at night so I'm up at that hour. I'll help you. You gon' make it. You are in God's hands." After a short pause, Josie continued: "You gotta remember," she explained to Margaret. "Pressure bursts pipes, so imagine what pressure in our minds will do. You gotta get support."

After each woman checked in, Trisha invited me to talk about my study. I gave my business cards to Betina, Margaret, and Trisha, who all said that they knew women who might qualify. They mentioned a woman who normally comes to group, "but she's a handful," Trisha warned. "She's fine one-on-one, but in a group situation, she acts out—like nobody's problems are worse than hers."

Because almost all of the women around the table were over 45 years old (past my pilot study's designated age cut-off), only one or two were eligible. "See, we're all older ladies," Trisha explained. "You don't get it together until your forties. In your twenties and thirties, you're still *out there*. You don't come to stuff like this much." It was one of the many moments in which WLWHA were not just interviewees but research contributors, making observations about our study design and unearthing inaccurate assumptions. Trisha was offering valuable insight into the difficulties our study was having recruiting women between the ages of 18 and 35, but she was also gesturing toward the transformative arc that many women in the community experienced during adulthood. Perhaps the HIV safety net attracted mostly those who knew their status and had accepted it with enough seriousness to ask for help and reveal themselves to others in a support group or a clinic. Perhaps the key was understanding what catalyzed women who no longer wanted to be "out there" in the sexualized drug economy or "out there" living seemingly normal lives but in debilitating isolation. When we expanded the Chicago study five years after my visit to this support group, we raised the age limit; invited black, Latina, and white women to participate; and aggressively recruited a number of women who *weren't* firmly ensconced in the HIV safety net, the richness of their experiences and their diversity deepening my understanding of transformative projects.

Two other women trickled in around 12:45. One was Laverne, a white woman whom I recognized from another AIDS organization I had recently visited. Josie told her that it was good to see her and observed that it had been a while since her last meeting appearance. Laverne's long black and gray curly hair was gathered in a large hair clip, and she was the only woman in the group wearing makeup. She checked in and expressed frustration that she was having so much difficulty navigating bureaucratic hurdles to receive public aid, a bridge she felt she needed until she could find steady work. Trisha reminded her that public aid was a blessing, as few people qualified. Laverne agreed and said that she was trying her best to remain patient and not do what she used to do—lash out at everyone in her path. She spent Easter with her father and siblings and described how good it felt to be with her family sober and able to contribute. She was careful to decline offers of money and other help, saying, "I heard in my head 'go ahead and take it.' But my internal dialogue was like, 'I know I need to make it without taking advantage of them.'"

"That's right, we're takers," Trisha interjected as the other women nodded in agreement, harkening back to her days on the streets. "When you're an addict, you take, you never give. We learn how to manipulate people, and we have to be careful of that when we're in recovery. We lie, do whatever."

"Because it used to be about me, me, me," Margaret added. "I wasn't thinking about anybody else. I didn't tell the truth as long as I got what I wanted. That's all that mattered."

Betina jumped in. "Like when somebody would ask you if you were [HIV] positive, I'd say no. As long as I could get that money, it didn't matter."

"Yeah," Trisha declared, "and when I was out there I would sometimes ask guys, 'Don't you want to use a condom?' They would say, 'No, you look clean.' As long as I got what I wanted, I was fine."

"As long as they were paying, that's all I cared about," Joanie added as the women collectively nodded at the gravity of what their lives once were in the sexualized drug economy. This would be one of many times when I was struck by how women sought to hold themselves accountable for their pasts.

Once everyone checked in, the women continued the conversation. They described how they were feeling about various life issues and heard advice and encouragement from one another. Their language was very much inspired by 12-step programs. God was frequently invoked as the women encouraged each other to have faith and know that their lives had meaning. Trisha described not going to church but watching it on television. "See, that's important too," Margaret affirmed as she gestured around the table. "Because God is using you to help somebody else." The women talked explicitly about how they counsel themselves using their "internal dialogue," very much aware that they were battling for their health and their lives, and they were consciously trying to win the war.

Trisha then suggested that we break so that she could escort Tammy to talk to the AIDS advocate in the nonprofit located upstairs about filing for Social Security. As the women broke into side conversations, Josie approached Margaret, promising to pray for her. "She [Margaret] needs a sponsor," Betina offered. "Well, here I am," Josie said to Margaret. Margaret expressed gratitude and commented that she felt so much better having attended the meeting. "I want you to read the third step again. Do you have an NA [Narcotics Anonymous] book?" Josie asked. Margaret said she did. "Well," Josie continued, "I want you to read the first three steps again and write a short paper on what they mean to you, how they affect your life." "Okay, that's easy, I can do that," Margaret responded, amenable to the impromptu homework assignment. "I just need somebody to talk to. I'm struggling."

"God knows it," Josie responded. "Here, let's pray." She rose to her feet and held out both hands for Margaret to grab. Margaret clutched Josie's hands, and Josie began praying eloquently, giving thanks "for the day, for survival, for hope and for what God has done and will do in Margaret's life. Walk with her Lord, help her know that there is support around her and that she is in Your arms."

For the next 15 minutes the women trickled in and out of the room, running errands in the neighborhood, visiting with the staff at the afore-mentioned AIDS nonprofit, and conversing amiably. When Trisha returned from upstairs she asked whether anyone needed bus passes. Trisha handed two transit cards to each woman who raised her hand, courtesy of the case manager working upstairs. For those once ensconced in the fast-money world of the sexualized drug economy, these small but important resources seemed invaluable as they tried, day by day, to get back on their feet.

I would visit a number of HIV support groups like this one over the course of my research; I learned quickly that these gatherings function partly as emotional booster sessions and partly as economic strategy circles, providing women with emotional tools, material resources, and spiritual support. Some women attended these sessions as many as three or four times per week, alternating between their HIV and Narcotics Anonymous support groups. Essentially, WLWHA had taken the model of the prototypical AIDS support group that was ostensibly designed to serve a white, mostly middle-class, gay male constituency and bent and shaped it to fit their needs as women, a disproportionate number of whom were poor and/or women of color. They networked, brokered resources for themselves and each other, held up mirrors, and affirmed that their transformative projects—despite their challenges—were well worth pursuing and maintaining.

As we sat next to a large tinted window, the women chatted, ate, and vented about their lives. Although no one outside was able to see in, I could see out. The street bustled with men and women waiting for buses, congregating in the streets, and going about their everyday lives. This room was an oasis for the women who were able, if only briefly, to let down their guard and discuss their mistakes, fears, and glimmers of improvement. They encouraged each other and looked collectively toward the future, navigating challenges in a context of constraint while attempting to heal from inequality's brutal injuries.

.   .   .   .   .

How does one remake a life? How does a woman diagnosed with HIV transition from believing and behaving as though she has a death sentence to interpreting and coping with HIV as a chronic yet manageable illness? When multiple stressors confront every aspect of her being—physical, emotional, economic, social—how does she halt the downward momentum and change directions? And how does this happen when there are limited resources and multiple disadvantages, when engaging an arsenal of personal reserves and "throwing money at the problem" may not be possible? This chapter explores how personal agency, sound public policy, and organizational resources come together to create opportunities for accomplishing transformational change. I will examine how and when effective transformations happen and will begin looking at how sticking points emerge that cause women to get trapped or backslide into prior patterns.

Michele Tracy Berger's *Workable Sisterhood: The Political Journey of Stigmatized Women with HIV/AIDS* is foundational for my development of the notion of a transformative project. She focuses on how black WLWHA with histories of drug addiction grapple with these intersectional stigmas and become politically engaged, fighting the AIDS epidemic on the local and national levels.[2] I build on her notion of life reconstruction, a micro-level process, to highlight how remaking a life is embedded within institutional, policy, and political contexts at the local, national, and international levels.

Engagement with the HIV safety net accounts for a sizeable portion of the variation between those who thrive and those who do not following an HIV diagnosis, with some noteworthy nuances and complexities. Specifically, as framing institutions, organizations within this network shape the form and tenor of women's coping trajectories and transformations by offering information and a framework for understanding what it means to have HIV, language in which to talk about one's condition, and tangible resources with which to begin restructuring one's life.[3] They also connect women to individual and institutional networks that prove vitally important.

The most effective framing institutions facilitate or nurture the mind shift needed for massive personal transformation. They help women internalize and operationalize the realization that they need to change course and adopt new strategies to better cope with major life events and injuries of inequality. They reengineer the feedback loop about the women's marginalized status by helping women confront the powerful internal and external messages they receive about their worth and value that are undermining and destructive. As a result, women rewrite their conceptions of themselves despite having a stigmatizing social marker like an HIV diagnosis. By coupling this work with actual material resources such as access to health care and modest but valuable economic support, beneficial framing institutions serve a critical function for women moving from crisis to stability.

While several organizations act as framing institutions within the HIV safety net, some framing institutions in women's lives are outside of that network. All told, the HIV safety net, and the framing institutions within and adjacent to it, provide a model for helping women address injuries of inequality.

In this chapter, we pick up where we left off in chapter 1 and analyze why and how women begin to strategize differently following years of physical, emotional, and economic distress. We revisit Trisha, Keisha, Beverly, and Yvette to continue following their trajectories and highlight the similarities and variations among them and the remaining Chicago study women. We will also hear from our final central storyteller, Rosario Salazar. As these women's stories illustrate, there are two important ingredients needed for transformative projects to occur: the cognitive shifts that determine for women that they must adopt new strategies to cope with their changing lives, and their use of relationships that are available to them through the HIV safety net and other framing institutions. While the previous chapter explored how the AIDS infrastructure came to be, the current chapter analyzes how the Chicago study women engage with it on the ground. Subsequent chapters will analyze the women's longer-term strategies and the "stickiness" of their transformative projects.

COGNITIVE SHIFTS

A serious health diagnosis can drive a person's identity into a state of flux. Individuals in these circumstances often undertake meaning-making and strategizing to achieve stability in the face of uncertainty.[4] Coping with a newly discovered health status is therefore a complex, multidimensional process that is presumably shaped by available resources and demands; the psychological and social dispositions of individuals; and the family, friends, and medical providers who constitute one's support network.[5] Unlike acute illnesses, chronic illnesses exhibit an unfolding or emergent quality that forces sufferers to continuously negotiate how they understand their conditions and reconcile these beliefs with their health-management behaviors. In the early stages of a serious health diagnosis, individuals generate preliminary illness-management strategies to achieve or maintain a sense of control and emotional equilibrium as they struggle with shock, anguish, anxiety, powerlessness, and fear of mortality.[6]

These dynamics might characterize how people cope with many kinds of crises, not just those related to illness. Psychologists describe cognitive reappraisal as an emotion-regulation strategy that involves changing the trajectory of an emotional response by reinterpreting the meaning of the emotional stimulus.[7] This two-step process begins first with recognizing one's negative response and then reinterpreting the situation either to reduce the severity of the negative response or to exchange the negative attitude for a more positive attitude. Emotion regulation addresses primarily an individual's perception of a situation, rather than directly altering the environmental stressors themselves. However, cognitive reappraisal could in fact be a precursor to resistance.

Cognitive reappraisal, the *internal* mindset shift that suggests that "things have to change," often takes place following an *external* pivotal event or set of interactions. For some of the Chicago study women, cognitive reappraisal occurred shortly after diagnosis. For others, it took years. Turning points, external events that affect women significantly, call into question the efficacy of their preexisting strategies for economic, emotional, and physical survival. Turning points stop the negative momentum, break up routines, and inspire deep reflection. In other words, the cognitive shifts that are critical for women's transformative projects take place through their interpretation of turning-point events and their assessment that they must fundamentally shift how they are conceptualizing, strategizing around, and tactically addressing their struggles.

Beverly referred to her cognitive shift as her "awakening." It occurred shortly before she was diagnosed HIV positive, as she awaited an available bed in a drug rehabilitation facility:

> When I was in jail waiting on my bed, I realized I left my apartment with somebody in there doing stupid shit [selling drugs and other illegal goods]. I was on the phone arguing with them, and the police officer told me, "Hang that damn phone up!" I'll never forget her. I looked at her like, "Who the fuck are you talking to?" She's like, "Did you hear what I said?" And I had a spiritual awakening at that moment. I looked at her and I looked at the

phone . . . and my first . . . [thought] was, "Pick the phone off the wall and go beat it in her head." And the Spirit said, "Then you gonna catch another goddamn case." And then I'm saying, how the fuck did I get *here?* Who is she *talking to* like that? You don't talk to me like that. Not me. And I'm like, "How did I get here?" God got a sense of humor 'cause it's like, "Uh, you didn't get an invitation." [Laughter.] It was like, how did I get here? Oh, playing the paper [selling stolen credit cards]. Like, what the fuck am I doing playing paper? And it hit me: the drugs.

Beverly clearly articulates the psychic dimensions of transformative change. She altered her emotional response to the police officer by reinterpreting the meaning of the moment. It was no longer about the officer; Beverly realized that her life was on a trajectory that put her in a place, in a status, that she never imagined for herself. The guard, Beverly realized, felt obliged to speak to her harshly because of where they were and how she was perceiving Beverly. She was in an institution where such treatment was normalized and accepted. She reflected on the events that brought her there and realized just how dire the situation had become. A deeper level of accountability became part of her thinking. Beverly began to make a plan:

In a quick five seconds, all this starts happening, and I realize that I had been fucking up my life. And it was like, "Okay, what I'm doing here? Okay, I'm waiting to go to treatment. Okay. When you get to treatment, you've got to do every damn thing the people tell you to do so that you never have to come back." By the time I got to treatment, I was so hungry, I was so thirsty, I wanted treatment so bad, 'cause I didn't want to have to go back. I was like, "I can't go back to this damn jail bed, got to sleep on this hard cot and the cold. What is wrong with you? You in jail, and somebody else is in *your* apartment doing hell. What is wrong with this picture?"

Beverly had been in detox four times prior to this incident, exasperating her mother Verna. What changed? This time, a harsh reality confronted Beverly, one echoed by several of the women with whom I spoke: although they had once believed they were master players in the sexualized drug economy, each became aware that she was in fact being played.[8] Beverly realized that it was she, not the friends and associates currently stationed in her home, who was paying a huge price for being in the drug game. It had to stop. When she entered the Open Gate drug treatment facility,

Beverly was clear she was there for transformation and that she wanted out of that life: "It was on the lake, and it was so beautiful and so peaceful. Oh, man, that was a beautiful place. So that's where I went in, with a new attitude, so that was a big difference." The facility introduced Beverly to people who could help her gain a new perspective on her health as well. Just as her own mother had weighed the gravity of one daughter's breast cancer diagnosis against another daughter's HIV diagnosis, Beverly gauged her own survivability relative to those afflicted with acute illnesses:

> While I was in treatment, I went to a funeral as strength, support for a girl whose aunt got Ebola. The disease ate her up. She didn't have any intestines. It ate up her neck. It ate up everything it touched. I was strong on my [drug recovery] program. And I went with her to that funeral and I came back and I said, "I can live with HIV." 'Cause this woman had four days before she died. She ain't got time to get nothing in order. And I was like, shit, I can live with the virus long as I don't get nothing else. I've got time. So I was like, okay, I can do this. I just gotta get some education. I gotta find out what it is I'm fighting. I gotta get on top of it. And that's what I did.

Over 60 percent of the Chicago study women described a noteworthy cognitive shift, a "wake-up call" moment that helped them realize that they had to manage their physical and emotional health in a radically new way and that they had to make a long-term commitment to doing so. I heard it expressed in any number of ways: "I got tired," "I got tired of being tired," "I was getting too old for this," "I didn't want to die," and "Enough was enough." Many realized that they wanted to "do better" for their families and themselves. Lupe, a 56-year-old Puerto Rican mother of four adult children who became addicted to drugs in law school, explained,

> I was smoking crack, and I'm sitting in South Beach, right in front of Club Madonna, and I saw a lady pushing a cart. And she was all dirty, like I've been. I'm sleeping in the street. [The lady] was nothing different than what I see every day. But this time, I saw something on top of her, it was like dark and white, like good and evil. I saw, like, an epiphany. I didn't know what I saw, but that scared the heck out of me, and I gave my drugs away and I walked out of there.

The cognitive shift for women engaged in the sexualized drug economy was often associated with what many in the addiction community call "hitting rock bottom." A frequent interlocutor during my research, I discussed with Phill Wilson, founder of the Black AIDS Institute, why the cognitive shifts I was observing seemed so pronounced among these women. He reflected:

> I think what HIV does, particularly among women or men in addiction, is—you can be in your addiction, but HIV basically says, "Listen." In your addiction you think, I *could* die, but HIV says, "Listen. You're *going* to die." And so then, you go, "Oh! Maybe I don't want to do that." And so, it's not that death is *possible*, it's like a reality check: It's *going* to happen, and it's going to happen soon if you continue using. So at this moment, *you decide.* Do you really want to die? And if you don't, what are you going to do?

In other words, such a cognitive shift was a response to a collision between the abstract and the concrete. An early death is an abstract notion that many people face, particularly when they are engaged in higher-risk behavior or living in a context of heightened physical danger. But an HIV diagnosis, particularly in the years prior to the strong presence of highly effective medications, crashes headlong into this abstract notion of death and demands that women see it as a very real possibility. The cognitive shift is an existential moment, a time when women are forced to step back and assess: despite the struggles and despite the pain, do I want to live?

Because I followed several WLWHA for more than a decade, I was able to observe some cognitive shifts that were much more gradual and not tied to drug addiction. Such reappraisals tended to involve grappling with what it meant to truly live, not just physically, but also psychologically, with HIV. During our first interview in January 2007, Yvette, whom we met in chapter 1, was adamant she was not going to disclose her HIV-positive status to her 21-year-old son Steven. She held the shame close, unable to loosen its grip:

> It's been time [to tell him]. I think I'm just being cowardly in not telling him. I think I'm just so afraid of his reaction . . . because he's been around [to see] some of my bad boyfriend choices, and I guess I don't want him thinking that I've made an even worse choice. . . . I'm afraid that he's going to think I'm just the most irresponsible mom that there probably ever was, even though I think I've accomplished a lot in my life and I still have many goals to try to accomplish. I still think that he'll think I'm so stupid, you know?

When we spoke three months later, Yvette's position had shifted. "I want to tell him," she declared. I could see her processing the issue, and I wondered what had changed. What caused her to start contemplating disclosure when she resisted so firmly just a few months prior? We were conducting the interview in a small conference room at LifeForce, the AIDS service organization that runs her support groups in part on Ryan White CARE grant funds:

> I want to tell him . . . I want to because, some of the people that I've met here at LifeForce, I like, you know? I want to have a barbecue, and I don't know very many people in Chicago. And so when [my son] sees like a transvestite and a gay woman, he'll say, "What in the world has my mom been up to?" You know, because I'm kind of straight-laced and go to work and have never been a partying type person. And then to bring people home like this, he'll say, "Where in the world did you meet them?" And, my answer for everything, "Oh, they're part of my book club." Well, I'm tired of lying. I'm tired of lying about little things like that because there's nothing wrong with coming to a facility like this. I'm doing real good for myself and in my life. So I just want to let people know. Yeah, I want to tell my family, some family.

Yvette's connection to the HIV safety net contributed to her desire to share her HIV status with her son, her contemplation around disclosing her HIV status reminiscent of the considerations around "coming out" weighed by LGBTQ individuals. Her connection to LifeForce has helped her forge ties with a new community, and one can see how Yvette is not quite fluent yet in the language used to describe the non-normative genders and sexualities of her new friends. Her connection to the HIV safety net is, however, encouraging her to reflect on the consequences of her silence and to grapple with how guilt and respectability are closely tied to her sense of herself as a mother. Yvette regularly declined visits to friends' homes if they had children or if she knew that she might be invited to eat from the family's dishes, despite her knowledge of scientific evidence demonstrating that these are not routes of transmission. "I can breathe a sigh of relief when I come here to LifeForce," she explained. The diverse community of people living with HIV/AIDS meets regularly to share recommendations about the best doctors, hear the latest news about the disease, and process their feelings.

Yvette's transformative project therefore would not happen overnight. I once asked what she imagined it would be like to tell her son that she is living with HIV. She said that the tears would flow, "And I don't want them to flow. I want to be able to sit down and talk to him without crying, and I don't think I will be." I asked Yvette what would happen if she cried. "Why is that a bad thing?" I asked. "I don't know," Yvette stated, lowering her gaze. "It makes me look even weaker than having HIV already does."

Moving from *dying from* to *living with*—what psychologists might describe as the transition from cognitive or behavioral escape-avoidance to coping through social support—was not simple for the women I interviewed.[9] Despite significant scientific advances and increased access to treatment since the mid-1990s—including effective drug therapies and better monitoring of viral loads and T-cell counts—the mental toll of the diagnosis still held many women in a state of emotional death. The longer life expectancies for PLWHA led to the ironic consequence that women now had to determine how to cope with the stigma for the rest of their lives. Moreover, many had spent their entire lives swimming upstream, battling personal struggles, familial wounds, and societal hurdles that constantly undermined their self-worth. Given these challenges, how did women embrace these shifts in their thinking and find ways to channel them into concrete life transformations?

FRAMING INSTITUTIONS

> I came into drug treatment November 1, 1999. One of the
> ladies says, "Chicago Women's AIDS Project is doing a
> Thanksgiving event. Do you want to go?" And I went with
> her. And from that, I went to their support group. I did not
> speak for a year, I just sat there. And then finally, I opened
> up. And then I took facilitators' training, and the rest is
> history.
> —Trisha

A cognitive shift, an epiphany, or an awakening is not the only ingredient necessary to launch a successful life transformation. Given the formidable environmental and personal hurdles that women face, positive thinking, self-efficacy, and personal motivation would not be enough. They also would need a deep and wide well of support.

Framing institutions can create the space for, and support, women's embryonic cognitive shifts. They can help generate forward movement by sparking new modes of thought. At the same time, women can enter these institutions after experiencing their own shifts in mindset, as reappraising their situations can inspire them to seek assistance. Framing institutions offer new language, adaptive skills, and practical knowledge that shape how we interpret new life conditions and determine whether we ultimately see a new life situation as a platform for growth. Framing institutions operate as intermediaries between our individual perceptions and actions and environmental forces and systems, positioned between the personal response to a new circumstance and the larger set of privileges and disadvantages that we experience due to our social status. Inspired by famed sociologist Erving Goffman, who defined frames as "schemata of interpretation" based on which individuals understand and respond to events, I interpret both institutions and individuals as active, agentic, and dynamic as they construct social reality.[10]

As evidenced in table 1, Chicago study women exhibited a high level of connectedness to the HIV safety net overall, with 82 percent affirming during our interviews that they visited or talked with someone at an HIV-focused organization, agency, group, or healthcare provider at least once every one to three months. Twenty-five percent of women in the Chicago study were using only healthcare services, seeing an HIV physician or nurse periodically for check-ins and bloodwork screenings to monitor viral loads and T-cell counts. A little more than half (57 percent) described themselves as more heavily engaged, seeing both a healthcare provider and visiting an agency where they received some kind of social support such as case management. Notably, 18 percent of Chicago study women reported no connection to the HIV safety net, suggesting that they were not currently connected to available healthcare or social services. The next chapter will explore this phenomenon in greater detail. Racial differences were also noteworthy, with black women, and specifically poor black women, utilizing social services along with healthcare services in greater numbers than their white or Latina counterparts.

Churches, prisons, and other bureaucracies in women's lives also served as framing institutions, circulating information, frameworks, language, and in some cases resources that framed the medical and social implications

Table 1 Women's Connectedness to the HIV Safety Net

	All (n = 84)	Black (n = 35)	White (n = 21)	Latina (n = 22)	Biracial (n = 6)
Connected to the HIV safety net					
Medical care only	21 (25%)	2 (6%)	7 (33%)	10 (45%)	2 (33%)
Medical care and social support	48 (57%)	27 (77%)	9 (43%)	10 (45%)	2 (33%)
Not connected to the HIV safety net	15 (18%)	6 (17%)	5 (24%)	2 (9%)	2 (33%)

NOTE: Figures are based on interviews with 84 Chicago women who participated in the snapshot study (see appendix A for further details). Institutional connectedness was determined by a participant's answer to the following question: "Do you visit or talk with someone at an HIV-focused organization, agency, group, or healthcare provider?" If the participant indicated interaction with one of these entities at least once every one to three months, she was counted as connected.

of HIV for women. As such, framing institutions can be beneficial or undermining forces, depending on how they frame issues. For example, a church that delivers damaging and shaming messages about HIV/AIDS operates as a negative framing institution. On the other hand, a church that offers hopeful and affirming messages and perhaps runs an AIDS ministry is both a positive framing institution and a part of the HIV safety net. Positive framing institutions help women confront internalized stigma; negative framing institutions reinforce it.

Thus, the role institutions play as framers, and their power to help individuals negotiate what Goffman called a "spoiled identity," should not be overlooked.[11] A change in an individual's social status and self-definition often results when a stigmatizing experience occurs or a characteristic interferes with or disqualifies one from full participation in normative roles, statuses, or social relations in a community. WLWHA often sought to reclaim "safe" moral identities by looking for social meaning in their diagnoses and by seeking to strictly control the conditions under which they disclosed their HIV status to preserve their social status and relationships.[12] We often imagine this as an internal process residing solely within the individual, as women reflect on a spoiled identity and make decisions based on their beliefs about how others might perceive them.

As my visit to Trisha and Josie's HIV support group meeting suggests, however, framing institutions can play powerful roles in helping individuals interpret and address spoiled identities. They use rules, norms, language, frameworks, policies, and support to shape thinking and behavior in response to a spoiled identity. What distinguishes many AIDS service organizations is their capacity to simultaneously embrace, challenge, and revise societally determined spoiled identities in the service of transformation at the individual and community levels. As women engage with the HIV safety net and bring their whole selves—injuries and all—to these environments, I witnessed how they often saw their role as healing themselves and in turn using their strength to help heal other WLWHA.

Information and Frameworks

Women funneled multiple and sometimes conflicting messages about HIV into a set of organizing principles, generating an approach they could adopt to cope with the disease. The experience of being diagnosed, and the healthcare providers involved in this interaction, shaped how women began to conceptualize what it meant to have HIV. Particularly for those who were asymptomatic at diagnosis, the social meaning of HIV often took on greater significance than any physical signs of illness. For example, Rosario Salazar, a 37-year-old Latina, was diagnosed in 2007 during a prenatal visit. She was relieved when her daughter was born HIV negative, but the turmoil of her own diagnosis remained. What would life be like now? HIV support groups helped frame how Rosario would come to understand her diagnosis:

> When they told me I was HIV positive, I didn't know how to feel. I couldn't cry. I couldn't do anything. I just sat there and was like, "Oh, wow." Then I was in denial. I was real negative about it. . . . A year and a half later, with the support groups helping me out, I'm in acceptance of it. Everyone around me is pretty much in the same shoes. So seeing that everybody else was doing okay, I had to be accepting of my own situation. Everybody else is maintaining jobs, doing the things that they are doing in daily life to try to maintain their households and things of that nature. So I said, "Well you know, hey, I guess, it's not really all that bad. If they can do it, I can do it."

In other words, support groups offered Rosario a framework for understanding HIV/AIDS as a chronic and manageable illness rather than a death sentence. Other women who have walked similar paths, and who were out in the world taking care of themselves and their families, provided models for interpreting the diagnosis for those just starting their transformative projects. Framing institutions were therefore important messengers of ideas that stayed with women. Beverly explained:

> At the residential treatment center where I was diagnosed, I had a great support system. So they just started giving me stuff I was able to read, and I could take time out and spend like five or six months just focusing on me, my disease, and where I was gonna go from here. I needed to know what I was fighting, what I was dealing with, how I was gonna do this. I just wasn't gonna lay down and let it get me.

Continuing the tradition established through early AIDS activism, framing institutions also armed women with information they needed to fight the disease, effectively turning "the shocked diagnosed" into informed patients.[13] Yvette appreciated that her monthly "Dedicated to Living" coed support group enabled her to connect with long-term survivors and share information about issues like aging with HIV. They routinely hosted pharmacists and physicians for their question-and-answer sessions. Yvette also valued hearing about fellow members' experiences with medications in honest and sometimes brutal detail. "So it's very informative. . . . I mean, they'll just lay it on the line," she commented. "And not that their experiences would be like mine, but if a certain thing happened to me, I could say, 'Well, they said they felt this too.'"

Perhaps one of the most powerful aspects of many AIDS service organizations is, however, their engagement not only with the health and social implications of HIV disease, but also with the myriad injuries of inequality that women face. In the support group described at the beginning of this chapter, HIV was just one of many topics covered. Women were engaged in conversations about substance use, family dynamics, economic survival, spirituality, and many other topics. There was an undercurrent in the conversation that suggested the women were also seeking to address gaps in self-worth: a desire to learn from the incidents and experiences in their pasts that had chipped away at their self-esteem. Women found these venues of support so attractive in part because of the opportunity for self-definition and self-expression: no bureaucrats were imposing directives from the top down. Rather, the women were assisting each other, often with the support of trained professionals who staff the safety net.

In this sense, positive framing institutions become sites where women who grapple with multiple -isms (racism, sexism, classism, etc.) turn their spoiled identities on their heads. Sitting around the support group circles, doing their first speaking engagements, and volunteering to join Ryan White planning councils gave women opportunities to convert their histories of trauma, addiction, and violence into experiential knowledge and to vocalize those experiences constructively. This knowledge becomes a form of social and cultural capital, a hard-won credential that parallels the formalized training of HIV researchers, clinicians, and policy experts, who are also powerful voices in the epidemic.[14] Even for women who do not have futures in the world of HIV/AIDS activism or power brokering, their experiential knowledge and newfound voices could be used closer to home as they engaged with friends and family members and, perhaps more importantly, internalized new perceptions about their lives.

Language

Framing institutions also generate a shared language among participants and reinforce social norms that shape discourse. In the support group co-led by Trisha and Josie, language was a key community-building mechanism for the women involved. Betina opened the meeting with a set of directives I would hear repeatedly in support groups: "Don't interrupt, and let everyone have their say. Don't break confidentiality. No one is better than anyone else." This created a space for all the women's voices to be heard.

The imprint of addiction recovery programs in the language shared by women utilizing services in the HIV safety net is unmistakable. Through regular support groups, HIV information sessions, and frequent contact with others who had drug addictions *and* were HIV positive, this lexicon helped women name, frame, and address significant events in their lives. They discussed balancing a sense of personal agency with spiritual surrender, acknowledging past mistakes, and learning to live healthier lives, often describing HIV and drug addiction interchangeably. They frequently invoked God and spirituality as a source of strength. In their dialogue, the women alternated between confession and forgiveness, talking openly about their pasts and candidly revealing their ongoing struggles to forgive themselves.

In our interviews, Beverly frequently used the phrase "So I just had to get some acceptance for it" when describing a frustrating situation in her life. "Living life on life's terms" was another frequently heard phrase. Moreover, the women described needing to "avoid people, places, and things" that threatened their progress, applying the language of drug avoidance to managing HIV and their post-diagnosis lives. As we saw with Trisha and Josie's support group, the women rehearsed redemption scripts, giving themselves credit for changes they were making but also identifying patterns of thought and behavior that failed to serve them.[15] Janine, a case manager at a community health center in Chicago, described this phenomenon: "The women, they really share a lot. How they are feeling, even if they are depressed; happy, if they're doing good; they'll let you know. I think the older they're getting, they're looking at things a little different than before. And that's a good thing. They realize if they could have done things differently, they would. . . . They really talk to you a lot about life."

Women did not simply learn the lexicon of HIV/AIDS; they helped to shape it. Since the beginning of the AIDS movement, activists have been mindful of the power of naming as a way to shift the discourse. I once sat in a research meeting with national activists and advocates who talked about the importance of the term *women living with HIV/AIDS*. The term *HIV-positive women*, some in the room argued, put the disease first in how they would be named and framed. They were women first, they reminded us, who happened to be living with HIV/AIDS. It was a part of who they were, but it wasn't all of who they were, or even the first thing that they saw within themselves. Women living with HIV/AIDS (or WLWHA) is certainly a more cumbersome term, but this example gets at the very heart of who the women are and how they want to be understood. Framing institutions are important sites where this is established.

The women circulated another discursive style in groups and in our interviews: rhetoric extolling the power of the individual. Hearing this so often in interviews and support group meetings encouraged me to reflect on the difference between *personal responsibility* and *agency,* terms that are bandied about in political discourse, self-help circles, and other venues. In political discourse on both HIV/AIDS and poverty, my two areas of research specialization, a rhetoric of personal responsibility is often applied to encourage certain behaviors and to justify punitive action should individuals fail to adopt them. For low-income women the message is clear: get off public assistance, go to work, and stop having children you cannot afford. Those engaging in behaviors understood to be at higher risk for HIV transmission also hear clear messages: engage in "normal" sexual activity (e.g., heterosexual, monogamous, marital) and do not use drugs. These constitute expected, "correct," and normative behaviors that one should adopt, and the implication is that anyone who fails to follow these directives may be deemed undeserving of assistance. The language of personal responsibility draws a moral line in the sand. But the rhetoric also assumes that each of us enjoys the same (or at least similar) options and opportunities for meeting our personal responsibilities; there is rarely a focused discussion of the structural or environmental factors that may heavily restrict one's options, movement, and behaviors. The discourse also presupposes that we all agree on the prescribed rules of human behavior. These behaviors are often presented as obligations, and when one fails to conform, the societal response can be swift and punitive.

Personal agency, on the other hand, might be thought of as individual power coming from within. It represents the deliberate and strategic deployment and leveraging of available options, leading to choices and behaviors that can fall inside or outside the lines of normative behavior.[16] Agency places individual action within an environmental context, and it can be highly restricted for those lacking resources and limited in power.

Transformative agency fuels the transformative project and represents a person's distinct and deliberate tactics for advancing from *what was* to *what can be*. Here I am relying on a definition of agency posed by sociologists Mustafa Emirbayer and Ann Mische in which they reconceptualize human agency as "a temporally embedded process of social engagement, informed by the past . . . but also oriented toward the future (as a capacity to imagine alternative possibilities) and toward the present (as a capacity to contextualize past habits and future projects within the contingencies of the moment)."[17] In other words, agency represents an individual's outlooks, decision-making capabilities, and experiential knowledge at work in the service of some kind of personal and perhaps even societal process, shaped by the past and with an eye toward the future. Through that process a person can progress from instability to stability, from silence to voice, from stigma to esteem. Transformative agency is therefore the moment-by-moment, day-by-day tool that women apply in building successful transformative projects over time. It is more dynamic than resilience or coping. To leverage agency in a transformative project is to use one's power, however limited, to create dramatic and positive change while confronting trauma, stigma, violence, and disenfranchisement, potentially shaping an individual's personal and even her community's well-being.

For many years, WLWHA were given "death sentences" upon diagnosis, and many around the world live in highly disadvantaged contexts that also reflect a kind of economic, physical, and social "death."[18] Under these conditions, achieving and sustaining transformation poses a monumental challenge and represents a significant accomplishment. Transformative agency enables an individual to acknowledge and embrace her own accountability in this process while battling stigma. Self-awareness lies at the heart of transformative agency, something arguably required to initiate changes that stick. As I observed women in their transformative projects, there seemed to be a fine line between shame and accountability. The HIV safety net helped by creating forums in which women could confront shame while simultaneously engaging in the soul searching involved in identifying their own agency and accountability regarding events that may have transpired. But unlike the rhetoric of personal responsibility, agency in general, and transformative agency specifically, carry the potential to generate protest and demands for political change.

Resources, Services, and Networks

The vast majority of Chicago study women have private or publicly subsidized health insurance that covers their HIV medications and medical treatments; most of them therefore reported minimal healthcare costs directly related to HIV. Living in a large city with a historically strong AIDS advocacy community, the women also had options for their healthcare needs. They could access care in Chicago's flagship hospital for PLWHA (known as the CORE Center), or they could visit one of the city's university teaching hospitals with major infectious disease clinics. They could locate their physicians at community health centers, or they could access care within various AIDS nonprofits across the city that housed clinical and social services under the same roof. One hospital even hosted a job fair and offered training to work for the census, expanding the reach of the safety net even further. As Beverly explained, when Ryan White HIV/AIDS program funds were at their most generous, some women were even able to locate the occasional provider who introduced them to alternative therapeutic services:

> So once I started educating myself, I started seeking out services. Then I ended up in a place called the Coach House. And the Coach House was a facility for alternative therapy and mental health for people living with HIV on the South Side. They provided alternative therapies, low-cost acupuncture, and massage. And at the time they had a juice bar. And then they had support groups, and they just had a lot of stuff. So I started going there for about a year.

HIV/AIDS carries a variety of other financial implications, however, largely tied to how women pursue resources for daily survival and address the disclosure question in the process. Low-income women who connect with the HIV safety net can discover that their economic situations actually stabilize following an HIV diagnosis.[19] They are often so disadvantaged prior to diagnosis that the institutional assistance for which they now qualify can offer increased financial stability. Although by the time I was conducting my research the eligibility requirements for Social Security disability assistance had tightened for people with AIDS, many women nevertheless qualified due to co-occurring health challenges. They relied on the HIV safety net's case managers and advocates to help them navigate this labyrinth of bureaucratic eligibility to gain access to Supplemental Security Income (SSI), Social Security Disability Insurance (SSDI), and other benefits.

The nonprofit and public institutions that women frequented for HIV support groups and social and healthcare services also often offered free subway and bus passes, stipends for facilitating support groups, and in some cases affordable housing and access to employment training opportunities. Chicago also has a food pantry dedicated to PLWHA that provides nutrition counseling and education. Trisha was ineligible for disability assistance, Medicaid, or Medicare because she is not a US citizen. However, she received $150 per month for chairing the local HIV Ryan White planning council and serving as the council's liaison to the HIV Prevention Planning Group, a network of AIDS service providers who gather monthly to share information. She also collected $35 stipends every other month for her work on the community advisory boards of two other AIDS organizations. Accepting a speaking engagement once a month or so added another $200 to her income. At one point, Trisha worked as a house monitor in a home for formerly incarcerated men run by another woman living with HIV, until they ran out of funding and Trisha no longer received the $500 monthly compensation. These small stipends added up and provided Trisha with dollars in her pocket and experience that she could add to her résumé: "I've done enough illegal in my lifetime. I'm changed, and I don't want to go back to that place. So I'm very grateful for whatever stipends I get . . . it's much more peaceful, and I'm not stressed." Trisha's HIV medications were subsidized through the ADAP, and she received medical care and saw a therapist for four and a half years at the Core Center. Her viral load was undetectable and had been for years.

From the epidemic's earliest years, the AIDS community prioritized housing as a key lever in health management. Scholars have extensively documented the detrimental impact of housing instability on health outcomes (and vice versa).[20] One of the most robust studies of housing among PLWHA demonstrated significant reductions in emergency room utilization and improvements in self-reported physical and mental health among the stably housed, including reduced depression and perceived stress. Rental assistance provided by the Housing Opportunities for People with AIDS (HOPWA) program has been found, in some cases, to improve the viral loads of PLWHA. David Holtgrave, a former CDC official who has been involved with the National AIDS Housing Coalition (helping to organize NAHC's Research Summit series) since the early 2000s, explained, "I think early on, it wasn't always understood by federal appropriators that housing is an HIV-related intervention or service. It was: 'Isn't that separate? How is this related?' I think the research has gotten stronger and stronger and bigger and bigger over time, demonstrating its importance." Added Ingrid Floyd, executive director of Iris House, a

New York AIDS organization that has been around for a quarter of a century, "Housing is a form of HIV treatment: if you are securely, safely, and stably housed, we know that you are likely to have better treatment outcomes."

Housing also served as a linchpin for the transformation Chicago study women created as they moved from *dying from* to *living with*. Jada, a black 43-year-old mother of two, was diagnosed with HIV in 1995. As she explained, housing through the HIV safety net has provided stability:

> Before the job I have now, I worked in a shelter for homeless women and children as a cook supervisor. That's how I found out about the place I'm living now. I live in a low-income housing development for single women with children living with HIV or AIDS. And it's a very, very nice building. Rent goes according to your income. When your children get 20, 25, you don't have to kick them out. They can also stay there with you. It has a computer room. It offers tutoring for the children, play time, laundry facility in the building, clean building, nice tenants. So . . . it's good. It's good for me. I waited two and a half years to get that apartment. So I'm in there and I'll be there. Since that's permanent housing, I'm okay.

The increased access to resources that Jada describes is consistent with scholarship that paradoxically finds improved quality of life post-diagnosis among many severely low-income PLWHA living in areas with robust AIDS services, due to their increased access to state and nonprofit resources.[21] "The most economically disenfranchised segments of society," Johanna Crane and colleagues write, "may be placed in a difficult position of experiencing AIDS both as a threat and as a means of financial survival."[22] I saw this time and again, starting with Dawn, as a modicum of economic assistance offered through the HIV safety net facilitated their movement from instability to stability and into transformative projects. Yet, rather than a relationship of dependency, I observed how the dynamic between women and the HIV safety net featured *inter*dependency. Women were often asked to contribute by leading or serving: encouraging fellow participants in support groups or even leading the meetings, participating in public education and advocacy work, or serving as peer support for the newly diagnosed.

Further, some women parlayed their connection to the safety net into jobs beyond the AIDS community. But Ingrid Floyd at Iris House emphasized that the goal was not simply employment but economic self-sufficiency:

We have a client who just finished culinary school, who's going to get a job. So, if you're ready to go back to work, we definitely help, but we work with you on how to do it. What's the best way, so that you get the training and make sure that you're making more than minimum wage? Do they offer health insurance? Will your health benefits such as Medicaid be impacted? We help people figure it out and weigh it out. We definitely are supportive of people who want to return to the workforce.

In addition to the changes in their economic survival strategies, for many women, the transition from *dying from* to *living with* also required changing their social networks. This can be a fraught transition as women leave behind relationships that were important despite the fact that they may have undermined women's physical and mental health. For example, we cannot overlook the fact that personally destructive drug worlds, like most other networks, nevertheless offered women a sense of community. Trisha expressed a sentiment that Dawn, Beverly, and many other women echoed: "The only friends I had were other prostitutes. And drug people. There were some drug dealers that looked out for me. And I miss them in a certain way, they have a little place in my heart. But that's—they got to stay right there. I have fond memories of them, but it can't go past that. No, I don't have anybody I keep in touch with." Trisha went on to describe her new network: "My—it's like a community, the AIDS community, people living with AIDS. We kind of all know each other, and there's a bond."

Framing institutions within the HIV safety net therefore introduced women to strong and durable ties as well as what sociologist Matt Desmond has termed "disposable ties," or the short-term relationships one forms with strangers, which prove instrumental for everyday survival.[23] Rosario lived in Phoenix House, an apartment building on Chicago's South Side housing 25 families affected by HIV/AIDS. The building's mandatory support groups "give me insights," and the tenant council meetings inspired Rosario to assume a leadership role. Soon, her new neighbors were helping each other. "The last time that I've been to a food pantry," Rosario commented, "is probably a year ago. With the friends that I have in the building, [we always help each other out]. If I needed some food, they'll say 'Okay, here you can take some of this food I have, and you just accommodate me later.'"

Paying rent of only $96 a month at Phoenix House, Rosario's newfound stability was a far cry from her previous experiences, in which she and a friend had unknowingly moved into an apartment building that was in foreclosure. She stayed for several months after a representative from the bank told her to vacate, until her things were removed because she was considered a squatter.[24] Rosario sent her son to live with his father and her daughter to live with her mother. Instead of moving back into her mother's cramped apartment, Rosario bounced around the apartments of various friends until her case manager found a spot for her in Phoenix House. Not only did this housing assistance alleviate survival stress, it also provided Rosario with a built-in support system.

A SYSTEM FOR ALL? FRAMING INSTITUTIONS AND DISPATCHES FROM THE MARGINS

Not all Chicago study women had close connections to framing institutions or the HIV safety net. The critique that the HIV services are not sufficiently attentive to the needs of women lingers. "We women kind of feel like stepchildren at LifeForce," Yvette commented. "Everybody is very nice to us, but a lot of stuff seems to be geared toward gay men. We once thought about boycotting the group."

First-generation Latina immigrants struggled to connect to the HIV safety net, largely because of structural barriers related to poverty and citizenship status. Because of their limited access to government resources, they must work even when ill. When asked why she does not participate in services beyond meeting with her social worker, Yaritza, a 53-year-old Ecuadorian immigrant, explained, "No, I only talk to [my social worker]. I don't have time because of work. It takes three hours to go to work in the morning, and then I take the bus and go to the other job. And the return is three more hours, and my day is already over." While these women have access to medical services, they do not enjoy the same kind of access to other pieces of the safety net, potentially stymieing their transformative projects. Long-term investments in their emotional and social growth, cultivated through support group meetings, visits to therapists, and attendance at events hosted by various AIDS organizations, are not possible. These women have to focus on their basic survival every day.

In addition to facing structural constraints, some immigrant women also contended with social dynamics and cultural scripts rooted in both the sending and receiving locations that position silence and isolation as survival strategies.[25] Chicago study women from Mexico, Ecuador, El Salvador, and Guatemala tended to move to the United States later in life, migrated with their husbands, and told almost no one about their HIV status. A number of them had histories of abusive relationships and had isolated themselves, or had husbands who isolated them, from social ties. Their sense of shame was so pronounced that they described disclosure of their HIV status to family and friends as impossible. They shouldered the burden of living with HIV on their own, the social death suffocating them like a fog. Yaritza elaborates on this sentiment: "I don't want to give [my family] those worries about my health, about my life. It's preferable that I face my life alone." With the large number of immigrants among them, this might explain why Latinas in the study overall were among the most weakly attached to AIDS services and largely did not experience dramatic transformative projects at the same rate as other women in the Chicago study.

Notably, we met some women—approximately 21 percent of them, based on our interviews—who seemed to still be "in the struggle" or "out there," to borrow Trisha's term, having yet to experience the cognitive shift that might encourage them to believe that they can move successfully from *dying from* to *living with*. Their stories mirror the difficult experiences of the women I described in chapter 1, but there were no turning points or cognitive reappraisals evident in what they shared. Unaddressed histories of trauma, serious co-occurring illnesses, ongoing substance use problems, and stymied personal motivation frequently interfered with the ability to make that shift or to effectively leverage framing institutions.

Some women described a feeling of disconnection from other women in the HIV safety net as their reason for not engaging deeply. They utilized healthcare services but had no desire to attend the support groups or activist events. Rather than developing a sense of community, they felt isolated because of perceived dissimilarities between themselves and other women.

After escaping her boyfriend Marcus's home, 19-year-old Keisha, whom we met in chapter 1, bounced from shelter to shelter: three months in one designated for young adults, another three in a shelter for PLWHA, and finally two months in a shelter for pregnant girls. Several stigmatizing situations weighed on her—a fresh breakup from an abusive relationship, her HIV status, homelessness, and a teenage pregnancy. In each new environment, Keisha negotiated those events and conditions. What would she disclose? To whom and under what circumstances? She found her first stop, Safe Space Shelter, to be unwelcoming because of her HIV status: "I was pretty low-key with my status. No one knew until one of my roommates saw one of my medications, Combivir, which is Magic Johnson's medicine. And she started going around the shelter saying, 'Well, that's the medicine that Magic Johnson takes . . . '" Her relationships with the other residents deteriorated from there. They made comments about her having HIV and incorrectly speculated that they could become "infected" from sharing a bathroom or food with her. "In order for me to just keep my calm, I moved out," Keisha explained, the violent incident from high school still fresh. "And that's when I went to Stepping Stone."

At the Stepping Stone residential facility, Keisha found a community of PLWHA, but they didn't have much else in common with her. The residents were older and many had histories of addiction. The facility also lacked staff with experience working with pregnant WLWHA, and she was placed on the fifth floor without an elevator in the building. From there, Keisha moved to Ashley's Place, a six-unit building for young pregnant women. Sharing a two-bedroom apartment with another resident gave her much-needed privacy and supported her needs as a pregnant woman. But without any other residents living with HIV that she knew of, she felt isolated again. As many of the girls living in Ashley's Place were former residents of the Safe Space Shelter, her HIV status circulated quickly. But this time, it didn't become a topic of tension. "They saw how I reacted when it first came out at Safe Space," Keisha commented. "They knew just to leave it alone."

For Keisha, coming to terms with her HIV status was a work in progress for most of the decade during which I followed her, and I believe that this was due in part to her early (and formative) negative experiences with institutions such as high school and the shelters in which she felt stigmatized and isolated. Her age and lack of drug history prevented her from fully fitting into the wing of the HIV safety net populated mostly by women who were in their twenties during the crack epidemic of the 1980s and 1990s. We discussed this at length when I asked if she found HIV support groups helpful:

> Not really, because it wasn't my age group. I couldn't say to the older women, "Girl, you right!" you know? I can't do it. . . . If I can be in a room full of teenagers, and they're all talking about being HIV positive, now that's what I would like. 'Cause maybe then I can say, "That was the same way I got it." I can't sit here and talk to a 40-year-old, 'cause I can't relate to that. So that's why I don't go. And most of them are all substance abuse, drugs and all that. I don't like that. . . . I really don't like being around people who've been on drugs.

But Keisha's isolation from a network of WLWHA sometimes caught up with her. While I was driving to work one day, Keisha called me from the hospital, sobbing. She had just given birth, and the reality that she was now a single mother living with HIV, along with the postpartum hormonal roller coaster, was settling in. Her mother was back in her life, but she would be working all day and could offer no help with the baby or to Keisha as she healed from a C-section. Keisha's mother called a cousin to see if her daughter and the baby could stay with them during the day, but the cousin refused, commenting that she worried about Keisha sleeping in a bed where the woman's son would sleep later. "She's afraid I'm going to bleed in the bed or something!" Keisha sobbed.

I visited Keisha in the hospital within hours of the call. Walking through the maternity unit, the doors of many of the rooms were open to reveal families visiting new parents and tiny newborns. I wondered who had come to visit Keisha and was confronted with her sense of isolation. What should have been a happy occasion was complicated because some of her family members saw her as contaminated and hazardous.

Keisha was in her hospital bed when I arrived, an hours-old baby Jordan lying snugly on her chest. She didn't seem at all like the person with whom I had spoken earlier. Chipper and relaxed, she stated that Jordan "needs to wake up soon so that I can feed him." I commented that she seemed to be doing better and she agreed. "I'm going home day after tomorrow, the doctor said I could. I'll be fine," she shrugged. The air of control that

Keisha presented during our first interview was back: she displayed not a wrinkle of fear. She picked over her dinner of baked chicken, salad, and Jell-O, commenting on how bad the food was. "I'm cool," she stated, "My mother will help. I'll be fine . . . I've even already learned how to give him his medicine." Keisha would have to give Jordan regular doses of medication to increase his chances of remaining HIV negative.

As I followed her I realized that Keisha resisted aligning too closely with the HIV safety net not simply because of age differences and her lack of connection to the dominant subculture within it. She was also struggling with the extent to which she wanted to be defined by her HIV status as a young adult: "I really support everybody like me. It's just . . . I don't want to put myself in that whole category as a 'positive' woman, female, African American. You know, I feel that I just don't want to be stigmatized [even more]. I feel that I'm already stigmatized like that." As a network of support, the HIV safety net appears to strongly value, and to some extent, expects that one view HIV as an important and accepted part of one's identity. However, Keisha's comment reminds us that the notion that a health condition—and a stigmatized one at that—must become a central aspect of one's identity is not a foregone conclusion.

As a result, Keisha's transformation from *dying from* to *living with* was much more incremental than those of many other women whom I followed. Rather than developing long-term friendships with other WLWHA, she relied on boyfriends and friends for support, many of whom moved in and out of her life and were not particularly well educated about HIV. She disclosed her status to a fast-food restaurant coworker with whom she bonded, who quickly spread the news. Keisha was then fired for coming to blows with someone at the job who made negative comments about her HIV status, an incident sadly reminiscent of her high school days.

Keisha's transformation was therefore marked less by a definitive turning point and more by a series of exchanges and incidents that moved her slowly along the coping trajectory: a case manager who provided a housing voucher and helped her find an apartment when she really needed it, the advice of her doctor who successfully guided Keisha to help her prevent Jordan from carrying HIV, and casual conversations with other WLWHA in clinic waiting rooms. In those moments, Keisha was able to gather important information that often moved her in the right direction, but without forging any long-term ties or adopting a strong identity as a WLWHA.

Are institutional connections a necessary condition for transformation? Women with substantial family support, relatively stable economic situations, and no histories of drug addiction were by far the most effectively equipped to move from *dying from* to *living with* without strong institutional ties. Maria is a 35-year-old Puerto Rican woman whose first love died of AIDS-related complications after a long battle with drug addiction. She utilizes the HIV safety net only for healthcare services. Her mother and long-term boyfriend, both of whom know her status, provide the emotional and financial support that she requires to cope with HIV and other challenges in her life: "I never did the support groups, because my doctor asked me if I would want to go, but I thought, no need to. Because if I felt like I wanted to talk to somebody, I could talk to my mom or my boyfriend about it. There was always somebody that I could let my fears out to, or if I just felt like talking about it, I can talk to them about it."

Relying heavily on very small networks of family and friends to cope with HIV and other injuries of inequality carries some risks. These individuals may not be able to offer the emotional resources or the most up-to-date knowledge about the illness, despite their best intentions. They may offer advice that is inappropriate, generic, or unrealistic because of their lack of experience. Intimate network members may be grappling with their own feelings about a loved one's HIV-positive status and the disruption it has created. "Invested supporters," sociologist Peggy Thoits explains, "therefore may minimize the threatening aspects of the problem, insist on maintaining a positive outlook, or pressure the person to recover or problem solve before he or she is ready."[26] This suggests that while Maria's strategy is effective, it has certain disadvantages.

The Significance of Class in the HIV Safety Net

Conventional wisdom might predict that middle-class women who are HIV positive reap even greater benefits from interacting with the HIV safety net than low-income women because of their ability to deploy cultural capital to advocate for themselves, as well as the larger quantity and quality of personal economic and social resources that they can combine with the institutional resources they can procure.[27] I observed nevertheless that middle-class women of all racial backgrounds engage with the HIV safety net very differently from their lower-income counterparts, apparently driven in part by the disparate economic implications of HIV for women as well as the social meaning of engaging with the AIDS community.

An HIV diagnosis appeared to heighten the sense of financial vulnerability for middle-income women while lowering this sense for low-income women who engaged with the HIV safety net. As discussed earlier, low-income women who accessed the safety net could often obtain healthcare services and in some cases economic assistance and housing services. In the pre-Obamacare era of data collection, middle-class women spoke at length about the potential of HIV to cause downward mobility should they lose their jobs or health insurance. HIV, after all, would be considered a preexisting condition that could make it difficult to secure replacement insurance. Unlike low-income respondents who looked to the HIV safety net for economic help, middle-class respondents believed that these organizations were unlikely to protect them from the financial risks associated with HIV. Barb, a 62-year-old white woman, was diagnosed in 1984. Her story is a cautionary tale that reflects a serious concern shared by many of the middle-class women I interviewed:

> I worked part-time while I raised four kids. Got a master's [degree] in biochemistry before I started regularly getting sick. I had a husband who made good money, worked for an insurance company, years of promotions, years of raises. Six months after I tested HIV positive, he got terminated. Our lawyer said it would be hard to prove it was my status. We lost our house. We had to get divorced so he could become employable again. He had been blacklisted until we got divorced, so I could not be on his health insurance at work. . . . He died of a heart attack. I think it was the stress. And then I went on Social Security—$674 a month.

Barb's story is unique among the women in our sample, as what she experienced is far less likely in this era of employment protections for PLWHA. HIV discrimination still exists, though, and the prospect of such an occurrence loomed large in the minds of middle-class respondents. Katy, a white 35-year-old married mother of one, described this sense of economic vulnerability. Diagnosed in 2010 while pregnant, Katy was sure that her job making $120,000 a year would be at risk should her status become known in the workplace: "I report directly to the president of my company. And I know how my company works. There is a law against letting someone go for HIV, but there are 15 ways to let someone go without saying it. I am the main provider for my family. We just had a baby. What would I do?"

For Katy, protecting her job means living in silence about her health status. She shared this attitude with the vast majority of the middle-class Chicago study women, fewer of whom reported revealing their HIV status than their lower-income counterparts. Katy described her reluctance to connect to the HIV safety net: "My doctor told me about a program pairing women with HIV together and also support group lunches hosted at the hospital. I don't need to tell anybody. I've never gotten myself there." Middle-class women often went to great lengths to hide their HIV status, failing to see how AIDS service organizations could help them, financially or otherwise. Katy therefore worked long hours, hiding the fatigue and digestive irritation that were side effects of her HIV medications. Because she had no social ties to the AIDS community, Katy did not operate in a network of people who might have suggested protective strategies to help her cope.

Like their wealthier counterparts, low-income women expressed fear of the stigma that could result from disclosing their HIV status. They often found that their economic survival *depended*, however, on disclosing to a broad array of service providers and other PLWHA. Privacy became a luxury that most impoverished women with HIV could not afford, and disclosure could generate institutional ties that proved very beneficial for economic stability. Poor WLWHA with few institutional ties or who chose not to utilize existing ties to the HIV safety net found themselves highly vulnerable economically.

Furthermore, to middle-class women, affiliations with the HIV safety net offered no status-enhancing effects of the sort that low-income women like Trisha and Josie experienced. Quite the opposite prevailed: WLWHA who were not viewed as "highly marginalized" by societal standards sometimes felt especially threatened and demoralized when participating in these networks. Deflecting stigma and reconstructing one's sense of self were critical for all WLWHA; such needs appeared to be intensified for those who, prior to diagnosis, lived with relatively fewer stigmatizing social characteristics. When HIV-positive status was at the center of an institutional relationship, these women had to negotiate whether and with whom they would associate and define their identities.

For example, Barb struggled as a social service client, which traditionally involves displaying compliance to appear "deserving" of services.[28] In their study of welfare administration in the United Kingdom, researchers found that front-line workers employ a pervasive moral categorization based on clients' perceived body language, demeanor, interactional style, expressions of gratitude, and capacity for aggression.[29] The economically disadvantaged, therefore, often learn how to present themselves to caseworkers and other front-line service providers. Barb's privileged status as a white woman who was once firmly ensconced in the middle class collided with her status as an HIV-positive client. The new reliance on the HIV safety net also required Barb to forfeit some of her privacy if she was to receive economic assistance:

> One of the major shocks to the system for anybody who comes from a middle-class or upper-middle-class background is that [service providers] are going to feel free to ask you these questions and think nothing of it, and more than one person. Because nobody with HIV, once you've had it for a while, has only one case manager. So you have to repeat the same soul-crushing, degrading stories to multiple people. You have no privacy, your whole life—you have to discuss the most private and intimate parts of your life with someone who's basically a stranger, to get services. You're no longer seen as a human being, "You're our client." Client does not equal human.

This harkens back to a point made earlier that for many women, having HIV represented a deep moral failing and demoralizing loss of respectability. For the middle-class women, few of whom have lifelong histories of trauma, an HIV diagnosis was unlike anything they had ever suffered. Meeting with me at the US Conference on HIV/AIDS in 2017, Dr. Bambi Gaddist described seeing this dynamic play out time and time again in her HIV prevention work with black women in South Carolina:

> Black women from higher socioeconomic backgrounds are also at risk for HIV, but we think only certain kinds of women are at risk. It's challenging to penetrate our walls of denial. It has been one of my biggest challenges,

when we're out, trying to educate and bridge barriers in thought: "I'm not the woman you're talking to, I'm not at risk." That based on my social class, my position, my man is not the man you're talking about. . . . We find it easier to focus on black women of lower socioeconomic status as the voice of women with HIV. They're the easiest to approach. But they're also women who are more likely to listen because they're struggling with other "realities" and they know it. However, we can never address the HIV epidemic in black communities until black women of social and economic means embrace this health disparity as they have breast cancer. Until then, it's always easier for people to target our attention on women and girls we want to believe need more help than we do.

I found the social distancing between middle- and lower-income women that Dr. Gaddist described widespread among the Chicago study women as well. Yvette was one of the few professional women who regularly participated in HIV support groups, although she noted that she had yet to find her perfect fit. The groups comprised mostly of gay men were helpful to her as they covered such topics as medically managing HIV and dealing with stigma. But she felt isolated because of her unique experiences with these issues as a black woman. When she started gravitating toward the women's groups, she faced another challenge. Because so many WLWHA are also poor or working class and perhaps former participants in the sexualized drug economy, the topics of conversation within these settings often involved access to resources and coping with both past and fresh traumas. The struggle of association for Yvette and women like her was in part that these organizational ties not only defined them as HIV positive but also placed them in the same space as women they perceived as worlds apart from themselves. Yvette explained what it was like for her to attend the women's group at LifeForce: "When I went into these meetings, they were drug-addicted women . . . I just didn't have anything in common with them. . . . Like I want to discuss, I don't know, some racist things that may go on at work, or a book I am reading . . . [it's] not that they cannot identify with it. But I don't know . . . our ideas . . . just don't click. They just don't."

As a government worker making $87,000 a year in 2007, Yvette had long struggled to reconcile her economic privilege with her HIV status. Her desire to discuss events at work that impeded her climb up the ladder, or the latest cultural artifacts of middle-class status, were largely sidelined by her group-mates' more pressing concerns. Furthermore, as Yvette revealed, the experience for some women linked them to a societal status and struggle that they may have fought to escape as black women who were newly minted members of the middle class. Yvette thought that this was why women who shared her socioeconomic status simply opted out:

> I think it's such a scary thought to be identified, especially if your life is going pretty well and you've pulled yourself up by your bootstraps as I have. And to be identified as, I don't know, a bad person or an irresponsible woman and . . . I don't know. I just think that it's so terrifying to be identified that people just stay away [from AIDS service organizations]. . . . As a matter of fact, I thought that if I run into one of my colleagues from work or somebody like that when I'm walking out of LifeForce, I would say, "Oh I volunteer here, I'm not going here, I volunteer here."

As a result, most of the middle-class women I talked with chose to forgo the institutional benefits offered by the HIV safety net rather than adapt to their norms. The social costs were too great, they reasoned, as these ties threatened the social status they were struggling to retain, foregrounded the stigma and shame that they felt, and sometimes required them to give more advice and support than they received. These women did not require the basic economic resources supplied by these organizations, and the social incentives were minimal. Thus most middle-class women in the Chicago study reported having very few ties to people or organizations associated with HIV and often described a sense of isolation.

While their deep investments in their privacy constricted movement through the HIV safety net, there were two noteworthy exceptions. First, middle-class women were much more likely to engage with AIDS service organizations as professionals than as clients, working as activists, advocates, or case managers. When they engaged in this work, they often had a much more complex and nuanced view of women whose lives were very different from their own but who shared their diagnosis. For example, as a middle-class white woman, treatment advocate Dawn Averitt was reluctant to disclose that she likely contracted HIV through a sexual assault that took place while traveling abroad in college:

For years there was this idea--and it still exists--that there are "victims." There are those that don't deserve this, and then there's everybody else. And for me, the discovery of the HIV community and the building of that family was the key to my survival. So I didn't want anything that distanced me from that. I didn't want to be differentiated in any way. And I felt really strongly, even from the very earliest days, [that] I never met anyone who deserved this. And so I couldn't bear the distinction.

Rather than allow their differences to divide them and reinforce hierarchies, middle-class women who worked in the AIDS community, schooled by activists and advocates who brought a decidedly intersectional politics to the task of AIDS organizing, tended to push against that. Many of the female activists of color were quite persuasive in arguing that clinging to those kinds of power hierarchies would be detrimental to WLWHA and their cause. Pat Nalls of the Women's Collective had this to say:

I was naïve about so many issues, and I quickly realized that if I had to live in some of the situations, the childhood trauma that a lot of the women . . . have lived through, shoot, it might be easier to stick a needle in my arm to forget about all that had happened in life. So I learned a lot from just sitting in those groups and hearing all of our experiences and what led us to where we end up. So, I guess I feel like I learned a lot. I became even more involved in gender issues. I learned a lot more about what makes people do what they do. You know, I think it's very easy for many of us to say, "Oh, well, why can't she just stop doing that?"

Black WLWHA working in the AIDS community also understood the value of their role as "middlewomen," to borrow a term from sociologist Mary Pattillo, professionally positioned between white-dominated power structures and black communities.[30] Linda Scruggs, who now co-owns a successful health consulting firm, previously worked as a liaison between patients and providers at John Hopkins hospital:

Being a community person [is important]. You're close enough to the community to be able to translate what the lady is saying, and what the provider or clinicians are thinking, to help it make sense to both parties. So I spent the first part of my career being that middle person. I wasn't a clinician, but neither was I an underserved woman. I don't come from the slums of DC, or Mississippi, or anything like that. So. . . I was a great gap person to figure out both spaces, and that leadership [experience], that's what led me into working with, and speaking on behalf of, other women. I, like many women, had been given a lousy opportunity to step forward.

Middle-class WLWHA who worked within the safety net were also able to use their cultural capital to expand the definition of what constituted AIDS care. In their roles, they could provide the kinds of experiences that might spark transformative projects. Linda would borrow the hospital van and use her own money to pay for the gas to take women from Baltimore to Washington:

> What I found was, the women I was working with had something unique to offer me, and I had something unique to offer them. What I had to offer women was a vision that they had not been afforded. I was able to say to women, "Come on, get in my car. Let's go see some other stuff." Because many women, when we look at living in the inner city or a rural community, they stay right there. And suddenly what I found was when I took someone to east Baltimore from west Baltimore, they didn't know they had that. Some providers at the hospital saw me doing something that nobody had done. I was taking these women out, my ladies in the doggone van, to go sightsee. I mean 40-, 50-, 60-year-old women had never been to DC, and Baltimore's right up the street. I was able to open doors. I think what I really wanted to do . . . I didn't want these women to hurt. Women were still dying . . . we were dying. And I was in my own space with my HIV, where, if we gotta die, what good can you do right now? So that's really what the safety net was, teaching women, you know, if you had a year, if you had two years, what would you wanna leave? What is your story?

The HIV safety net, through the interventions of the women working within it, was expanding from its early days to help women see possibility. Women like Linda knew that offering services could be effective, but they really wanted to use the resources of the safety net to help women heal—to heal them from the traumas of prior experiences and the marginalization that many had experienced their entire lives.

Middle-class women engaged with framing institutions in another way that should not be overlooked: they received assistance through one-on-one support in private and highly confidential settings that was less visible, but just as important, to their well-being. They frequently referenced pastors, therapists, and private doctors as the main institutional actors who were helping them come to terms with and manage their health status, many of whom were not part of the AIDS service community. Their transformations were less about massive overhauls of their lives but still required support as they moved from believing and behaving as though they had a death sentence after the shock of diagnosis to treating HIV as a manageable chronic illness. Whether through expansive networks in AIDS organizations or more individualized care in the quiet moments in a therapist's office, institutional ties still created opportunities and spaces for a range of women to remake their lives as WLWHA.

Negative Framing Institutions and Perverse Safety Nets

It is noteworthy how often jails and prisons served as framing institutions; a number of the Chicago study women were diagnosed there. Given the disproportionally high rates of incarceration among black and brown people, these institutions cannot be overlooked as key sites where prisoners, as well as those employed within these systems, circulate information, frameworks, and language about HIV that reaches large numbers of people of color and travels back to communities. Stevie (black, age 44) described being told by the prison nurses who diagnosed her not to disclose her status to her fellow inmates because of the stigma, and she witnessed a fellow inmate be ostracized when her status was known. Those early impressions lasted long after Stevie left prison, and her shame festered.

Ironically, prisons also operated as a perverse safety net, offering some Chicago study women their strongest connection to healthcare services when they were *dying from*.[31] Tina (black, age 28) described being "incarcerated for doing something stupid." During her sentence, she had a physical exam, complete with blood work. Reeling in disbelief after the HIV diagnosis, Tina faced other medical issues. She was diagnosed with cervical cancer, an indicator that her HIV infection had progressed to AIDS. After surgery, radiation, and a series of other treatments while incarcerated, doctors began treating her for HIV, prescribing Sustiva and Combivir, which Tina continued taking consistently throughout and after being incarcerated. Sadly, it was the most consistent healthcare that she had received in years, and it likely set her on the path to long-term management of HIV.

These perverse safety nets arise through our systematic refusal to establish stronger and broader protections against certain injuries of inequality and our zeal to put in its place tools to surveil, contain, and punish marginalized populations.[32]

.   .   .   .   .

Insofar as HIV/AIDS remains a life-threatening disease, it might be surprising to learn that three-fourths of women in the Chicago study described some kind of transformative project that helped them stabilize their lives. Physical challenges abided, due largely to the side effects associated with their medications and other co-occurring illnesses, and the women still grappled with stigma and other negative consequences of HIV. Moreover, 85 percent of the Chicago study women reported personal annual incomes of less than $20,000. These women therefore faced the stress of living on meager incomes, on paychecks from the low-wage labor market, Social Security Disability Insurance, or a patchwork of informal income sources.

The majority of the Chicago study women nevertheless understood HIV as a chronic but manageable condition rather than as a death sentence. They credited framing institutions with motivating them to engage in self-care: to visit their doctors regularly, manage their diets, take prescribed medications, reduce and manage stress, address drug addiction problems, and learn about symptoms and medications. In part, positive framing institutions also—through information, networks, and a common language—created spaces in which women held themselves and their fellow WLWHA accountable. They simultaneously grappled with the external events that traumatized them and the efficacy and consequences of their responses to those traumas. This later positioned them to be able to offer a more expansive analysis of the events and conditions that shaped their lives and to reflect on both the personal and the political strategies and tools that they wanted to use in the future. Coupled with the fact that almost all of these Chicago-based women have access to healthcare services and medication, some of their greatest vulnerabilities were somewhat ameliorated.

The distinct social meanings related to HIV made coping an ongoing process. Feelings of internal shame and external stigma could throw women off course at any time. Learning to live with HIV required not only managing the emotional turmoil and physical symptoms of the disease, but also examining and coming to terms with prior experiences of pain and marginalization that may have led to exposure to HIV.

Framing institutions, therefore, both positive and negative, helped women understand their worth. This was critically important because for so many WLWHA, the movement from death to life hinged in part on recalibrating their value outside of the sexualized drug economy, which had a very different system of currency that often depended on a woman's sexual value. Trisha and Beverly had to reimagine what they could contribute to the world, and the HIV safety net gave them not only the space but also the tools to do that.

Because the women's backgrounds and circumstances differed, the motivations that drove their transformative projects differed as well. For some, transformation was partly about atonement. Not only had they been injured throughout their lives, some had injured others and had to address and repair those offenses to feel redeemed. For other women, transformation was about financial and social mobility, moving from constant crises in one's economic and social circumstances to stability, or at least minimizing the crises. For still others, transformation was a liberation project, one that broke the psychological shackles that bound them to abuse, addiction, and deep pain and allowed them to find freedom in their lives. Finally, transformation was about healing, recovering from deep injuries to the psyche and finding a place of inner peace—in other words, recovering from the physical and emotional costs of living with HIV/AIDS.

4 The HIV Safety Net Meets the Test-and-Treat Revolution

In September 2017, I attended the US Conference on HIV/AIDS, a gathering of activists, advocates, service providers, researchers, clinicians, and policy specialists hosted by the National Minority AIDS Council. Part ideas exchange, part pep rally, part networking marathon, the conference offers participants a chance to hear about the latest scientific breakthroughs in the epidemic, share best practices to take back to their organizations, and catch glimpses of the politicians and celebrities who address the crowd. The conference theme, "Family Reunion," reinforced the notion that the AIDS community sees itself as a unified force, although no one would deny that tensions and dramas persist. There is, however, an underlying bond and energy that is unmistakable. Members of the crowd shed tears during video montages capturing the past and continued devastation of the epidemic and mourned when the names of lost friends and loved ones were invoked. Between plenary speakers, a DJ spun the hottest music as activists and advocates danced and erupted into spontaneous rhythmic club clapping. The group was there to draw on its collective strength, acutely aware that in the previous year, with a presidential election that did not go as most had expected, the gains that have been made toward securing affordable healthcare access, LGBTQ rights, and other relevant policies were under attack and new vulnerabilities were likely to surface on the political landscape. For now, both death and life were held in the room, as contributors to the HIV safety net eyed the future.

Decades of labor and struggle had produced remarkable results. The 2017 conference boasted a particularly exciting development: the promotion of the U = U campaign. More than two decades since the widespread adoption of antiretroviral medicines in the mid-1990s, several major breakthroughs in AIDS treatment had emerged. Scientists discovered that if PLWHA begin taking ART when their immune systems are relatively healthy, as opposed to delaying therapy until the disease has advanced, they have considerably lower risk of developing AIDS or other serious illnesses.[1] Moreover, researchers found that when taken as prescribed, ART can lower patients' viral loads, making them 96 percent less likely to sexually transmit the virus to others.[2] The CDC estimates that diagnosing PLWHA and ensuring they receive prompt, ongoing care and treatment could avert 90 percent of new HIV infections in the United States.[3] The CDC then declared in 2017 that "People who take ART daily as prescribed and achieve and maintain an undetectable viral load have effectively no risk of sexually transmitting the virus to an HIV-negative partner."

Given these advances in treatment, the next frontier in the fight against HIV/AIDS is therefore helping PLWHA achieve viral suppression, reducing the number of HIV particles or "copies" in one's blood below a certain threshold. Having an undetectable viral load does not mean that the virus is completely gone or that one has been "cured," but it suggests that the virus is under sufficient control. At the conference I attended, a large banner proclaimed the new message of the AIDS community: "Undetectable = Untransmittable," the slogan of the U = U campaign.

Would the end of AIDS come this easy? In the 1980s and 1990s, people literally died waiting for what we now have: a biomedical tool for treating HIV and preventing its spread to others. The success of this tool hinges, however, on one important ingredient: commitment. U = U requires PLWHA to be tested, visit their doctors, and take their medications consistently. They must overcome the side effects, logistical burdens, stigma, and psychological struggle of daily medication adherence. U = U also means asking individuals who may have struggled to maintain healthy commitments in the past to adhere to a fairly structured and regimented practice, despite all of the other complexities in their lives (which we have explored in previous chapters). At the same time, U = U demands a commitment from the larger society: medical care and medications must be accessible and affordable. HIV stigma must be reduced to encourage more people to be tested and seek treatment. Moreover, we must continue to enact robust preventive interventions. When this fails to happen, as we saw in chapter 1 in the case of Austin, Indiana, the epidemic can quickly gain a foothold in a community and become a serious public health threat.

Yet another component must fall into place if we are going to see the end of AIDS. My research strongly suggests that our individual and societal commitments to ending the AIDS epidemic will not succeed without a robust and sustained HIV safety net to serve as a crucial intermediary. In this chapter, reflecting more than a decade of fieldwork, I present the cases of four women whose experiences shed light on why focusing solely on "getting pills into bodies" is likely to fail. These cases illustrate that the HIV safety net has played and must continue to play a critical role in medication uptake and adherence. I invoke the HIV safety net in broad terms, as I gesture toward not only the medical providers who prescribe the pills and measure the viral loads and T-cell counts but also the advocacy, social service, and other organizations that have proven to be highly instrumental in encouraging medication uptake and adherence. Unless we recognize the important role a comprehensive HIV safety net can play in leveraging one of our most promising scientific discoveries, our best opportunity to end the AIDS epidemic will go unrealized. We may even cultivate an undetectable divide whereby individuals and communities with the necessary economic and social resources are able to fully embrace and implement the message, while those without get left behind. The HIV safety net is the bridge between those two worlds. If U = U is successful in reaching PLWHA, it could radically change the epidemic and what it means to live with HIV.

DAWN'S STORY: GETTING DRUGS INTO (FEMALE) BODIES IN HISTORICAL CONTEXT

Undoubtedly, some of the most important tools that make it possible for PLWHA to live longer lives are the medications themselves. Women have been pivotal players in ensuring that treatment science and the development of life-saving medications do not leave them behind. "When we start describing what the eighties and early nineties were like [with respect to HIV/AIDS treatment]," said treatment activist Dawn Averitt, "it's a little like talking about horse-drawn carriages versus the motorized vehicles of today." Dawn Averitt (not to be confused with Dawn Stevens, whom we met in the book's introduction) was diagnosed in 1988 as a 19-year-old college student. A middle-class white woman from Stone Mountain, Georgia, she had learned about HIV while witnessing gay friends of hers at New York University (NYU) succumb to the disease. When her own lymph nodes grew to the size of golf balls and stayed that way for months, she visited a series of physicians for a battery of tests. She asked her doctor to give her an AIDS test, assuming that they could quickly rule out the disease. "He said he wouldn't test me," Averitt recalled. "We got into this back-and-forth about it being expensive, about him not wanting it on my family's record, and he said, 'And there is no point, *is there?*' Kind of a leading question like, 'Have you been doing something that we should know about?' So we had this very animated back-and-forth and eventually, he just said, 'Fine, I'll give you the test.'"

Two tests confirmed her diagnosis. Averitt's doctor instructed her not to tell anyone because of the potential repercussions. Her family saw the news reports about the public humiliation that Ryan White and his family had suffered, and they worried that Averitt's father would lose his job and the family's health insurance. "So my parents, brothers, and I spent a number of years largely keeping it a secret. And in that moment, the doctor kind of locked us into this closet of shame, where nobody could know."

Eager to make the best of what she believed to be her life's last years, Averitt left NYU to finish her bachelor's degree at home in Georgia and landed a job working for US Senator Sam Nunn. When ACT UP activists descended on the then senator's office to protest, she dared not share that she too was living with HIV. Her T-cells were dropping rapidly and she was prescribed sequential monotherapy, a very early drug approach. "I remember saying to the doctor who put me on my first treatment regimen, 'If I get my T-cells up over 500, does that mean I can stop?' And he said 'No, you'll be on this for the rest of your life.' And it made my life very finite in that moment. Because we all knew these drugs weren't working that well."

Determined to find a way to channel her fear and fight her sense of isolation, Dawn turned to the one friend to whom she had disclosed her status, who worked as a receptionist at the AIDS Survival Project in Atlanta. Perhaps Dawn could apply for work there. She showed up to her interview:

> I knew very little about HIV at the time, except that I had it, and more T-cells were better than . . . [fewer] T-cells. But I memorized the opportunistic infection chart that Project Inform had developed. And I went in, in my pumps and pantyhose, and frantically went through every infection, which ones were viral, parasitic, bacterial, and fungal, for my interview with them. They were like "You're a nut job! What happened? Why are you here?" This beleaguered interviewing panel of five queens, as I lovingly and adoringly refer to them, [later] said, "We were just sitting there staring at you, trying to figure out if you'd been sentenced to community service. Like, why were you here?" And I had to say in the interview, for the first time, to people I didn't know and didn't have a trusted relationship with, "No, I have HIV."

Averitt was hired as a treatment resources specialist and put in charge of the organization's library. She began reading every medical journal, newsletter, and communiqué from the NIH and FDA that she could get her hands on. "We didn't have Google and computers at that point. And I'm making photocopies of all the articles and three-hole punching them and putting them into binders and shelving them on this wall of over 300 binders that I have organized by conditions, treatments, alternative therapies, side effects, and toxicities. So the learning curve was extraordinarily steep." Averitt was developing the knowledge as a lay person that would make her formidable in conversations on HIV treatment, while she soaked up her new world of peer support.

Averitt attended several pharmaceutical advisory meetings and in 1993 wrote a grant proposal to start a new nonprofit called the Women's Information Service and Exchange (WISE). WISE sought to address the treatment information and advocacy needs of women, inspired by those who were coming to Averitt at the AIDS Survival Project "wearing floppy hats and sunglasses, sliding up to my desk, and discreetly asking if there was treatment information focused on women." Nevertheless, Averitt found that she was a lone voice in her first treatment advocacy meeting. "I was in this room with, I'm not joking, 19 gay white men from New York and California. I was 24 or something. I looked around the room and said, 'Who's representing women here?' And they all rolled their eyes and said, 'You are, sit down.'" She sat among them and studied the sea of acronyms and scientific terms, eventually earning her place among treatment advocates. At the time, this was a wing of the AIDS community widely considered to be elite, a highly educated group of mostly white men who, as "lay experts," worked closely with the scientific researchers, FDA and NIH officials, pharmaceutical company representatives, and clinicians who were trying to unpack the science of the epidemic:[4]

> I became a part of that group partially because they just needed a HIV-positive woman. And also because I love the science. And so those were my early days of indoctrination into research and clinical trials and what all of this science would mean eventually for the lives of real people. . . . I learned what I learned from these guys who came from every walk of life, all different kinds of careers, who were basically doing nothing more than just trying to stay alive.

Dawn Averitt and other female treatment advocates understood the fundamental truth once stated by Katrina Haslip: AIDS looks different in women. Without their advocacy, the clinical trials, drug discoveries, and other scientific tools used to confront the epidemic might not exist or have the same level of efficacy for female patients. But once the pharmaceutical lifeline for which Averitt and other treatment advocates had been fighting finally existed, they faced a different fact :

> It was a little like a relay race where you had been racing as hard as you could to get this baton to the next runner. But when the protease inhibitors hit, we realized we got the baton (FDA approval) there, but we had not set up another runner. We had not tied the communities together: treatment and services. We were all working for the same thing on some level. But hardly anybody [in the treatment world] had really thought about what *access* was going to look like. And what treatment was going to *mean*.

The discovery of ART would raise a whole new set of questions about the access and affordability of the medications, but also about the social meaning that people ascribed to them and how they would prioritize them in often complicated lives.

PATHS THAT COMPETE, PATHS THAT CONVERGE:
DIFFERING APPROACHES TO HIV/AIDS CARE

Approaches to fighting HIV/AIDS have historically fallen into one of three categories: biomedical, behavioral, or structural. Biomedical interventions emphasize the use of medical technologies to reduce the number of new infections and treat PLWHA. While the AIDS community has sought biomedical solutions from the beginning of the epidemic, it was not until the advent of ART that effective tools that could serve as primary weapons against AIDS were available. With the latest scientific discoveries confirming the efficacy of these drugs, biomedical approaches have gained even greater prominence in the coordinated response to AIDS.

Prior to and even after the discovery of effective medications, considerable focus on fighting the epidemic has targeted behavioral inventions. Public health campaigns and community messaging promote safe sex through condom use (or abstinence), limiting the number of sexual partners, using clean needles (or no needles at all), getting tested, and taking prescribed medications. Behavioral scientists and public health officials have led the creation and evaluation of programs promoting these messages, targeting both the general public and the groups most affected by the epidemic. Behavioral interventions have varied significantly in tone and effectiveness, but they encourage individuals to change behaviors that may cut their lives short. Support groups, case management, peer educators, and other tools fall into this category.

Structural interventions offer a third approach to the AIDS response. These target the social determinants of health, what the CDC identifies as the "complex, integrated, and overlapping social structures and economic systems that are responsible for most health inequities."[5] Social determinants unquestionably help to drive the AIDS epidemic. They represent the sum of the experiences, constrained options, and barriers that confront people daily and chip away at or sometimes overwhelm physical and mental health. Within the social environment, physical environment, and the health services system, it is well documented that race, class, gender, and sexual inequities contribute fundamentally to the root causes of health problems and the opportunities and resources needed to prevent and treat poor health.

Structural interventionists therefore seek to attack the drivers of the AIDS epidemic by targeting the systematic ways in which social and economic inequality directly and indirectly increase the risk of infection and deleterious post-diagnosis experiences.[6] The Ryan White CARE Act, Housing Opportunities for People with AIDS (HOPWA), and the Affordable Care Act (ACA), which aim to improve healthcare access and affordability, are perhaps the closest we have come to structural interventions in the epidemic given their scale, but these interventions still fall short in addressing the root causes of HIV as an injury of inequality. Scholars working in the social sciences and humanities have been at the forefront of bringing social, political, historical, and cultural analyses to bear in understanding HIV/AIDS prevention and treatment pathways, evolving AIDS policy, the politics of scientific research, and the HIV safety net both in the United States and abroad.[7] They join like-minded activists and advocates in challenging the field to create interventions that confront social structures, prejudices, and biases and interrupt some of the historical and political processes that shape the experiences of marginalized populations within the epidemic.

In 2012, the US Department of Health and Human Services issued new guidelines recommending ART for both adult and adolescent PLWHA, regardless of CD4 count or viral load. Before then, many physicians prescribed medication only when the disease had advanced and patients had low CD4 counts, as the medical consensus was that inconsistent medication adherence could build the body's resistance to treatment. If a doctor and patient were not confident that a patient could adhere to the daily protocol, the physician would not prescribe ART, waiting until T-cell counts and viral loads had reached a certain threshold.

Known as "test-and-treat" or "treatment as prevention," the new approach entailing earlier initiation of ART would become the harbinger of U = U and is now widely considered the best available strategy for prolonging lives and stopping the AIDS epidemic in the absence of a vaccine or cure. If treatment as prevention is the public health strategy for ending the epidemic, U = U is the message to PLWHA that they can fully restore their lives. It also definitively places biomedical interventions at the forefront of the AIDS response. Ensuring that PLWHA connect to and sustain their ties to medical care over time has therefore become the central focus in AIDS treatment and prevention efforts. In 2011, Dr. Edward Gardner and colleagues developed the concept of the HIV care continuum, or "treatment cascade," to highlight the steps required for individuals to fully benefit from combination ART. The Gardner cascade has the following stages: diagnosis of HIV infection, linkage to care, retention in care, receipt of antiretroviral therapy, and achievement of viral suppression.

At the global level, in 2014 UNAIDS released the 90–90–90 plan, with the goals that by 2020, 90 percent of all people living with HIV will know their HIV status, 90 percent of all people with diagnosed HIV infections will receive sustained ART, and 90 percent of all people receiving ART will be virally suppressed. In 2011, the CDC estimated that of the 1.2 million PLWHA in the United States, an estimated 86 percent had been diagnosed with HIV, 40 percent were engaged in HIV medical care, 37 percent had been prescribed ART, and only 30 percent had achieved viral suppression.[8] In other words, only 30 percent of Americans with HIV were thought to have the virus under control. Through the HIV Care Continuum Initiative, established in 2013, President Obama directed federal departments to prioritize addressing these gaps as part of the implementation of the National HIV/AIDS Strategy (NHAS), unveiled in 2010 and updated in 2015. In 2016, 48 percent of PLWHA in Chicago had undetectable viral loads.[9] While this is far from the city's target of 80 percent, this represents a noteworthy and steady climb. David Ernesto Munar is the former head of the AIDS Foundation of Chicago and is currently president and CEO of Howard Brown Health, one of the largest LGBTQ health organizations in the country. He joined the coalition of activists and advocates who originally encouraged the creation of the NHAS and said this about the 2015 update:

> The updated strategy was basically written along the Gardner cascade. And so the idea was that these were the outcomes that were going to be evaluated: testing, linkage, engagement, viral suppression. That's a shift. It changed the way services are delivered because the primary metric is not "Are people using your services? Are people happy with their services?" All these are different kinds of possible metrics organizations could be using to assess their services. However, the metric, "Are your clients virally suppressed?" goes to the heart of impact. Programs that support clients in achieving viral suppression address the whole continuum of care, directly

interrupt transmission, and provide the better possible HIV-related health outcomes for those living with HIV.

Twenty years since the advent of ART, the biomedical approach reigns supreme. Challenging the false distinction between the "biomedicalization" of HIV prevention and treatment and structural approaches, sociologist Barry Adam writes:

> Perhaps the most striking, but inadvertent, lesson to be drawn . . . is that all biomedical prevention technologies are also social interventions, whether that is explicitly recognized or not. [These technologies] are clearly strongly dependent on "adherence," a term often associated with patient recalcitrance and management, but which glosses the very large realm of how interventions fit with everyday exigencies, cross-cutting demands of home and workplace, available options, economic resources and interpretative frameworks of the people who are to adopt these technologies.[10]

Although many of the Chicago study data were collected just prior to the issuance of the 2012 federal guidelines recommending test-and-treat, the stories in this chapter will reveal how taking daily medications is indeed a socially constructed event. A woman's relationship to medication, we learned, is largely about intersections—intersections between the medical and the social, between the body and identity, and between scientific knowledge and women's lived experiences. The women's stories suggest the need for a broad base of support to ensure that test-and-treat and eventually U = U can be fully realized. Women pointed to the critical role of the HIV safety net in helping them confront denial, medication side effects, the isolation of illness, and the multiple barriers in their paths as they attempted to move from *dying from* to *living with*.

NAINA'S STORY: CONFRONTING DENIAL
THROUGH THE HIV SAFETY NET

Naina Khanna was 25 years old when she was diagnosed in 2002. For reasons both practical and symbolic, two years passed before she next visited the doctor to check her T-cell count and viral load. At the time, she was among millions of young adults who lacked health insurance, so she was unsure how she would pay for her medical care. Having been diagnosed outside of the US, Naina also worried that accessing HIV services would create obstacles to future health insurance coverage due to preexisting condition exclusions. Furthermore, deep denial paralyzed her. She felt perfectly healthy. How could she possibly have a life-threatening illness?

In 2004, Naina's then boyfriend encouraged her to visit an HIV doctor, as the couple had done some research online and learned that she might be less likely to transmit the virus to him if she were on medication. "A lot of times," Naina explained over lunch with me at the 2016 International AIDS Conference in Durban, South Africa, "women make decisions because of people we love, and so, that was a big motivator for me. My partner wanted to know what my viral load was and if I needed to be on medication." Expecting to hear that everything was fine, Naina was shocked to discover that her T-cell or CD4 count was only 120, well below the acceptable threshold of 500 for PLWHA. Naina had AIDS.

A treatment advocate at the clinic disclosed that he too was HIV positive and advised her to start medication immediately. As Naina recalls, her mind was flooded with questions and an overwhelming sense of fear:

> I was very unprepared for that information, and it was delivered to me by this white man sitting in a room in a hospital in New York, and he's trying to run through my treatment options with me on the same day I get an AIDS diagnosis. And in his hand, he was turning this model of an HIV molecule around, showing me where the different medications attached to HIV. I just could not hear a word he was saying. I had just been given an AIDS diagnosis. It was just like Charlie Brown, "wawawa," so then I asked him, "What if I want to have kids, what do you recommend for somebody who wants to have kids?" He didn't know. He didn't have the information. He'd been on medication for years, but he didn't have any answers for me as a woman. So basically he said, "Well, if you're not going to start medication, there's nothing we can really do for you." So I left and didn't go back.

After the encounter at the clinic, Naina battled for months with the reality that she had an AIDS diagnosis, drifting between denial and panic in the profound state of distress that I have described as *dying from*. Finally, she moved to California in 2005, in part because she heard about the mobilization of WORLD, the organization that Rebecca Denison founded in

1991 (discussed in chapter 2). Naina was hungry for a connection to other women facing the same challenges and wondered if her fiery passion for social justice would find a home at WORLD. Shortly after arriving, she met the woman who would become her "framing agent," an individual within a framing institution who is instrumental in facilitating the conceptual shift that helps a person launch her transformative project:

> When I came to WORLD as a client, I got a peer advocate. She was a Latina and Native American woman who was also living with HIV. Through her support, she was just amazing. She came to my house one day—she knew that I was kinda struggling with the decision around starting meds and one day she called me and said, "I just got a great little new pamphlet in the mail about the medications. It explains them all and the side effects, and it breaks them down really well. I think you might be interested." And she was like, "Do you want to come look at it?" And I said, "No I can't really make it in there," I had all kinds of excuses, whatever, I was busy, I didn't have the transportation. She said, "No problem, I will drop it off at your house, in a sealed envelope. I'll put it in your mailbox. It will be there when you get home tonight." That's what she did . . . that's the kind of support that peer advocates at a community-based organization can give—who really understand women dealing with disclosure issues and stigma. She understood me culturally more than that white guy in New York, understood my concerns around the stigma, around disclosure, around my health, around my body, around what healing meant for me, all of that, being willing to come to my house. That's the kind of support that gets women into [health] care. And that's what ultimately got me into [health] care, taking medications, being healthy, and so, it's really going through that whole process.

As Naina's story illustrates, the medical and the social aspects of treating HIV are co-constitutive and interdependent: focusing on one without attending to others produces uneven results. It can take years for someone to commit to lifelong medical treatment, to acknowledge that she is now forever tied to a set of pills, and to accept an HIV-positive social identity. Naina's story reveals the important relationships that she viewed as critical for her adoption of a medication regimen. First, we see another clear example in which connection to the HIV safety net had lifesaving results. After Naina's first cognitive shift, which inspired her move to California and connect with WORLD, her relationship with this framing institution led her to start taking HIV medications. And for Naina, this transformative effect extends beyond her own life. What many AIDS organizations have come to understand is that moving women along the HIV care continuum toward consistent treatment can generate broader transformations.

In 2006, Naina started coordinating a speakers' bureau program at WORLD. She was drawn to WORLD because of its commitment to empowering women to become leaders in the fight against AIDS: "I read a lot of stuff online and realized that my experiences were really not unique. A lot of women were dealing with stuff that was much worse, and facing many more barriers than I was with my relative amount of privilege. Yeah, so, I felt like I needed to work in HIV. That's how I got involved." She became a valuable part of building the organization's advocacy and policy work. "We always had the understanding that advocacy work and leadership development work for [WLWHA] had to be done in a way that's really supportive and holistic to honor the whole woman," Naina explained. Now executive director of a national membership body of WLWHA called the Positive Women's Network-USA, Naina represents the national and even global advocacy that emerges out of framing institutions, organizations that provide women with the space and tools they need to launch transformative projects.

Second, Naina's story illustrates the relationship individuals have with the medications themselves and their intertwined social meanings. As one AIDS activist stated, "I had to get okay with the fact that I would have to take these meds every single day for the rest of my life, whether I wanted to or not." The seemingly simple task of suppressing HIV in the body through daily medication is complicated by very reasonable concerns about the side effects and the long-term impact that these drugs may have on the body. As Eve (black, age 31) described:

> When you have HIV, you get a lot of symptoms from your medicine. I go through sometimes really bad nausea, throwing up, irritable bowels. . . . So juggling those things. And then sometimes you feel like food is just, you can't eat. And then there are some days where you feel like every two hours, you got to eat something because you just feel like you haven't eaten at all. So it just depends on how the day is, you have to deal with this stuff all day long, throughout the day, while you're trying to do what you got to do.

Women reported nausea, vomiting, diarrhea, fatigue, weight gain, weight loss, and muscle cramps associated with their medications. Because some had yet to experience symptoms or illnesses directly related to HIV, the side effects of the medications were often their most visible and debilitating physical reminders of illness. As Beverly shared, "One of the side effects of the medication is depression. So we have to be careful and we have to be attuned to that, if you want to survive well . . . so I have that mental note. Okay, three days in a row, if I'm depressed, then I need to address it." Many Chicago study women in fact chose not to use HIV medications because of the side effects, especially prior to the test-and-treat era, when the guidelines for adoption were much more fluid.

When women in the Chicago study invited me to attend their medical appointments, I witnessed firsthand how infectious disease doctors made their pitches to try to get their patients to maintain adherence. This revealed perhaps the third important relationship associated with test-and-treat: the one between PLWHA and their healthcare providers. In Naina's case, the lack of rapport with the first treatment advocate undermined initiation of medication. Dani's story highlights another dynamic.

DANI'S STORY: CONFRONTING THE ISOLATION OF ILLNESS THROUGH THE HIV SAFETY NET

The most effective HIV doctors I observed were well aware of the importance of patients' relationships with the HIV safety net for medication adherence. Chicago study participant Dani Russell (black, age 44) invited me to accompany her on a chilly Chicago morning to a routine appointment at the Ruth M. Rothstein CORE Center.[11] Founded through a partnership between the Cook County Health and Hospitals System and Rush University Medical Center, the CORE Center has provided outpatient care for PLWHA and patients with other infectious diseases since 1998. The large red brick structure, with picture windows that scale the side of the building and invite in plenty of natural light, was designed with patient input and serves as a one-stop center for treatment. Patients can receive primary care, laboratory testing, pediatric services, dental care, specialty consultations and screenings, pharmacy services, and mental health care all under one roof. The facility also offers social support services through case management and support groups, prevention and education programs, and opportunities to participate in research.

I was sitting in the main lobby when Dani emerged from the elevator. She had arrived early with her father and settled him in the waiting room on her doctor's floor, his cane leaning against the chair beside him. Dani is her father's primary caretaker, so I was not surprised that she brought him to the appointment as she previously expressed concerns about leaving him home alone. They had been to the CORE Center three times in the previous two weeks. All of her doctors were there (her psychologist, neurologist, primary physician, and gynecologist). She had three major health concerns: HIV, high blood pressure, and the aftereffects of a brain aneurism she had suffered in 2005. That day's appointment was with Dr. Matthews, a neurologist who would assess Dani's memory loss and the intense numbness and needle-prick feelings she had been experiencing in her hands and feet for months.

After about ten minutes, a nurse invited Dani and me to the patient service area while her father stayed behind in the waiting room. Dr. Matthews entered a few minutes later. A youngish white male with a warm and professional bedside manner, he greeted Dani and listened as she introduced me and explained that I was "doing a study about her." He offered me a seat in the examining room, took a seat at the small desk with a computer, and asked Dani to sit in the empty chair next to the desk. After Dani updated him on the problem with her extremities, he asked her several questions about when the numbness in her hands and feet were at their worst (when she is sleeping) and how bad the memory loss had become (significant). With her memory loss, Dani's elderly father was increasingly taking on the role of her care provider despite his own health challenges, and he had recently worried aloud that Dani would forget to provide his medication.

Dani climbed onto the examining table, and Dr. Matthews began the physical exam. He used the sharp end of a safety pin to test Dani's feeling in her palms, fingertips, and feet. She could often feel the pin pricks but seemed unable to feel pricks in portions of her wrist. Dr. Matthews would order some additional neurological tests to accompany Dani's routine three-month HIV bloodwork. He also suggested that he see her later in the week at his other office, where he could conduct some more sophisticated neurological testing. He would look into ordering an MRI for Dani as well. Her neurological problems, he suggested, could be a side effect of her HIV medications or a lingering symptom of her aneurism.

Dr. Matthews then looked up "her numbers" on the computer to assess the status and progression of HIV in her body. Her CD4/T-Cell count was 960: "Great," he commented. Her viral load rendered Dani "virally suppressed," the status most prized in the HIV continuum of care. The lasting effects of her brain aneurism and the high blood pressure would be greater concerns now. Multiple health challenges are quite common among PLWHA. In fact, having observed several appointments between the women and their doctors, I often noticed both parties assigning greater urgency to non-HIV health challenges, demonstrating the far-reaching definition of AIDS care.

"What have you been doing about your blood pressure?" Dr. Matthews asked. "What has your primary doctor suggested?"

"I'm not sure," Dani commented. "I haven't been in to see Dr. Gupta in a while."

"Well, let's go see if she's available now," Dr. Matthews suggested, leveraging the comprehensive nature of the CORE Center's services to draw another physician in for consultation. He left the room and returned to announce that Dani's primary care doctor could see her now. He asked whether she had any additional questions and we said our goodbyes. We returned to the main waiting room to collect Dani's father and headed for Dr. Gupta's suite a floor above. We joined a group of patients sitting in Dr. Gupta's waiting room. In just a few minutes, Dani and I were escorted to the examination room by Dr. Gupta herself.

As we sat down, Dr. Gupta turned to the computer to access Dani's records. "So how are you doing?" After Dani commented that she was fine except for her blood pressure, Dr. Gupta responded. "I know you're taking your HIV meds," she commented, "because your numbers are great." Dani commented that the previous month, her dentist had not been able to treat her because her blood pressure was too high.

"In January," Dr. Gupta commented, "your blood pressure was fine. Are you taking your blood pressure medicine?" she asked.

"Yes, definitely," Dani answered. Dr. Gupta crossed over to the other side of the small examining room, grabbed a blood pressure cuff, and wrapped it around Dani's thin arm.

"With your aneurism," Dr. Gupta commented, "your blood pressure scares me. 140 over 90."

"It was 160 over 100 in the dentist's office," Dani offered.

"This is odd," Dr. Gupta commented, "if you are taking your blood pressure meds, your numbers should be better. What are you eating?"

"I eat everything," Dani commented. She went on to confess to binge eating when waves of depression wash over her. "I know I should stop it."

"What's going on in your life?" Dr. Gupta asked. "How is your father? What about the boyfriend that was buying you all of the gifts?" I was impressed by how much Dr. Gupta knew about Dani's life outside of the examining room.

"My dad is fine," Dani answered. "He's the same. The boyfriend, he's on his way out."

"What about going back to support group meetings?" Dr. Gupta persisted. "Seems like you could use them. You've gained ten pounds since I saw you three months ago. You were so thin when you came to me that I was happy to see any weight gain. But now I think it's getting out of control with the eating. With your blood pressure up and down like this, we gotta do better with that."

"I'll do better," Dani promised, "And I'll think about going back to group."

Dr. Gupta wrote a prescription for a higher dosage of blood pressure medication. "Try this," she said, "But do better with the eating. And go back to group."

As Dr. Gupta demonstrated in her interaction with Dani, treating patients requires her to think holistically about their lives and leverage the social support services of the HIV safety net. Dr. Gupta knew that Dani had recently moved out of Wheeler House, a residence for PLWHA, to take care of her father. She had quit her job in office administration to oversee his health, distrustful of anyone else who might care for him and without the resources to hire the kind of high-quality care that she wanted for him. And Dani was carrying an even bigger secret: although her father had waited within the walls of the CORE Center with her on numerous occasions, Dani had never disclosed to him that she was living with HIV. It is possible that with his older age and health challenges, he had not made the connection with the mission of the institution. But it is also possible that he was fully aware that his daughter was living with HIV, tacitly agreeing to maintain a strategic silence between father and daughter. Regardless, sensing that Dani was adrift and that it had consequences for her health, Dr. Gupta prescribed support group attendance alongside a new medication, encouraging Dani to make a deeper connection with the HIV safety net.

·   ·   ·   ·   ·

The system of AIDS care in many of America's major cities has improved greatly since the early years when Dawn Stevens (whom we met in the introduction) was diagnosed in 1985. Many AIDS organizations have been encouraged to partner with medical providers to deliver comprehensive medical and supportive services. For example, when Rosario was diagnosed in 2007 during a prenatal care visit, she was immediately "moved into care." A case manager accompanied the clinical nurse who delivered the news and immediately framed the information: "It's not a death sentence. You're going to be fine if you take your medicines. We're going to provide you with a doctor. This doctor is going to make sure that you get medicines to take." Within days, Rosario was meeting with an HIV specialist, and her viral load has been undetectable ever since. "I was in A-1 health before, and after the diagnosis, I actually maintained that," Rosario said proudly. "I don't have any symptoms attributed to the virus. I eat right, I exercise, and I go see my doctor every four months."

While case managers often provide sounding boards to women in crisis, their main objective is to connect their clients to the right combination of services so that they stay, to borrow a frequently used phrase, "linked to care." As we saw in chapter 3, these services can be transformative for women. However, the AIDS community has a very clear strategy in mind: the goal is to eliminate or minimize any barriers that prevent women from visiting their doctors and taking prescribed medication. As Annette, a case manager in Chicago, describes,

We have even driven people to the CORE Center. . . . If somebody needs medical care, we'll drive them. We've given them bus passes . . . whatever it takes to get people their treatment. We have a list of healthcare providers. We have a list of homeless shelters. Woman comes in and has a child and needs shelter. Where can we send her where they're not separated? Where can we get them referred? They don't have any winter clothes. Where can we send them? We don't leave any stones unturned.

The HIV safety net is not, however, this robust everywhere it is needed. Further, given the numerous challenges women face, sometimes even dedicated assistance fails to keep women linked to care and adherent to their medications. Among the biggest threats to the promise of U = U are the disconnects—involving systems, organizations, and individuals—that prevent women from fully benefiting from the current state of AIDS care.

TANYA'S STORY: WHEN SYSTEMS FAIL AND WOMEN'S BURDENS ARE TOO HEAVY

Tanya Sharpe (black, age 40) is a mother of four children, ages 21, 18, 17, and 15. She resides in Phoenix House, an apartment building for PLWHA run by a nearby church. Although this is a building that Rosario, who lives there with her three children, praises, Phoenix House has suffered for years under the weight of poor institutional staffing and meager funding. The building's high incidence of case manager turnover means that temporary social work students are routinely assigned to Tanya's case, a steady rotation of well-meaning but inexperienced neophytes examining the intimate details of Tanya's life. In addition, Tanya trusts few staff members to keep information confidential, so she does not take full advantage of the services offered at Phoenix House. "[The executive director] knows all of us," Tanya explained. "She knows our ups and downs 'cause she interacts with us. So she's caring. But the rest of these people, no. They shouldn't be in and out [of our case files] because all they do is gossip back and forth. . . . I hear them . . . they have no respect for our [support] groups. They walk in and out. . . . It's no respect here."

Tanya's story reflects what can happen when a breakdown in the safety net meets a client facing multiple barriers. An individual with severe and deeply rooted injuries of inequality will challenge even the most effective organizations; indeed, institutions that are struggling can actually operate as *negative* framing institutions by making it more difficult for women to reconcile with their HIV status and stay linked to care. When we met in 2005, Tanya's 17-year-old son had recently been arrested. He stood accused of stabbing a male acquaintance of his girlfriend. Tanya was convinced he did not do it and spent much of our first meeting asserting that the evidence against him was weak. Getting involved with an older girl "who ain't about nothing" had been his downfall, Tanya believed, exposing him to a caliber of people that Tanya wanted him to avoid. The girlfriend was, however, a regular visitor to her son's jail, frustrating Tanya's efforts to convince him to break up with her. Tanya was very frustrated with her son's naïveté; she frequently told him that he needed to be more careful.

Tanya's world effectively came to a halt with the incarceration of her child. Her mind grappled with the unimaginable, the violence to which he could be subjected and the possibility that there would be no end to the nightmare. Seeing her son ensnared by the system became all-encompassing for Tanya. She slept little in the nights before our first interview and spent her days on the Internet researching the law and hunting for a lawyer. Just days before our first interview, she hired an attorney who reportedly assured Tanya that winning her son's case should not be a problem as the police had questioned the 17-year-old without a parent present. This lawyer was sent by God, Tanya believed, and she was even surer of this when, during our first interview, her youngest daughter interrupted us to tell Tanya that her son was on the phone, reporting that his lawyer said that he should be getting out soon.

Tanya's challenges did not stop there. Diagnosed with bipolar disorder at 16, she had been struggling ever since with her mental health. HIV prevalence is much higher among women suffering from mental illness; the mental instability and limited power that this diminished and stigmatized social standing produces makes them vulnerable to drug addiction and risky sexual experiences.[12] Tanya told me she occasionally heard voices and was on medication. Her physical health since her HIV diagnosis in 2002 had also been challenging, as Tanya often felt extremely fatigued and could not get out of bed. She had had suicidal thoughts and once tried to slit her wrists with a dull knife. Tanya's youngest and second-oldest daughters, both teenagers, "monitored her," taking turns sleeping to watch their mother. The girls had few friends, and Tanya believed this was because they were too narrowly focused on caring for her. Moreover, Tanya speculated, the girls probably wanted to avoid the embarrassment of bringing friends to an "AIDS house." The neighborhood boys on the corner had already asked them, "Which one of ya'll has AIDS?" after observing the family head into Phoenix House. With tears streaming down her face during our first interview, Tanya described feeling as though she "let her kids down" by becoming homeless, contracting HIV, and not "taking care of the family." Her oldest daughter harbored considerable anger toward Tanya about their family's state of affairs and spent most of her time at her boyfriend's family's house. She had even taken to calling her boyfriend's mother "Ma," deeply wounding Tanya. Between sobs she whispered, "I tell her, I pay for you to have a roof over your head and take care of you. And yet you call this woman 'ma'?"

A month after our first interview, I called Tanya to set up an observation session. Bad news burdened her voice. The lawyer she hired had done nothing for her son's case. "He should have been out, at least on bail if not with the charges dropped months ago, but his lawyer hasn't done anything. I've called other lawyers and they all agree that he should be off the case and that it's bad. But they all want money too." As Tanya sought counsel in a sea of lawyers who seemed to make their money collecting poverty-stricken clients, her 17-year-old son remained in an adult jail.

Despite the crisis, Tanya invited me to attend her next doctor's appointment at the Westside Family Health Center, a community clinic in the Lawndale area of Chicago. Tanya arrived with Rae, her second-oldest daughter, who was five months pregnant, in tow. They had been fighting that morning, Tanya explained, about Rae's boyfriend. With her eldest daughter spending all of her time at her boyfriend's parents' house and her son arrested after dating a girl that Tanya didn't like, it felt like yet another one of her children was slipping away. Whether their behavior was simply teenage rebellion or desperate attempts to escape the instability of their home, Tanya's children appeared to be struggling under the weight of the family's intersecting injuries.

After waiting a stunning hour and a half past our appointment time, Tanya and I were finally called in to see the doctor. Tanya introduced me to Dr. Patel, the primary care physician who had diagnosed her as HIV positive three years prior. After Tanya explained that she was participating in a research study, I took a seat in the corner of the room. Tanya climbed onto the examining table and Dr. Patel checked her heartbeat, breathing, pulse, and blood pressure. He said things seemed normal and asked her how she was doing. Tanya explained she was finding it difficult to sleep and was stressed about her son. He seemed familiar with the situation and asked Tanya when the boy might be released. "How are your daughters?" he asked. Tanya gave a brief summary: Her oldest daughter was still living with her boyfriend. Rae's baby was due in a few months. Her youngest daughter was "doing fine."

Dr. Patel then moved over to the desk where he pulled out Tanya's medical file. "Your numbers," he said with deep concern, "aren't so good. Stress will wreak havoc on your immune system. You have to find ways to deal with what is going on without sacrificing your health." Tanya nodded, taking in the message. The three of us sat in a knowing and heavy silence in the examining room: until Tanya knew that her son was okay, taking care of herself would be the last thing on her mind.

Nevertheless, Dr. Patel pressed on, explaining to Tanya that she was dangerously close to developing AIDS. He would conduct another round of bloodwork to observe her viral load and T-cell count. "Are you interested in getting back on your meds?" Dr. Patel asked. "Because if not, this is going to continue to be a problem. I am going to call Dr. We [Tanya's HIV doctor] and tell him that you are going to get back on your meds. Tanya, you have to do this. Your numbers aren't good."

Tanya nodded, without protest. She looked exhausted. Dr. Patel asked if there were any other issues. Tanya shared that she had a cold she could not get over, and Dr. Patel moved close to listen to her lungs with a stethoscope once again. "It's your immune system," Dr. Patel concluded, driving home his point. He asked if Tanya was still seeing her psychiatrist. When she revealed that she had stopped both keeping appointments and taking her psychiatric medication when the crisis with her son started, Dr. Patel shook his head, looked Tanya straight in the eyes, and told her he was worried about her. "Tanya, we need you to take care of yourself. Your son and daughters need a healthy mom. Please, we know what we have to do, you need to do it. Please." Dr. Patel asked Tanya if she had any more questions, and our 20-minute appointment came to an end.

Over the course of our interviews and check-ins weeks and then months later, I observed Tanya struggle in a high-stress state, *dying from* the serious issues with her physical and mental health, family stressors, and the weight she carried on her shoulders. Every time I interacted with Tanya, I left feeling as though I was watching someone walk on rickety floorboards that threatened to give way at any moment, plunging her into an abyss. Phoenix House appeared to be ill-equipped for the challenge. Her relationships with the staff continued to deteriorate. She reported that she was told that her family was likely to be evicted because Rae's now newborn son would put the family over the occupancy rate for their unit. Tanya was deeply upset and wanted to take up the matter with the church advisory board that oversaw Phoenix House. "They sell you a dream," she said about Phoenix House. "When they see you got a sore, they constantly pick at it." Given all her challenges, no transformative project appeared to be on the horizon.

It is a nebulous term for some: *social determinants of health*. But as Tanya's story demonstrates, poverty, family crises, unaddressed mental health issues, a broken and inefficient criminal justice system, and weaknesses in social support networks can be devastating to health. These issues, which confront significant numbers of PLWHA, can severely undercut even the most promising of medical advances and scientific discoveries.

HOLES IN THE SAFETY NET AND THE PERIL OF THE UNDETECTABLE DIVIDE

With the emphasis on the biomedical tools available to treat HIV, on getting drugs into bodies, many AIDS activists and advocates worry about the potential for a slow walk away from the social support and other holistic services of the HIV safety net, despite their documented success. They are frustrated by the assumption that the only institutional relationship that test-and-treat requires is the linear one between patient and physician. After reciting the names of AIDS organizations that had recently closed, Naina Khanna explained that "we're seeing a dismantling of a lot of the community infrastructure . . . and a changing landscape for women in particular. Peer-based programs, support groups, and stuff like that have been really underfunded. There is the idea that just getting folks into care, making sure they have the medical care they need, the treatment they need, is enough." AIDS activist Linda Scruggs explains,

> I've heard some colleagues in the government refer to the social piece of the CARE Act as the fluff. . . . Quality of life is a priority and key to why we wrote the CARE Act originally. But the support services that were the priority in the CARE Act are now the least important part. That is the "medical model" that we now live in. Most of our communities don't know how to live in a medical model. That's not gonna speak to the whole, all the issues. So it's that gap space.

This is not to suggest that AIDS advocates completely reject biomedical approaches. There is some acknowledgment that behavioral approaches have limitations, while structural interventions are hard to engineer. SisterLove founder and public health advocate Dázon Dixon Diallo had this to say:

> There's not a real conflict in terms of biomedical versus behavioral [approaches], because the evidence is pretty clear around the efficacy of the biomedical and [the limits of] behavioral interventions. With all the efforts that we've done, even with the testing and counseling just in the US over 30 years, we're still seeing roughly 45,000 to 50,000 new cases a year. So all we're doing is holding firm. We're not making enough headway. And if the rate of infection is still going up among certain populations, then we need something else. And the truth of the matter is, there's not a single virus out there that we have conquered solely through behavioral [interventions].

What many activists and advocates envisioned in the current era of the AIDS response, especially those who work heavily with communities of color and women, was an even *tighter* relationship between biomedical, behavioral, and structural interventions. While test-and-treat currently drives global strategy, the social realities of PLWHA and those at higher risk cannot be ignored. The social burden of HIV and its related challenges can completely undermine an individual's ability to address the medical burden of the disease. Dázon continued:

> It's taken us years to have biomedical options, but you know what? You can sit a whole row of pills in front of somebody, but if you haven't educated and offered the opportunity and the support to stay adherent, then you're missing the boat. So there's a way to look at these—the [bio]medical, behavioral,

and social—as *combined* interventions. To look at the three as a way of expanding the arsenal that we have, and to know that there's no one intervention that's going to work alone. . . . An individual person has to assume some agency to decide to get tested and why and when. And when they get linked to care, to show up, and to stay in that care and to take a pill every day or take a set of medicines every day, and to get their virus under control and to stay that way. *At every step of the way, there has to be some level of social engagement.* And there have to be some safety nets built in, and there has to be an easy level of navigation in the health system. The whole thing has to be put together in order to stay virally suppressed, which is the *clinical* outcome at the end of the day. But the *quality of life* outcome at the end of the day requires a whole lot more.

Observing the effectiveness of the HIV safety net firsthand made the examples of its gaps, failures, and shortcomings even more frustrating. Because the AIDS community had identified a model that worked reasonably well, it was difficult to witness instances in which the gains were not evenly distributed and the benefits not experienced by those who desperately needed them. Anthropologist Alyson O'Daniel and others have captured the variable experiences of women's access to resources, especially in the South.[13] Back at the Women's Collective in Washington, DC, Pat Nalls described in stark terms what happens when women don't have the resources and the space to address inequality's wounds in the wake of declining or nonexistent access to services:

> We used to give women a card to go to the grocery store, get some food . . . but we don't get that anymore in our grant. . . . So then, the next thing you know, they're coming in and they're asking us, "Can I have some of the cleansing wipes?" That's to do survival sex work. They will even tell you the corner where they will be, or you'll see them there. . . . Or we'll hear "I met this guy, and he said me and my kids could stay with him." We know what that means, right? . . . People are gonna have sex to have a place to spend the night. . . . People are gonna have sex without a condom while taking no medicine. They're going to put food on the table before filling a prescription that requires money for a copay.

Clearly, an underemphasis on the structural and behavioral approaches to AIDS care—one that deemphasizes issues of inequality, trauma, and the necessity for social and at times material support—has the potential to undermine the efficacy of the biomedical drives of test-and-treat and U = U. It also limits opportunities for women to launch transformative projects by not generating the space for the work of cognitive shifts and positive framing institutions to take hold.

.   .   .   .   .

Clearly, a great deal of work *can* be accomplished through a U = U approach that embraces the community-based supportive services for WLWHA. The structural, cultural, and material elements of the HIV safety net are not supplemental; they are *vital* to the very important public health goal of helping PLWHA achieve viral suppression. My research challenges an AIDS response that focuses solely on the medical management of the disease—healthcare interactions dedicated exclusively to tracking viral load and T-cell counts and prescribing ART—at the expense of reducing the scope of the HIV safety net. To achieve the desired medical outcome of viral load suppression, the pathway along the HIV healthcare continuum—diagnosis of HIV infection, linkage to care, retention in care, receipt of ART, and achievement of viral suppression—is best paved with attention to the social dimensions of women's lives and an HIV safety net that addresses these elements. As such, the HIV safety net remains an important site of activity in a new and highly medicalized era of AIDS.

5 Thriving Despite

> I was in church one day, and a woman who lived near my
> family years ago came over and asked me, "What happened
> to that sister of yours that used to get in all that trouble?"
> I said, "That would be me." She said, "Oh, that was you?"
> I said, "Yeah, that was me." She said, "Oh, okay, you
> got yourself together, huh?" I said, "Yeah, finally I got
> myself together and life is good." She said, "Well, you
> look good."
>
> —Beverly

If transformative projects are to succeed, they must be sustainable over time. After stabilizing their health and escaping immediate crises, transformed (and transforming) women confront what may be their most significant test: firmly establishing their new survival strategies to support their remade lives. How do women maintain this trajectory and even thrive following significant and notable transformations?

A systematic and deliberate process sustaining a new modus operandi involves generating and operationalizing a new identity and self-narrative; (re)claiming productive social roles within families, communities, and other social groups; and/or identifying a strategy (or set of strategies) to create economic stability. It may involve deeper political engagement, as women leverage the skills they learned from the HIV safety net to confront a variety of social ills. As Verna's daughter observed in the chapter's opening quote, sustaining a new modus operandi, like other components of the transformative project, is notably interactive: women are not only grappling with the difficult internal work of coming to terms with traumas of the past and building their futures; some are also being held account-able for the behaviors, struggles, and circumstances from before their transformations. They are renegotiating their status in the world and how others will come to see them as WLWHA.

Sustainability is the characteristic that best defines a successful trans-formation. Women's newfound life approaches will be challenged—by cir-cumstances, by the people in their lives, and from within—over many years. A momentary period away from behavior that risks economic, men-tal, or physical health is not sufficient to qualify as a transformative project. Returning to prior strategies such as silence, avoidance, denial or tactics such as self-medicating or high-risk behavior when new difficulties arise or when circumstances make it tempting undermines a transforma-tive project. One must instead adopt a framework and set of strategies for navigating inequality, and the instability and volatility it produces, that is tested and proves effective over time. While effective strategies ideally generate upward mobility, women also define success as achieving a state of stability that significantly reduces "drama" or economic, health-related, or social breakdowns in their lives.

Transformation, or *thriving despite*, is therefore an act of resistance.[1] Women who succeeded in executing transformative projects did not allow themselves to be reduced to the trope of "AIDS victim." They wanted to participate, to be included, and to have every right to live and love just like anyone else. They would not cede their status as mothers, even if they had made mistakes. They would not forgo the possibility of intimacy, despite living with an infectious disease. They would not surrender oppor-tunities to dream and pursue advancement, even when their systems of education and career development failed them. They transformed their post-diagnosis lives, not to adhere to an externally driven standard, but to remake themselves from within. They transformed themselves because they wanted new relationships with their children and other family mem-bers. They transformed themselves because, despite struggle, pain, and injuries, they wanted to live. They transformed themselves because they had grown tired—tired of the vicissitudes of the sexualized drug economy and other soul-sucking gauntlets. They transformed themselves because

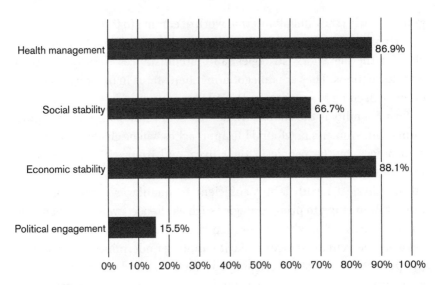

Figure 3. Transformation indicators for snapshot study respondents (*N* = 84).

they finally approached an intersection between their hopes and a structure that could lend support: the HIV safety net.

How do we know when transformation has taken place? As a social scientist, I am trained to identify certain measures or indicators of the social phenomenon of interest. In the course of speaking with women, certain guideposts became apparent, and I note them in figure 3. This list is not exhaustive, and I based my assessments on the women's self-reports and my research team's observations. Nevertheless, my approach outlines the major life domains in which we saw women move from severe crisis to stability, from *dying from* to *living with* to *thriving despite*.

First, I looked for evidence of a significant change in health management. For each respondent, my team and I analyzed whether she understood HIV or other health conditions she might be experiencing as a serious medical issue that could be managed. We looked for signs that she was proactively managing her health. Was she visiting her doctor regularly, taking medications as prescribed, and following advice pertaining to diet, exercise, sleep, and stress management? What were her doctors saying about her viral load and T-cell count, and were the numbers moving in the right direction? Had she achieved viral suppression (i.e., was her viral load at undetectable levels)? Did she describe other beneficial health outcomes that had taken place over the last several years? According to our criteria, 86.9 percent of the 84 women in the snapshot study experienced a transformation in health management since receiving their HIV diagnosis. Not all of them were virally suppressed when we interviewed them, but their doctors had indicated to them that their numbers were heading in the right direction.

Second, we looked for evidence of significant improvements in the size and quality of each respondent's social support networks over time. Did she have a community of supporters, and was she providing non-draining support to others? Did she describe her relationships with family members, friends, and romantic partners as healthy and supportive, even when conflicts arose? Was she involved in an intimate relationship that she deemed mutually beneficial? Alternatively, had she embraced being single as a choice rather than a consequence of her HIV status? Had she embraced her sexuality as a WLWHA, and had she discovered ways to constructively address a previous history of sexual trauma? According to our criteria, 66.7 percent of the snapshot study women experienced some significant shift or set of shifts in their social relationships after receiving their HIV diagnosis.

Third, we looked for evidence of significant improvements in each woman's economic situation. Was she economically stable, perhaps as a result of a steady job or monthly disability benefits? Or did she experience serious material instability in her day-to-day life and when challenges arose? To be sure, improving one's economic situation does not necessarily eliminate economic difficulties. A startling 70 percent of the 84 respondents in the Chicago study who participated in our one-time interviews reported annual household incomes of less than $20,000 per year, and 85 percent reported incomes below $40,000 per year. Women in this disproportionately impoverished group faced serious material hardship. Nevertheless, while looking for shifts in women's economic situations we were particularly interested in capturing gradual movement away from economic survival strategies and decision-making that greatly undermined physical safety, physical health, or mental health and toward strategies that could bring greater independence from others and greater month-to-month financial stability. Fifty-six percent of our respondents were moving in this direction thanks to government assistance (typically a combination of disability benefits, subsidized housing, and subsidized healthcare). Some were working in low-wage jobs and counted on the Earned Income Tax Credit and food stamps to maintain their financial stability. Others had higher-paying careers, so we looked for signs of stable employment and access to private insurance while trying to determine whether those women were jeopardizing their health to maintain their jobs. In all cases, we looked for some level of month-to-month financial stability to cover basic costs and strategies for accessing resources that did not increase health risks. According to our criteria, 88.1 percent of the 84 women we talked with experienced greater economic stability after their diagnosis, due largely to their involvement with the HIV safety net.

Fourth, we looked for evidence of increased political and civic engagement. This was typically linked to participation in the HIV safety net. Because political and community engagement are likely to change over time as life events draw one into other activities, we looked for histories of post-diagnosis participation as well as current participation at the time of the interview. We asked each respondent whether she served as a peer advocate or employee of an AIDS-related organization. Had she led a support group or participated in public speaking to educate people about HIV? Had she served on a community advisory board in an AIDS organization, or on a Ryan White planning council? Was she engaged in any AIDS activism and advocacy work? According to our criteria, 15.5 percent of the snapshot study women experienced deeper political engagement after launching transformative projects.

My team and I combed through transcripts for the presence of these indicators of long-term transformation. If there was significant evidence that three of the four improvements had taken place and were sustained over time (defined as twelve months or more), we considered a woman's transformative project a success. We recognize that this is a very crude measure and a moving target; transformation is best conceptualized as a dynamic process that can move in many directions, rather than as a destination reached on a straight line. Therefore, we also wanted to understand the following: When challenges arose regarding health, finances, relationships, or community engagement, were women's problem-solving strategies fundamentally different from those they followed prior to transformation, when they were *dying from* various health, social, economic, and community stressors? Did women come to resist environmental pressures and avoid coping strategies that could undermine their own physical, mental, or financial health? Were they confronting longstanding or newly emerging injuries of inequality in ways that were fundamentally different from how they had responded previously? And did the presence of institutions help women's abilities to overcome challenges?

Of the 84 women whom we interviewed as part of the Chicago study, 51 described significant shifts in at least three of four areas of their lives that we explored in depth: health management, economic stability, social relationships, and political/community engagement. In previous chapters, we learned in great detail how women made such changes, with our central storytellers giving us in-depth accounts of these processes in action. We will now consider in depth how each of the four indicators of transformation manifested itself in women's lives over the long run. Given the previous chapter's discussion of women's physical health and their health care experiences, we begin by looking at women's emotional well-being and identity reformation.

(RE)MAKING PEACE: IDENTITY (RE)FORMATION, WORTHINESS, AND ACCEPTANCE IN THE TRANSFORMATIVE PROJECT

Transformative projects are about inner work and outer work. The cognitive shift in which women decide that "something has to change" is only one part of the inner work of transformation. Transforming women also revise assumptions and challenge beliefs they may have held for decades. They develop the ability to question the internal and external voices that tell them that their deaths are imminent, that they are unworthy of love and care, and that silence is the best and only strategy for coping with pain. Transforming women create new tapes in their minds, new messages to help frame and emotionally work through the injuries of inequality they have suffered and may continue to suffer. Women do not condone the structural and interpersonal violence to which they have been subjected. Nor does transformation involve accepting blame for circumstances and events over which they have no control. I observed, however, that when women found ways to confront, process, and interpret injuries they have suffered and to broker some level of peace with themselves and the events that have occurred in their lives, they were much better positioned to navigate future struggles.

Self-acceptance is a critical element of the transformative project. Black feminist scholars have noted that in a society that routinely traffics in anti-black and misogynistic messaging, self-acceptance holds radical potential.[2] It is linked to self-love and self-care, which can be interpreted as acts of social and even political resistance in a population that has been maligned and regularly battles shame. Beverly described her process, revealing a great deal about the early motivations that contributed to the woman we met in chapter 1 and how she changed into the woman who could tell her fellow church member, "I got myself together, and life is good":

> I knew I had the power, but I did not know to what extent. See, because I had come up in a household where my spirit was attacked on a daily basis. So I didn't come up with good self-esteem because I had a sister that was conditioning me, telling me I was ugly on a regular basis. So as I grew up, I grew up thinking that. So I moved in that way. So if you think it, so it is. Had I been told something different then maybe I would have lived a different life. My perception of the world would have been different. So it wasn't until after I grew up suffering mentally from that, moving in a way that a person with low self-esteem moved. Because when you suffer from low self-esteem, then you move in that way. Instead of you going for the best, you just settle for less because you don't think you can get what you truly want. Not even trying, because you don't think that's even an option for you, so you just settle for anything. That's a process that takes place over time. And if we don't ever find a way out of it, then consequently, a lot of people will live in that and stay in it for the rest of their life. Fortunately for me, I was able to get out, get some healing, get some real sense of my whole life from start to finish and just everything that has taken place and the part I played in it. . . . I understand that most of my life, I moved in brokenness. I was broken. I was . . . I was wounded . . . my spirit was wounded. So I moved like a wounded soul.

Beverly's reflections peel away a new layer of the meaning of *dying from*. The double blow of early sexual abuse and her sister's taunts, the fascination with the fast life and Beverly's need to attract the "big players" in the neighborhood, and living in an environment that conditioned her to "settle for anything" because it would be the best she could get: these were injuries that began externally and later became self-inflicted. Challenging and reversing that pattern would take years of work: in rehab, in the support group network, and with a private therapist. "I haven't arrived," she explained, affirming the notion that the transformative project is a process, not a destination. "I don't think I'm going to arrive in this lifetime. I'm just going to stay on the road."

One's sense of worthiness lies at the heart of any transformative project, and this becomes particularly vexing for black and brown women who battle intersectional stigmas. Phill Wilson offered a provocative quote that resonated with me as I watched some of the Chicago study women struggle with their coping trajectories:

> The part that keeps me up at night is worrying whether "we," meaning black people, believe enough that A: our lives are worth saving and B: we believe in our own efficacy to do it. I think our fundamental challenge is, are we worth it? Are we worth the effort: am I willing to work that hard to save *my* life? Am I willing to work that hard to save *your* life? And here's the difference. And this is a very, very, important issue on the race question: the white boys in 1984 were willing to work that hard. Because they *knew* that their lives were worth it; they knew it. Everything in our culture and their upbringing, everything told them that their lives were worth it; and there was not a price they weren't willing to pay to save their lives.

Spirituality often played an important role in the process by which women remade their identities. As Lupe (Latina, 56) explained, "I used to be in prison. I used to be a very violent person. I've got bullets in my body. I've got stab wounds. But when God came to my life, I just put it at God. I don't react no more. I never let things upset me like that." Beverly agreed:

> For me, after 11 years clean, you understand that it's not about the drugging. Drugging was only a symptom of the problem. It was the person that needed . . . that had issues dealing with . . . emotions and feelings. So I have to stay centered, stay balanced, doing what I need to do to stay spiritually toned and fed so I'm peaceful. So it takes more than just my recovery meetings to get me there. It takes my church, it takes my spiritual food, it takes me reading.

Unfortunately for Keisha, the process of gaining acceptance was marked by disappointing setbacks. She met Jacob, a white man who lived in her neighborhood, and their friendship soon blossomed into a romantic relationship. But in the decade during which I followed her, Keisha also developed a drinking problem, which began affecting her adherence to her HIV medication as she missed doses. News that she was pregnant caused Keisha to make changes. She stopped drinking immediately. "Don't get me wrong, I had the urges," Keisha explained, "I mean, it was horrible that I would actually have urges." When I visited her while she was pregnant with her daughter in 2016, Keisha was slowly growing into the belief that she was worth the fight for a better life. By the end of the study, Keisha was consistently taking her HIV medications, she and Jacob had married, and they were happily raising their new daughter. During our final interview, ten-year-old Jordan, whom Keisha was carrying when we met in 2004, wandered into the kitchen where his mother and I were speaking, kissing her on the cheek before heading outside to play basketball.

(RE)MAKING SOCIAL RELATIONSHIPS

Women's engagement with the HIV safety net tended to change over time, from intensive daily engagement with framing institutions at crisis points to periodic interactions with medical providers for routine care. After a period of robust participation in the HIV safety net that included heavy use of support groups, long-term residencies in housing facilities for PLWHA, or regular participation in AIDS advocacy work, their reliance on these institutional networks shifted as their lives evolved. Many essentially "graduated" from intensive case management while ideally maintaining their connection to healthcare. They found other forms of long-term institutional social support, often through churches.

Women who maintained multi-year connections to weekly HIV support groups were often also in recovery for drug and alcohol addictions, as meeting attendance was viewed as an ongoing and even lifelong part of the recovery process. Others lived in residential buildings for families affected by HIV/AIDS and thus came into contact with members of the

AIDS community regularly. Rosario is one of these women: "Now I go to the support groups for just a stress reliever, just to kind of talk generally about whatever we have on our minds. It's like a venting tool. You can go, and you can talk, and feel comfortable around your peers, and be able to say whatever it is you need to say, and leave it there."

Janine, a case manager at a community health center in Chicago, expressed a similar view. For her, a successful transformative project frequently involves individuals gradually shifting to a focus on social networks outside of the HIV safety net. She explained the transitional nature of her relationship with clients:

> I believe that it depends on where the woman is in her life. I had a client that I just knew would never work. I thought, "There is no way she's going to go and get a job." She always maintained her medical appointments. She maintained her case management appointments, but it just seemed like she was just so comfortable with going to support groups, making her case management appointment, and just spending her time with her family. She was getting Social Security benefits. And then she said, "I got a job!" So you never should assume, but always keep it open that it is a possibility.

Women also had to recalibrate and renegotiate their relationships with family members, friends, and acquaintances who were now witnessing significant changes. Disclosure, the revelation of a personal detail such as one's HIV status, is a dynamic process. Women often disclose over a long span of time, to a few people at a time. Many began by living in post-diagnosis silence—hiding their medications, perhaps even avoiding medical care altogether. One thing that surprised Beverly was the acceptance that people extended to her when she finally revealed her HIV status: "When I found out I had the virus, I didn't know what to expect, how people were going to act. So I prepared for the worst . . . but it didn't turn out that way." Long-term survivors in particular saw their HIV status recede into the background in their relationships with their families. Charlene said, "Just living with it for so many years, it's just something that's a part of me. They're used to it." Similarly, Rosario had this to say:

> I have very supportive friends. I have a best friend who I've known 20-plus years and we have been just really tight. I mean this has actually brought us closer, because I told her about my diagnosis. She's getting married in July,

and I'm in her wedding. Yes, my friends have been so supportive of me. They call me, check on me. I have male friends as well, who call me and check on me to make sure that I'm okay.

This is not to suggest that HIV stigma is a thing of the past. In this book, we have encountered many stories about the ignorance and prejudice that remains associated with HIV/AIDS. But as the epidemic has evolved, new treatments have become more effective and available, and public figures like Magic Johnson have continued to thrive; the public's views appear to be slowly evolving in turn.

(Re)Making Motherhood

Among the most complex relationships women described were those with their children. Less than a handful of the women's children were also living with HIV, a testament to the significant work that has been done over the past 30 years to dramatically reduce perinatal transmission in the United States. In the epidemic's earliest years, as we heard from Pat Nalls and others, women were confronting their own mortality and determining who would raise their children if they were to succumb to the disease. Yvette reflected, "I thought I would die within like three years [of getting diagnosed]. When my son Steven graduated from grade school, they had some little kiddie graduation. And I was the only one in there crying, because I thought, 'Well, they probably think I'm overreacting but they just don't know, this may be the only graduation that I see my son at, you know.'"

As these mothers watched their children grow up, defying estimates of how long they would live, they had to contend with yet another challenge as long-term survivors of HIV. Many like Yvette worried that the disease undermined their credibility as role models, making them questionable paragons of sexual virtue and parental authority. Yvette and I conducted our final interview in 2014, when I arranged to visit her in Washington, DC. Now 47, she had moved back to the East Coast a year prior, seeking a stronger support system. Her son, now 28, had recently moved back in with her after a stint in California. She was still working for the government, albeit in a different role, making over $100,000 per year after decades of climbing the ranks. Her viral load was undetectable. She hadn't connected much with the AIDS community after her years of participating in the support group scene in Chicago, but she very much enjoyed the company of her sisters back east. She still had disclosed her status to only one sister, but she had taken the big step of telling her son:

> I finally told him. I cried through the whole thing. I wasn't boo-hoo crying, but you could hear it in my voice. You could hear the quiver in my voice. And so, he says, "Well ma, you know, I wished you would have told me earlier. It's okay, everything's still exactly the same." I think it mattered a great deal because I didn't expect him to say that. And I see that he takes great pains, whenever we go out to dinner, to drink from my straw, which irritates the hell out of me! I hate it, but he does it. And I'm like, okay, if that's his way of accepting it and saying, "I'm okay with you," then I just let him. I'm fine with it. But it's not sanitary [laughs]! I'm a germaphobe!

Others used their HIV-positive status to deliver teachable moments. Rosario learned that her eldest daughter's father, with whom she had an on-again, off-again relationship for years, tested positive for HIV. He had died of what she believes to be AIDS-related complications just days before our interview. Although she did not share these details with her children, she has used her status as a tool to teach her children about protecting themselves:

> My kids have actually taken it very well. I've talked to them about it . . . So I don't really see a change in their attitude about that. I think that they're so eager to learn more about it because I am suffering with it. So they want to be more aware and teach someone else about it. So my daughter, especially, she's so eager to know more about it, so I always show her my T-cell count and viral load whenever I go to the doctor. "This is me, and you know that you don't want to be in the same predicament as me, so you want to take steps in order to protect yourself." We go through that whole scenario every day, and my son, too. . . . It's actually a tool, a kind of a scared-straight type of deal, to kind of keep them focused. STDs, HIV especially, this is something that cannot be toyed with.

Women with histories of drug addiction were seeking to (re)establish their credibility and reclaim the moral high ground as parents after sometimes years of being inconsistent, absent, or troubled. The long-term impact of pre-transformation lives on children was one of the hardest things for the women we interviewed to acknowledge. Despite their willingness to peel back the curtain and wrestle with histories of sexual trauma, addiction, and survival sex, analyzing and talking about the imprint their periods of struggle may have had on their children was almost an impossible truth to bear.

An important part of their transformation therefore involved deciding how to address the impact of their pre-transformation lives on their children and other family members. This was a decidedly gendered phenomenon. While men may have to account for absenteeism or an inconsistent record of caregiving, women are likely to be subjected to even more scrutiny and judgment due to gendered expectations placed on them as mothers. Gwen (black, age 56), who had once used her adult daughter's basement as a party space during her heaviest days of drug use, was still working to gain back her daughter's trust. "It hurts like hell," she said, referring to her loss of parental authority and the emotional distance between them. "I'm not going to say it don't hurt, it hurts. But I'm not going to let my kids' [anger] get me back to drugs and alcohol. I fought, I fought too hard to get where I'm at." Beverly was adamant about not allowing her adult daughter to hold her absence or struggles over her head to manipulate her: "Because a lot of people can't accept the fact that I might have been using ten years ago, but I did an about-face and now I'm at another point in life."

(Re)Making Intimacy and Overcoming Sexual Trauma

What does sexual autonomy look like for women living with HIV/AIDS? How do they exercise sexual agency? Discussions of the sexuality of WLWHA often frame the issue in terms of risk reduction and sexual responsibility. While this is critically important for public and individual health, this emphasis has at least two consequences. First, the romantic and sexual lives of WLWHA are often medicalized, and the important social dimensions of their intimate relationships are often overlooked. Second, if not approached carefully, conversations about risk reduction can demonize the sexuality of WLWHA by constructing them as deviant and dangerous, especially if they continue to have sexual lives. For example, Stevie (black, age 44) described being horrified at "carrying the package," believing that she was forever sexually undesirable and vulnerable to stigmatization and rejection. We also talked with women like Charlene, who were celibate because, as she put it, "I don't want to meet somebody and tell them I'm HIV positive, so I'd rather just not deal with it."

However, the vast majority of women with whom we spoke were either in relationships, dating regularly, or just coming out of romantic involvements. HIV had not foreclosed the possibility of an intimate life. Rosario and her boyfriend were about to celebrate a year of dating when we interviewed her. She disclosed that she was living with HIV in the first three weeks of their relationship. "At first it was kind of hard for me to tell him about my status," she explained. "But I found myself being comfortable enough to tell him, and we've actually been very close. It's actually been good. He's been one of my support systems as well, as far as the emotional thing. He's great in my life. He loves my kids." Taking precautions to prevent transmission is an important part of their relationship. "I keep condoms, dental dams, all kinds of prophylactics in my drawer. There are never times when I don't use them. I know my situation, and I don't want to pass it on to anyone else."

The message of U = U, undetectable = untransmittable, offered even greater potential for women's sexual lives, an opportunity that some described as removing the biohazard symbol that they imagined was tattooed on their foreheads. But even with tools to protect against transmission, the road to sexual acceptance was difficult. When Chicago study women were diagnosed, they pondered whether they would find romantic partners who would not shun them because of HIV. As Rosario explained, "I always think, I have this disease, is it going to come between what we've established between each other? So I have that in the back of my mind. Sometimes I do worry. . . . So I guess I just have to kind of play it by ear. If he really wants to be with me, he will. Time will tell, that's how I deal with it."

It was therefore not unusual for the women we interviewed to date individuals who were part of the HIV safety net, living in the same designated building for PLWHA, fellow members of their HIV support groups, or co-residents in drug recovery programs. Such dating was discouraged by staff members, who were concerned that individuals should focus solely on addressing their health and other challenges and that relationships born in these environments often created drama and tension. Nevertheless, almost one-third of the Chicago study women interviewed

disclosed that they met their first partners after launching their transformative projects through the HIV safety net. For example, Beverly met
a man on a cruise for PLWHA and they were married within a year. They
divorced shortly thereafter: "Once we got married, he thought I would
change my mind and move to Florida with him."

As women came to terms with the diagnosis and experienced disclosure over time, many learned how best to have the conversation and grew
more comfortable doing so. For example, Yvette struggled from the beginning with disclosing her status to men she was dating. She found it so
stressful that she withdrew from the dating scene for years. In 2014, she
shared a different experience:

> I recently got a boyfriend after I don't know how many years. I'm so excited,
> and there was no quiver in my voice [when I told him]. There was no crying.
> It was just a straightforward conversation.... I think something within me
> over these last few years has made me come to accept it really as a medical
> condition and so, "Don't be so embarrassed and don't be so stigmatized. Just
> talk about it." I told him, "Do your research. If you decide that you don't want
> to get involved with me, I understand, and it's cool." He said, "No, I don't think
> this will change anything. I'll do like you asked, and I'll do my research. I'll talk
> to my doctor. But I really don't think this will change anything." You know,
> because I hadn't kissed him. I don't think I had hugged him or anything. I like
> telling people . . . right away so, you know, so if we do become intimate in any
> way, even a kiss. . . they won't blame me. I just like getting it out of the way.

The women who seemed to struggle the most with their sexual lives,
perhaps not surprisingly, were those who had experienced sexual trauma.
Engaging in sexual activity with an intimate partner could be challenging
given the walls that women built and the ways in which they often separated sex from intimacy during their pre-transformation lives. Historian
Darlene Clark Hine describes a "culture of dissemblance" in which black
women's attitudes and behaviors under systems of gendered and racialized violence offered the appearance of openness and disclosure but actually shielded their inner lives and selves to protect them from oppressors.[3]
Krishna Stone, a longtime staff person at the GMHC in New York, characterized it for me in even starker terms: "People have sex for a variety of
reasons, and if they are able to experience pleasure in the process, they are
fortunate."

We learned of Gwen's history of molestation at the hands of her uncle and godfather in chapter 1. She spent years in the sexualized drug economy, and her experiences with dissembling made intimacy difficult:

> My mental state now is better, but sometimes with my boyfriend, I'll go off on him. If sex is a certain way, especially the oral, I'll like just go off on him for no reason. Don't touch my head, because now you're forcing me. He's like, "But I don't understand." In the streets they could do it, but he couldn't do it. I didn't give a damn in the street because, you know, I'm gonna block this shit out of my mind. I want this [drug] bag. Okay, you want to hold my head, you go ahead. But sometimes it flares up when I find myself with him. I guess I look at him, he should have more respect. I don't know. Sometimes my mental state sexually goes and comes. I'm getting better at it.

As women worked through the pain of their traumas, they sought to stop dissembling as they communicated their needs in the pursuit of intimacy and pleasure. In these encounters with her boyfriend, Gwen is trying to gauge—moment by moment—the degree of control she can exercise to do what she will with her body. She is also learning what it means for her mind to be fully present with her partner during sex. Gwen sees a therapist and regularly attends Narcotics Anonymous support group meetings:

> I'm learning today. The relationship me and [my boyfriend] have is never forced, it's not being forced up on me. He's not threatening me. He ain't threatening to hurt my family, my mom, or nobody. When we know we're going to have sex, I have to focus. I go and sit, and I tell myself, "You need to enjoy. You're not six, you're not twelve. You're a grown woman. This is not your uncle, and this is not your godfather." I just finished one step forward in the program and that step helps you, what we call, clean out all your secrets, your resentments, your sex. And it's taught me, even though I let it destroy most of my childhood and my adulthood, today my uncle and them are dead. They can't hurt me no more, and every man ain't out to get me. Every man ain't out to use me sexually. So emotionally it's coming along. I'm making some progress. I'm learning.

Historian of science and black feminist scholar Evelynn Hammonds writes, "Silence, erasure, and the use of images of immoral sexuality abound in narratives about the experiences of black women with AIDS. Their voices are not heard in discussions of AIDS, while intimate details of their lives are exposed to justify their victimization."[4] Unlike the sympathetic portrayals of HIV/AIDS among white gay men and their devastating losses of love and intimacy that began to emerge in the 1980s through popular culture, the overall silence around the loss of love and intimacy experienced by WLWHA is striking. It prevents us from seeing these women in ways that both recognize their sexuality as part of their humanity and help us understand how intimate ties influence other domains in their lives.

For her part, Beverly described attending the funeral of her ex-boyfriend Ricky, whom she believes transmitted the virus to her. She underscores the pitfalls of what Jenny Higgins and colleagues critique as "the vulnerability paradigm," which suggests that women are universally oppressed and men form a powerful, monolithic group in the AIDS epidemic:[5] "I know he didn't do it intentionally. I know that he loved me and wouldn't have done anything to hurt me." Beverly remembered noticing the change in his body; he had lost a significant amount of weight when she ran into him once after their breakup. She reached out to Ricky's mother before the funeral, and she revealed that Ricky died of complications due to AIDS. He was just 25 years old:

> I was really in love with him. He was really in love with me, too. But he was at a point in his life where he was hustling. . . . I remember him telling me that he was tired all the time and he thought it was because of me. [Laughs] . . . He went down [died] quick because once he found out [he had AIDS], it was like he kind of had a nervous breakdown, and he just gave up. It was just really hard. And it was so unfortunate because he died in 1996. And there was beginning to be meds . . . but there wasn't a lot of information available. And then he was a heterosexual man, too. So he probably couldn't bear it, the stigma of that, you know. It was more than he could deal with. But it was . . . it was heavy.

A cadre of black feminist theorists have convincingly argued that a paradigm that reduces women's sexuality to a focus on sexual risk and trauma is quite limiting and negates the complexity of their lives.[6] In these examples, we see how sexuality is intricately woven into women's lives post-diagnosis as they move from, to borrow from Hammonds, a "politics of silence" to a "politics of articulation."[7] Intimacy, love, desire, and sexual pleasure are important aspects of identity that must be negotiated, sometimes with histories of trauma and loss vying for control over thoughts and emotions. Moreover, because sex has been fraught in the past for so many, what we heard from the women were their attempts to put themselves— rather than their partners, their addictions, or the messages they had absorbed—at the center of their sexual experiences. As women renegotiated their intimate relationships and sexual scripts, they were able to see themselves as sexually desirable despite their HIV status. Sexuality, therefore, became yet another important landscape for women to determine what it meant to move from *dying from* to *living with*. For Beverly and others, this was not about ignoring or apologizing for sexual desire but finding ways to express it in a manner that was affirming, pleasurable, and kept their sense of self-worth intact.

(RE)MAKING ENDS MEET: THE ECONOMICS OF TRANSFORMATION

In the pre-ART era, when post-diagnosis life expectancy was limited, many PLWHA dropped out of or reduced their participation in the labor force.[8] With the advent of ART in the mid-1990s, although many hoped to return to work, doing so was difficult due to uncertainty regarding the efficacy of ART, potentially debilitating medication side effects, the possibility of losing disability insurance, difficulties transitioning into the labor force after a long absence, the effects of long work hours and work stress on health, difficulty managing medical appointments and elaborate drug regimens while working, and the fear that disclosure might jeopardize one's job.[9]

With the increased efficacy of ART, Chicago study women who were working at the time of diagnosis for the most part stayed in the labor force. Many of the issues mentioned above remained, but leaving jobs became less feasible or desirable as women contemplated longer life expectancies and the reality that an HIV diagnosis does not alone constitute immediate eligibility for disability benefits. Women therefore focused on organizing economic survival strategies that would be conducive to their overall health, whether basing their employment decisions on securing health insurance, finding employment outside of the sexualized drug economy, or applying for Social Security Disability Insurance benefits due to a co-occurring illness.

When Beverly completed her drug rehabilitation program, her career as a trained hairstylist was long behind her. She would need to put together a new economic plan: "When I got clean, I had to change how I was making money." She turned first to a network that had proved to be quite helpful: the HIV safety net. It has been an especially effective source of employment for people with challenging or limited job histories, whose experiential knowledge provides a useful resource for HIV prevention and treatment peer education and support. One year into her visits to Coach House, Beverly began volunteering there. She became a paid employee, a case manager, in 1995.

As we learned in the previous chapter, in the biomedical era of AIDS work that relies less on grassroots community engagement, many of the opportunities akin to what Beverly accessed at Coach House are going away. However, it bears noting how volunteering and later working for an AIDS organization facilitated economic mobility for someone who desperately needed a chance.[10] With only a high school diploma, Beverly then realized that she needed more education if she was going to advance; "Whatever I was gonna do, I needed some education to do it." She earned an associate's degree and found a mentor at the community college who then helped her pursue a bachelor's degree. Within just five years of being hired for her first paid job after leaving jail and rehab, Beverly had earned two post-secondary degrees, all while serving other PLWHA as a case manager. Beverly then worked as a case manager for seven years at one of the flagship HIV/AIDS organizations in Chicago, providing technical assistance to other AIDS service organizations, speaking at schools about HIV prevention, and engaging in political advocacy work. She bought and renovated a townhouse on the South Side and sought investment properties as she observed the slow gentrification of the area. Harkening back to that young girl who was rudely awakened while helping her mother write checks on a shoestring budget, Beverly was entrepreneurial and strategic.

When I met her in 2005, Beverly was making over $65,000 a year as a government public health employee. She was also taking evening classes toward a master's degree in public health that she completed over the course of our interviews. Beverly networked heavily within and outside of the AIDS community, always thinking about her next professional step and connecting others to resources. "Whenever somebody has the virus," she explained, "my friends call me. I have one friend whose brother has the virus and they needed help and they called. I help people get whatever they need."

Beverly was also working with an attorney to achieve the one thing she deemed crucial to sustaining her transformative project: clemency from her criminal convictions. "I am tired of having a glass ceiling. And I know in my heart of hearts that I've been passed over for a few jobs because of my background. Because they would hire me and then when they'd fingerprint me, they'd tell me something else, somebody else was selected, so you know what that's about. Even if I get a PhD, I might still encounter that." When her petition for clemency was denied, Beverly decided to fulfill a lifelong dream and in 2012 moved to California. Twenty years since her last conviction, Beverly's criminal record was not an impediment in California and she was free to pursue her passions. She became a social worker, pursuing a master's degree in the field that was funded by her employer. This would complement the master's in public health that she completed in Chicago. Building on over two decades of experience in the social services, Beverly has found a new cause to champion, child welfare.

I observed time and again that HIV itself was not holding women back from economic mobility. In the current era of ART, many of the physical challenges had been alleviated and women could conceal their HIV status or decide that it simply wasn't relevant to share. As Beverly explained, "We aren't sleeping together, so I don't really see why it's relevant. I'm functioning—better than most of the employees in there—and it doesn't affect my job."

Rather, for a large subset of WLWHA, the very circumstances, histories, barriers, and behaviors that increased their risk of infection also made them less employable. As Layla (white, age 41) explained, "It's real hard finding a job. Not because I have HIV. I have a record. I have a felony. It's six years old now, and they usually don't want people unless their felonies are like seven years [old] or more. And even then it can be an issue." Moving from fast money to slow wages had significant drawbacks. While women were leaving behind the physical risks and emotional tolls attached to labor in the sexualized drug economy, finding economic stability in the "legit" economy was not always easy.

Some survival strategies were in fact still putting women at risk physically, and the economic instability was a serious health threat. Homelessness, returning to the drug game, and sex work could all lead to risky sexual and drug entanglements that might yield resources in the short run but that could quickly set women back into a state of *dying from,* something that members of the HIV community working on the ground understood all too well. Indeed, many saw the economic stability question as the next frontier in HIV services. Naina Khanna of PIN–USA explains, "I wouldn't necessarily argue for building a separate system for employment. But I think there are ways that the Ryan White Act could institutionalize, in every jurisdiction they fund, a vocational rehab coordinator who's a link to the workforce development world. It's very necessary."

(RE)MAKING AN ACTIVIST: THE POLITICAL
POTENTIAL OF REMAKING A LIFE

Transforming women frequently transform their environments. Whether confronting a family member about AIDS stigma or doing a speaking engagement, women described the positive influence they were able to exert on the lives of others as their transformative projects matured. As one Chicago study woman explained: "Just about everybody that knows me knows that I'm positive. Especially if I see them doing stupid shit that puts them at risk, that's usually the time that I have 'the talk.' I don't want them to hear [about my status] from somebody else, or just see me on TV doing stuff [around HIV]." A small but important segment (15.5 percent) of the women we interviewed were actively engaged in AIDS political work in Chicago. Gwen has taken several classes on HIV offered by LifeForce and was excited about an upcoming trip: "The seventeenth of this month, a busload of us are going to the state capital to visit lawmakers and advocate for funds toward HIV/AIDS."

The HSN is responsible for cultivating a cadre of female AIDS leaders domestically and abroad. As director of the Policy and Data Division of HRSA's HIV/AIDS Bureau, Antigone Dempsey is one of the nation's top Ryan White HIV/AIDS Program policy officials. She offers her perspective as a WLWHA rather than in her official capacity at HRSA. She joined her first

HIV support group just days after being diagnosed in 1990 at the age of 22 in her hometown of San Francisco. "I tested positive on a Saturday, and I went in that Monday night to the support group. I was in recovery for alcoholism, and I knew that I needed to be with people going through what I was going through." Antigone quickly moved up the ranks, from group facilitator to executive director of a new community-based HIV organization, to serving as a national voice on HIV/AIDS policy for youth. She was motivated in those early years by the warmth of the community and "a drive I felt to do something. Like, maybe I won't die if I have a role, and I'm able to make an effort. I didn't realize until later that I was negotiating with God or a higher power."

The goal of the Positive Women's Network (PWN) is to elevate this local work to the national and international stage, to train women to see themselves as political activists. In 2007, a small delegation of WLWHA from around the country, including Naina Khanna, attended a global YWCA conference on HIV. They were impressed with the delegations from South Africa, India, and other countries that had created national networks of women living with HIV and were holding their governments accountable to address their concerns. The United States needed a stronger policy advocacy voice for WLWHA, the US delegation reasoned, one that deliberately centered the voices of the women of color and the low-income women who constituted the majority of WLWHA in the country. Transgender women were also included in the conversation from the beginning, joining the convening of 28 WLWHA from across the country who would become PWN-USA. The group agreed to stand for principles that prioritized the needs of the most marginalized among them, with staff leadership and a board of directors that would reflect that commitment. As founding executive director Naina explained, "Class privilege, whiteness, racism, cisgender privilege, none of that should determine who gets to lead and whose voices matter."

The budding PWN-USA was called into action almost immediately. In the run-up to the 2008 presidential election, the larger AIDS community secured commitments from then candidates Barack Obama and John McCain to create a National HIV/AIDS strategy (NHAS). As activists and advocates began discussions about a draft plan, PWN noticed that WLWHA did not have an organized voice at the table. Shortly after Obama's election, PWN submitted the first-ever set of policy recommendations to a sitting transition team written entirely by WLWHA. Members of PWN were appointed to the Presidential Advisory Council on HIV/AIDS (PACHA) and advocated for black WLWHA to have a seat on the influential body.

PWN member Gina Brown became the second black woman living with HIV in history to be appointed to PACHA. She too is a transformed woman: she has become one of the most influential and well-networked AIDS activists in the country after recovering from crack addiction. Gina earned a master's degree in social work and serves on several local and national advisory boards. Sitting on PACHA during the Obama administration, she lent her input during the crafting of the second NHAS. "It was amazing," she said. "You knew that when you were speaking, the government officials in the room had the ability to bring it to President Obama and to his staff and that things were going to happen."

PWN partnered with other AIDS organizations and racked up several policy wins that are clearly aligned with what we have learned about WLWHA. They advocated for PACHA to pass a resolution on the needs of women in the epidemic and successfully advocated for President Obama to issue an executive order in 2013 creating a federal interagency working group on HIV, violence against women, and gender-related health disparities. The updated NHAS released in 2015 noted violence and trauma in the lives of WLWHA and included metrics for trauma-informed care. These gains were in part due to PWN's work as a local organizing partner for the 2012 International AIDS Conference in Washington, DC. The conference featured a historic plenary address by founding PWN member Linda Scruggs entitled "Making Women Count: A Comprehensive Agenda." In the address, Scruggs detailed her own transformation from *dying from* to *living with* to *thriving despite,* revealing her experiences with sexual and physical violence and the sexualized drug economy. The organization followed the presentation with a press conference featuring the latest research on WLWHA and the voices of more PWN members.

The injuries that so many WLWHA had experienced were finally gaining the political visibility necessary to move the conversation forward and influence policy. As AIDS policy expert Dr. Vignetta Charles observed,

PWN started with . . . 28 members, and now they're at like 3,000. There was a point where it came together, and we all felt it in the field. Suddenly PWN was everywhere and present, and there was no more forgetting women [in the epidemic]. . . . Federal partners ended up paying attention, and then resources followed. There were a lot of steps in between there, but I think it was a pivotal moment for an issue to be raised to the level of an International AIDS Conference plenary with Linda talking about her experience in a way that could not be ignored. And then the press conference. Resources followed. So that, I think, was a pretty critical moment.

This demonstrates a final component of women's transformative projects: becoming politically engaged and transforming their communities. Despite the biomedicalization push that threatens to reduce HIV/AIDS to a medical issue requiring only medical solutions, organizations like PWN maintain an unrelenting focus on attacking inequality and arguing for both policy and programmatic solutions to address trauma experienced by both communities and individuals. From the world stage at international AIDS conferences to passionate debates in meeting rooms in which the AIDS community is hashing out policy positions, these women are pushing the bounds of AIDS work. The intersectional social justice frame stands as both a companion and a counterweight to the biomedical and behavioral focus in growing amounts of HIV/AIDS work. Its proponents think critically about the structures of power that perpetuate entrenched inequality and how they might be upended, taking on issues such as HIV decriminalization, criminal justice reform, voting rights, and healthcare reform. Reminiscent of the ways in which the Black Panther Party's health activism—such as fighting for access to medical treatment—was an extension of its earlier forms of advocacy and organizing, these broader forms of advocacy and organizing among WLWHA are extensions of their early health activism.[11] As the individual agency captured in chapter 3 moves to a collective agency through political engagement, WLWHA are reshaping the conversation and the future of the epidemic.

CHUTES, LADDERS, AND SAFETY NETS: NAVIGATING VOLATILITY AND ONGOING INJURIES OF INEQUALITY

Just months after I visited the support group described at the beginning of chapter 3, Trisha suffered a massive stroke. It was a devastating setback, hobbling her ability to walk, talk, drive, and accomplish other tasks. Her various commitments in the AIDS community would have to be sidelined. Unable to live alone, Trisha left her small apartment and moved in with Darla, whom she met through their connections to AIDS organizations. She interrupted her education at the local community college, one course shy of her associate's degree, and attended speech therapy several times a month. In many ways, this would be yet another time at which Trisha was beginning again; the last time was when she went into treatment with nothing to her name: "Nothing. I took a holey pair of slippers and started my life over." Trisha's story reminds us that even after women transform their post-diagnosis lives, they still experience challenges and crises. Some endure further injuries of inequality, especially in the absence of larger structural interventions.

What we should note, however, is that we saw over time changes in women's coping strategies that were informed by their own cognitive shifts; their access to the HIV safety net and its resources, communities of support, and information; and new tools with which to overcome future obstacles. Their new ways of moving in the world reflected new strategies for self-love and acceptance, navigating relationships, and sustaining themselves financially. What we also saw, from the local to the national levels, were the ways in which WLWHA moved from *dying from* to *living with* and even *thriving despite*, expanding their voices on the national and global stage to confront HIV and related issues of inequality.

Inequality Flows
through the Veins

TRANSFORMATIVE LESSONS FROM
THE AIDS RESPONSE

In communities around the world, there are women whose lives are remarkably similar to those of the women we have met in this book. They are stigmatized because of some undesirable social characteristic, deemed unworthy and undeserving of our care and concern. Their lives may have been relatively stable before the crisis arrived. Or they may have suffered from a host of physical, emotional, and economic traumas. While some may be tempted to disregard these women or ignore their potential, it would be foolhardy to do so. We lose valuable political voices, mothers to children, partners to those looking for loving relationships, and teachers to those of us trying to understand important issues. We lose valuable members of our nation and even the world when we choose to ignore, stereotype, or reduce women to the circumstances they face or the choices they make, especially when those choices are so limited. Many of the personal transformative projects I have described benefit the greater good, and their contributions would be lost without the courage of the women who carried them out.

SIX KEY ANALYTICS

I've presented six core concepts or key analytics for thinking about women, inequality, and the AIDS epidemic: injuries of inequality, *dying from* to *living with* to *thriving despite*, the sexualized drug economy, the HIV safety net, framing institutions, and the transformative project. The injuries of inequality that women endure are rarely happenstance or void of context; they are historical, social, and political. They result from the proximity of individuals and communities to state, institutional, and interpersonal violence that results in systemic harm. I am very deliberate about my use of the term "injuries of inequality" rather than "social determinants of health." I want to emphasize the bidirectional relationship between inequality and health and center the root causes of these injuries: growing economic, social, and political inequities that exact devastating consequences on the lives of those with limited power.

I sought to capture how women process and interpret the shock of an HIV diagnosis alongside past and present traumas, their in-progress attempts at upward mobility, or both. Physical and psychological wounds can hobble women for decades—stopping them short from getting tested for HIV, wrestling them to the ground when they need to visit a doctor or take the day's dosage of life-saving medication, and grabbing them by the throat just when their voices need to be heard. As women suffer both the physical costs of HIV and its experienced, anticipated, and internalized stigma, we have seen how they often sink deeper into physical, emotional, or economic distress, essentially dying from the injuries of inequality they have sustained.

Such experiences do not take place in a vacuum. Structural conditions form the backdrop to the AIDS epidemic in the United States. A series of public policies, budget cuts, and economic divestment drained job opportunities, physical and mental health services, and other resources from many of the communities in which the women in this book came of age. Residential segregation and a sharp spike in mass incarceration were injuries in and of themselves, designed to marginalize, contain, and control low-income communities. The sexualized drug economy, from the rural town of Austin, Indiana, to the bustling city of Chicago, created temptations, norms, and social exchanges that accelerated the spread of the twin epidemics of HIV and drug addiction. Make no mistake: the sexualized drug economy is a racialized, gendered, and classed ecosystem with participants from all walks of life, but it metes out its harshest consequences to those who have the fewest resources and the least amount of power. Women do not control the rules of this game, and the high risk of physical and sexual violence places them at a clear disadvantage. There are ongoing debates about the complexities of sex work, as many in the AIDS community and beyond recognize the potential for individuals to engage in this kind of labor in ways that are not exploitative and are based on purposeful and economically rational decisions on the part of sex workers.[1] However, we saw time and time again among the Chicago study women that their engagement was often linked to drug addictions that were quite damaging and significantly restricted their agency.

Social networks constitute the routes along which HIV travels, raising or lowering the likelihood of acquiring HIV depending on the structural vulnerabilities or protective buffers of one's network. In other words, policies and practices of inequality materialize in our networks, become instantiated in our bodies, and are manifested through our health outcomes. These injuries of inequality—seen and unseen—too often go unaddressed, creating fertile ground for new injuries to occur. It is neither accident nor coincidence that the individuals, families, and communities most affected by the AIDS epidemic have historically been the most marginalized and stigmatized, with the fewest resources available for erecting a protective shield.

While poverty certainly drives the epidemic, not all WLWHA contend with it. Interviews also revealed that silence between women and their partners, and even between women and their healthcare providers, can act as a powerful accelerant fueling the spread of HIV. As Dr. Bambi Gaddist observed during our interview, "Women will come in my office, young women. They're really bright, they're really talented. But when you talk to them about their relationships and their sex lives, you see the other person that was sent out in the world without armor, and how they stumbled into HIV."

Perhaps one of the most disturbing patterns that my research uncovered involves childhood sexual trauma, the unspoken and unseen engine of the AIDS epidemic among both women and men. One in four Chicago women who participated in our one-time interviews (28 percent) revealed that she had been raped or molested before the age of 25, and two-thirds of the women with histories of drug addiction reported sexual abuse while young. These numbers likely underreport the true rates, given the difficulties involved in disclosure. The trauma of sexual violation in childhood and early adulthood is etched into the psyches and bodies of women from a variety of racial and socioeconomic backgrounds as they navigate the world. Until they address such trauma, many survivors feel the original violation makes them unworthy of love, validation, safety, or acceptance. Women carry that stigma with them as they seek out relationships and survival resources, and it shapes their core beliefs and decision-making regarding sex, drugs, and their own agency. This suggests that concerted attention devoted to ending childhood sexual abuse and offering extensive support to survivors are necessary upstream HIV prevention interventions.

Dying from can therefore best be characterized as an existential struggle. When our analyses of individual behaviors and experiences become inextricably linked to the structural, historical, and situational contexts of people's lives, we can extrapolate larger sociological and epidemiological lessons while appreciating individual complexity and distinctiveness. From the girls they were to the women they have become, women have suffered because of the rigid dichotomies and quick assessments that we typically apply to questions about who is deserving or undeserving of care, assistance, and additional chances. If we succumb to the lure of such superficial judgments, we miss lessons and we miss opportunities.

I am nevertheless hopeful. By analyzing the lives of over 100 WLWHA, I have also revealed how public policies and institutions—which implement programs, distribute resources, and facilitate everyday social encounters—can play surprising yet critical roles in sparking personal transformations. To be sure, the most comprehensive approaches to confronting injuries of inequality would demand systemic solutions, overturning existing economic, social, and political systems that drive the contours of the epidemic. What the AIDS community has created is a hybrid of biomedical, behavioral, and systemic approaches that do not upend existing power structures but nevertheless provide important tools to help women address their injuries and hopefully prevent new ones from occurring. It is an incremental approach to confronting inequality, but its significance should not be overlooked.

Noted poverty scholars Kathryn Edin and Luke Shaefer have advocated using a kind of litmus test to assess policies that respond to the needs of marginalized populations: Do the policies integrate and engage individuals as valued participants? Do they provide dignity?[2] The HIV safety net does both. Here we have seen how the framing institutions and policies that comprise it are helping women generate new strategies to navigate and challenge the entrenched, ever-present environmental hurdles and widening social inequalities that initially put them at risk of acquiring HIV. Positive framing institutions counteract the cold indifference often associated with organizations that target marginalized populations by offering information, frameworks, language, resources, and networks that help women reframe and redress difficult circumstances. When we examine the stories of these women over time, we see how much of their personal growth, as well as improvements in their health and material circumstances, were driven by their own skills and determination as well as the social institutions that met them along the way. In the best of circumstances, gaps in institutions were made up by, and supplemented with, effective, supportive, and loving relationships with family and friends.

THE TRANSFORMATIVE PROJECT AS A STRATEGY FOR CONFRONTING INEQUALITY

In this analysis, I have sought to challenge how social scientists have traditionally thought about mobility. While we can understand the focus on important indicators such as income, education, and wealth, I have captured another kind of mobility: the transition from *dying from* to *living with* HIV and even *thriving despite* injuries of inequality. The transformative project is marked by significant and sustained movement away from severe and ongoing economic, emotional, and physical crises to greater stability in those important areas of social well-being. It lays out a path along which personal agency and cognitive shifts intersect with stabilizing institutional supports and responsive public policies. Transformation offered some women enhanced social status and even economic mobility.

Most importantly, though, it generated improvements in the basic level of well-being many women had previously experienced, with better housing and income stability, improved physical and psychological health, and socially supportive relationships. This increased stability should have positive implications for the children and families of WLWHA down the road. This basic level of stability and social well-being is foundational for women, enabling them not simply to cope but eventually also to confront injuries of inequality. The transformative project therefore offers a framework for improving women's social well-being that has policy relevance, political potential, and theoretical utility.

The vast majority of the women interviewed for this book have known about their HIV status for more than five years. Thirty-three percent of Chicago study women who participated in our one-time interviews had known about their status for five to ten years when we recruited them, and 57 percent had known for 11 or more years. Therefore, this study captures the experiences of long-term survivors of HIV/AIDS and analyzes the longitudinal impact of the disease. This suggests that the transformative project is guided partly by time and that the patience of service providers, family members, and the women themselves may be tested as the process slowly unfolds. As we observed, it often took years for women to fully launch their transformative projects. Further, transformation is a process, not a destination.

Time alone is insufficient, however, to generate the transformative process. As women moved from *dying from* to *living with* HIV/AIDS, we watched and listened as they built strong partnerships with their physicians, followed prescribed medication and self-care regimens, attended drug and alcohol rehabilitation programs, and sought support within the HIV safety net to manage their T-cell counts and viral loads. Notably, all of this was made possible by the affordable and relatively accessible healthcare system in Chicago and the state of Illinois that provided women with much-needed medical attention and supportive services. It is hard to imagine such transformations of women's lives without the backing and encouragement of this substantial network of care. Their sheer will and initiative would not have been enough to address the practical challenges they faced. And we met some longer-term survivors, like Tanya in chapter 5, who were struggling even though some resources were available to them. For women who were continuously wounded by economic, social, physical, and psychological challenges, the HIV safety net could do only so much to help. It did not generate or facilitate transformation for all, and it would be unrealistic to expect it to do so.

What are the barriers to transformation? First, an individual's ability to generate, embrace, and operationalize a cognitive shift and implement the notion that "something has to change" has to come from within. As each individual is the source of her own transformation, she must come to terms with the idea that change is necessary, beneficial, and possible. An individual must also believe that she is worthy of an opportunity to effect change in her life. As we have seen, women sometimes struggled for years because they fundamentally did not believe that they were worthy of a second chance. Others held on to the belief that their adopted strategies for coping were sustainable. It was not until they hit the emotional or physical limitations of their coping strategies that women embraced the notion of transformation.

Second, regardless of the desire to generate significant change, when one must make difficult survival choices, any transformative project can be undermined and weakened. Even the women who demonstrated the most significant life changes were nevertheless navigating within tight spaces, as the economic and social constraints of their environments challenged meaningful social mobility. Third, transformations are extremely difficult in the absence of the supports needed to help women stabilize their lives. Imagine what would have taken place if the Chicago study women had not had the HIV safety net to provide assistance. Imagine how many women around the country and the world desire such a monumental life shift but cannot find that kind of assistance where they reside.

As I wrote this book, I often thought about the privilege of having a second, third, or even fourth chance to recover from tragedy. I wondered about the women who had not made it, who died before they could remake their lives. I returned to the troubling irony presented in the introduction of this book: that the resources that gave these women the support they needed came only *after* they were diagnosed with a potentially deadly infectious disease that threatens public health. We do not distribute opportunities for redemption and transformation equally in our society. Given what we have learned about the combination of internal and external factors that are necessary for remaking, it appears that even the chance to change course in one's life is a commodity shaped by the vicissitudes of inequality.

THE END OF THE AIDS EPIDEMIC? KEY TAKEAWAYS FROM AND FOR THE AIDS RESPONSE

As we ponder the purported beginning of the end of HIV/AIDS, the moment can be characterized by both optimism and consternation. Great strides have been made in the scientific understanding and social acceptance of this dreadful disease, not to mention considerable political progress. In 2015, the CDC announced that annual HIV diagnoses in the United States fell by 19 percent between 2005 and 2014, with steep declines among heterosexuals, PWIDs, and African Americans.[3] Annual HIV diagnoses declined by 24 percent among African American women, by 16 percent among Latinas, and by 9 percent among white women over this period.[4] In the 1980s, additional life expectancy for a 20-year-old newly diagnosed with HIV was twelve years. Today, that number is 53 years for a young person on ART. As of July 2017, of the 36.7 million PLWHA around the globe, 20.9 million were accessing ART, up from 15.8 million in June 2015, 7.5 million in 2010, and less than one million in 2000.[5] Although much work remains to be done, leaders genuinely believe the "end of AIDS" is possible.

The HIV safety net is an essential part of the HIV/AIDS response. The broad network of care makes it possible for us to leverage the medical and scientific advances that have taken place over the last several decades. The precipitous decline in the number of children born with HIV is due in no small part to the services offered through Part D of the Ryan White CARE Act, in addition to the critical work of scientists and clinicians determined to end perinatal transmission. Low-income PLWHA are more likely to achieve undetectable levels of HIV in the blood if they receive care at a Ryan White–funded facility.[6] The CARE Act directly touches every layer of the system, from states to cities to clinics and community health centers, shaped by the priorities set by local planning councils. It is a payer of last resort for healthcare, ensuring that PLWHA have medical assistance. On the twenty-fifth anniversary of the passage of the Ryan White CARE

Act, Republican Senator Orrin Hatch, who cosponsored the bill after losing a close childhood friend to AIDS, described the policy as "a landmark
piece of legislation. It is public health legislation of the highest sort. Its
purpose is to alleviate pain and suffering . . . and it is one of the finest
pieces of legislation to come out of the Senate."[7]

The AIDS model of care has also become a blueprint. In 2018, Senator
Elizabeth Warren and Congressman Elijah Cummings proposed legislation to respond to the country's growing opioid crisis that was explicitly
modeled after the Ryan White CARE Act.[8] Dr. Helene Gayle had this to
say during our interview:

> I think that HIV response was one of the pioneers in demonstrating that you
> really have to look at the social determinants of health, not just healthcare
> and access to healthcare, to drive change in health status, particularly for
> poor communities and communities of color. If you're not looking at jobs,
> education, transportation, neighborhood safety, any of these other issues,
> you're not going to impact health just by bringing in better and more sophis-
> ticated healthcare. And so I think HIV, more than any recent public health
> issue, really demonstrated that model.

From a pure public health standpoint, the HIV safety net continues to
be vital. We cannot forget that HIV is an infectious disease, costing lives
and millions of dollars in treatment. The average annual cost of HIV treatment was $19,912 in 2006 dollars and $23,000 in 2010 dollars; estimated
total costs per person over a lifetime hover around $400,000.[9] Our ability
to stem the tide of the epidemic by preventing new and costly infections
will depend on helping PLWHA achieve viral suppression so that they are
less likely to transmit HIV to others. As I have demonstrated in great
detail, viral suppression through the successful management of HIV is as
much a social, economic, psychological, and even political achievement as
it is a biological one. If we ignore the contexts of women's lives when we
talk about viral suppression, we are unlikely to end the epidemic.

This is a global fight. Many of the dynamics around *dying from* to *living
with* that I have outlined in the book are replicated cross-nationally, but
the economic disparities and variation in political responses across countries mean that the HIV safety net has very different scopes and scales
depending on the context.[10] Nevertheless, an assessment by sociologist

Sanyu Mojola about the epidemic in Africa bears striking similarities to observations made in this book: "Adding a social-structural layer to the individual-level interventions reflects a recognition that individuals do not operate in social vacuums, but rather make decisions in environments that enable or disable particular kinds of actions."[11]

Back in Scott County, Indiana, the rural community grappling with one of the largest HIV outbreaks in Indiana's history, building an HIV safety net has become the strategy for addressing its public health crisis.[12] Officials noted that what happened in Austin, a white rural community, could happen in any place touched by the dire combination of a drug epidemic, poverty, and a weak care infrastructure. To help PLWHA reach viral suppression and reduce the risk of transmitting the virus, public health officials, under the advisement of such entities as the CDC and the New York State Health Department, which have extensive experience with the HIV safety net, began building Austin's institutional infrastructure. Beyond tackling the immediate facilitators of the epidemic through the emergency needle exchange, officials aggressively recruited individuals to join the state's Healthy Indiana plan to obtain health insurance.[13] In addition, they opened one-stop centers to help people secure birth certificates and other identification needed to gain access to the healthcare system, offered addiction rehabilitation services, and expanded testing services. There was also transportation assistance and help paying for medication refills. Struggles continue as the city's economy remains quite depressed, the demand for drug addiction treatment still outpaces the supply of available spots in rehab programs, and it remains a challenge to ensure that residents living with HIV/AIDS consistently take their medications. But the number of new infections has significantly declined, and a large percentage of individuals are virally suppressed.

A key takeaway is therefore the importance of continuing the supportive services aspects of the HIV safety net through policies such as the CARE Act, Housing Opportunities for People with AIDS (HOPWA), the AIDS Drug Assistance Program, and the Affordable Care Act. One hopes that the growing evidence supporting such interventions continues to guide policy.

But in addition to the services, what structural and cultural elements have made the HIV safety net so effective? How can we make a similar infrastructure accessible to more people in need of support? While we cannot duplicate some unique aspects of its history, several useful strategies are potentially replicable. Some require significant financial investment, while others are quite inexpensive.

Members of the AIDS community had several key insights. Some pointed to the financial structure of the HIV safety net. From her office in Washington, DC, Kaiser Family Foundation policy expert Jennifer Kates explained that part of the appeal of the Ryan White CARE Act for lawmakers is that "every state gets money. Everyone has a piece of the pie. And no one wants to lose that." Ideally, the political success and funding structure of the policy should bode well for its continued existence.

Others pointed to the linkages between government resources and community input. PLWHA have a strong voice in the coordinated AIDS response, and this was built into the structure through the work of activists. David Harvey, the first executive director of the AIDS Alliance for Women, Infants, Children, Youth, and Families, commented during our interview:

> The HIV safety net in this country is the gold standard [of care]. . . . The federal dollars were allocated in ways that required community planning. As much as people struggled with the process, as much as people fought within it, you know local public health folks hated having to convene all these community people, because it was often full of conflict. But the community planning nature that was required for how these dollars got spent is another unique factor that resulted in people being educated, empowered to get involved, and contributing to a social movement. Without it, we would not have had the success we have had with the CARE Act as a whole.

The emphasis placed on the voices of people most affected by HIV/AIDS in policy creation and service delivery is noteworthy on several levels. We saw how the focus on peer-led services centered women's experiences and offered leadership training and job opportunities so that some service recipients had the opportunity to become service providers. Embodied in the HIV support group and case management model of care, women could articulate and address some of inequality's injuries and traumas on their own terms. This proved to be a highly effective strategy for helping women move from *dying from* to *living with*. Antigone

Dempsey, a WLWHA and director of the Division of Policy and Data within the HIV/AIDS Bureau at HRSA, describes the Ryan White program in this way:

> I see it makes a difference, beyond helping people get care and treatment. It goes much deeper than that, especially in working with women. It's helping them figure out who they are and that they are a lovable person, that they are of value, and they should be loved and cared for. To me, that's the heart of the Ryan White HIV/AIDS program. It's helping them find their value because we're talking about people who've been told for generations that they're not worth anything, that they don't know anything. But it's like, no. People know so much. And then seeing what can happen when there are resources targeted to make all that happen.

We don't typically imagine public policy serving that purpose, especially one that operates as a safety net for marginalized individuals. But women brought their experiences as some of the earliest care providers as well as some of the earliest patients to the conversation. They became politically engaged, combining, as sociologist Steven Epstein describes, "grassroots politics with a self-conscious redefinition of the boundaries of expertise."[14] Notably, women did this by both borrowing some of the strategies of the gay male activists before them and working alongside them, as well as by creating new strategies that centered their experiences as women seeking to address the unique intersectional inequalities they faced. They pushed back against the social inequities and power dynamics that were being reproduced both outside of and *within* the safety net. They challenged the scientific definition of AIDS and demanded that policymakers recognize that "AIDS looks different in women." When they felt that they weren't being heard, they established their own organizations with women at the center of the mission and pushed existing organizations to be more expansive in their services for women. They created national and then global networks so that women could find community, and they challenged the world to see how patriarchy, sexism, and racism shape the global pandemic. And they fed these experiences back into the policy world to ensure that women coming behind them had access to life-saving medications and services, social support, and community-building opportunities.

In short, women demanded to be heard and seen as full participants in and contributors to the AIDS response. Linda Scruggs explained: "We learned how to be leaders in our community. To be clear, when I started doing this work in the 90s, it wasn't about being a leader. It was about helping myself and other women. . . . But that safety net was about creating for women a place to have open and honest conversations, without judgment of their providers, without the thought of repercussions for having their own choices and their own thoughts."

As a scholar who attends various AIDS policy, research, and program advisory meetings, I am struck by the way in which the HIV safety net community-based approach is operationalized in these venues. In my previous experiences researching poverty and social policies targeting low-income women, I had been to countless meetings in which scholars, foundation leaders, and government officials conferred for hours about poverty. However, we never seemed to acknowledge that the only people in the room who were living at or near the poverty line were those silently moving around the space as part of the catering and cleaning staff. When I started conducting HIV research, the difference was stark. Alongside the policy officials, researchers from top-tier institutions, and representatives from large AIDS organizations, women living with HIV/AIDS are at the table lending their voices. They are from various racial backgrounds; some are cisgender and some are transgender; some have a wealth of economic resources and others live on shoestring budgets. But I quickly realized that it is unheard of *not* to have WLWHA included to speak for themselves. They offer their experiential capital and often bring deep knowledge of the scientific and policy issues under discussion, a continuing thread of early AIDS activism in which PLWHA demanded seats at influential tables when their lives were being discussed.

David Harvey highlighted another, perhaps surprising, aspect of the HIV safety net that he deems to be critical:

> I point to the nature of conflict itself within the community, the infighting that happens. The activists versus the policy wonks who wear blue suits. The infighting between sectors of the HIV community: gay white men, black women, gay black men, trans[gender folks], kids, youth, I mean, you name it, there are struggles within. But I think that the nature of the conflict itself is what gives the movement its social influence. Our conflicts drive results. There is an energy that comes from conflict, that's harnessed to drive progress. And without it, I don't think this movement would've been successful.

How can conflict drive, rather than derail, progress? Intracommunity conflict is well-documented in the story of AIDS activism, captured in historical archives and tense scenes from documentary films such as *How to Survive a Plague, United in Anger, Nothing without Us,* and *Black Is, Black Ain't.* In the course of my own fieldwork, I noticed the frequency with which activists and advocates "called things out" in meetings, panel discussions, and our one-on-one interviews, attacking the racism, sexism, classism, homophobia, and transphobia operating within the AIDS community. For example, in a 2017 statement by a collective known as the Racial Justice Framework Group, AIDS activist and filmmaker Marco Castro-Bojorquez put the challenge to his white colleagues thus:

> Would you be able to work in settings where sometimes you would not have the last word, or craft the strategy, pace and tone of projects? Would you be able to learn how to share political imagination, work, and freedom and not be the one in charge? . . . By embracing racial justice, you must learn how to accept discomfort, take risks, and stand side by side with us: leaders of color that work with integrity and have a vision to get things done.[15]

Much work remains to be done to undercut the inequality that still exists within the movement. But the willingness of activists, advocates, scientists, service providers, and other members of the community to openly, passionately, and constructively disagree with each other likely improves the collective work of the movement. "To this day," David continued when we spoke at the headquarters of the National Coalition of STD Directors, "there are tensions, and infighting, and arguments about how money gets spent. And who has more influence, or not. Or who is well represented, or not. About who's speaking for whom. Those were all very big issues from day one in the HIV community." These tensions persist and get worked out by the members of the community as they catch each other's blind spots, push against the –isms and phobias, and fashion a broad tent to improve the lives of people who are deeply affected by HIV/AIDS. This harkens back to a key point made by black feminist legal scholar Kimberlé Crenshaw. The most one could expect, she writes, "is that we will dare to speak against internal exclusions and marginalization, that we might call attention to how the identity of 'the group' has been centered on the intersectional identities of a few."[16]

I would add some additional observations to explain the success of the AIDS response, influenced by my previous experience studying another safety net, the welfare system.[17] First, the HIV/AIDS epidemic, and the individuals and communities most affected by it, transformed public discourse on health and introduced a comprehensive framework for understanding social well-being that incorporated not just physical health, but the freedom to live without stigma and the chance to start anew after receiving devastating news. This is a crucial point and an important feature that distinguishes HIV/AIDS from many other health issues.[18]

More specifically, much of the political animus against people living with HIV/AIDS is arguably rooted in hostility toward the sexuality and sexual lives of society's most marginalized. Although HIV can be transmitted via blood, semen, vaginal fluids, or breast milk, throughout the history of the disease (and of course prior), there have been overt and covert attacks on the sexuality of gay and bisexual men, black and brown women, transgender individuals, and the poor. These groups share a public narrative that their sexuality is inherently deviant, lascivious, and out of control. From stereotypes of black women as sexually available and highly irresponsible "crack mothers" to those of gay men as hyper-promiscuous and hedonistic, these controlling images seek to flatten the humanity of those struggling with the disease and its underlying causes.[19] As sociologist Trevor Hoppe has demonstrated, this politics of disgust toward the sexual lives of large swaths of the AIDS community has informed policy conversation on HIV/AIDS since the early years, giving way to policy prescriptions grounded in surveillance, containment, and even criminalization.[20] Barry Adam writes, "It is probably fair to say that no one objects to the control and eradication of the causative agent(s) of AIDS, but AIDS control policy has always been much more and has inevitably raised the question of the supervision and regulation of sexuality."[21] To counter this, AIDS activists engage in a politics that does not downplay but affirms sexuality and challenges assumptions that it is inherently deviant and problematic. The push translates into calls for non-stigmatizing, non-judgmental, and non-punitive AIDS service delivery, including sex-positive messaging and a focus on harm reduction that WLWHA embrace.

Second, the HIV/AIDS services community has started to advance the notion of trauma-informed care, driven in large part by the lives of women, and especially women of color, who elevated the conversation by identifying and articulating traumatic events as barriers and factors in certain health outcomes.[22] While definitions vary, Elizabeth Hopper and colleagues describe trauma-informed care as "a strengths-based framework that is grounded in an understanding of and responsiveness to the impact of trauma, that emphasizes physical, psychological, and emotional safety for both providers and survivors, and that creates opportunities for survivors to rebuild a sense of control and empowerment."[23] This framework has a natural fit within an HIV safety net that has been operationalizing much of this work for decades, as highly marginalized groups such as gay and bisexual men of color, transgender individuals, women, and low-income patients have demanded similar approaches to care. In 2018, HRSA identified trauma-informed care as a "Special Project of National Significance," elevating its visibility and funding.

Third, the AIDS community simultaneously leverages privilege and marginalization to build and sustain its political clout and access to resources. Gay white men used their racial and male privilege; economic, social, and cultural capital; and growing political influence to solidify a place for HIV/AIDS on the list of domestic policy concerns. They kicked opened doors and walked into rooms of influence and power ready to fight for their lives. From the outset of the identification of HIV/AIDS as a social problem affecting their communties, gay white men were able to shape the conversation, and subsequently, their destinies. The historical commitment to the issue of HIV/AIDS within LGBTQ communities is foundational for the safety net.

While women, gay and bisexual men of color, poor people, transgender individuals, and those who have multiple marginalized statuses may not have wielded the same level of economic and political influence or social privilege as their affluent white male counterparts in the movement, they too have shown serious and ongoing commitment to the issue and have put their bodies on the line to advance the cause. As we have witnessed throughout history, these populations have been granted less freedom to shape the conversation around their destinies, and their struggles are often diagnosed, targeted, and disciplined by forces outside of the community. But these groups have nevertheless found ways to offer crucial contributions to the AIDS conversation and the political, policy, and institutional responses, even when it meant fighting back against inequities within the AIDS movement. They have challenged us to redefine what an AIDS activist looks like to ensure that future histories of the epidemic include their voices. This integration and collaboration between privilege and marginalization among groups affected by HIV has been key to the power of the movement.

What is also significant about the HIV safety net is the way in which it allows women to negotiate their relationships with other women, deepening transformative projects. Sitting together in support groups, in clinic waiting rooms, and in community planning meetings, women from different walks of life have opportunities to reimagine their relationships with each other, to begin viewing social ties to other women as central to their well-being. Some Chicago study women certainly engaged in social distancing from other WLWHA, particularly around dimensions of class. Middle-class women largely kept their distance from the AIDS community in Chicago unless they were service providers themselves, forgoing their access to a community in favor of privacy and autonomy from a public AIDS identity. We saw some of this intersect with racial differences as well, as fewer Latinas interfaced with the HIV safety net, perhaps in part due to the immigration status of some. Nevertheless, I saw a fierce commitment among those active in the AIDS movement to not allow themselves to be divided from other women by mode of transmission, a respectability proxy, or other categories.

Finally, I would point to the significance of storytelling in the AIDS response. Its centrality cannot be overstated as a defining characteristic of the HIV safety net. It is one of the most important tools for community building as PLWHA seek out and provide support to each other. For Rebecca Denison at WORLD, storytelling was the bedrock of the newsletter. "I believe that people learn through stories," she explained. "I remember the names of opportunistic infections because I remember the stories of the friends who had them. I remember the names of medications because I remember the stories of the people who took them. I don't remember them because I read medical articles; I remember them because of those things." Storytelling is also important in the delivery of HIV/AIDS services as case managers and other providers draw out clients' stories in order to determine what barriers might prevent them from being retained in healthcare.

Storytelling also serves as a tactic to gather political support and to mobilize action in the epidemic. PWN's Naina Khanna explains:

> Storytelling is huge. It's a huge part of our movement. Mary Fisher at the Republican National Convention sharing her story. Ryan White's story. HIV has always been about sharing stories. Storytelling is healing, especially for survivors of trauma, and most people with HIV are survivors of some trauma. . . . Building sisterhood, creating supportive environments that address things beyond HIV . . . you cannot have a meeting of women living with HIV who don't know each other without going through a pretty extensive "check-in." . . . And the notion that you would fund organizations [to encourage storytelling], that you would train service providers [to facilitate it], and that you would bake that into the ethos is an important part of what [the HIV safety net] means to people.

Storytelling represents a way for people within the safety net to both connect and contribute. Offering life lessons through sharing one's story or encouraging someone along in the coping trajectory by drawing out her story is part of the cultural fabric of AIDS service delivery. I witnessed throughout the course of my fieldwork how women telling their stories of struggle, stigma, and trauma is part of the cathartic process of coming to grips not only with living with HIV but also with important life events prior to and since the diagnosis. In appendix A, I grapple with the downsides of this approach, and we observed in chapter 3 how this approach is not attractive for women who value privacy above all else. Nevertheless, time and time again, I saw storytelling operate as an essential element of the transformative project. It is how women constructively reckon with their injuries of inequality.

Given the high level of surveillance, scrutiny, and judgment that marginalized populations often experience in their everyday lives and especially through their interactions with systems (healthcare, criminal justice, welfare, child welfare, etc.), it is in fact revolutionary to build a movement and a service infrastructure around the notion of revealing. I saw firsthand how the welfare system encouraged women to reveal as little about themselves as possible, lest they share a data point (a boyfriend or job that could be a hidden source of income) that could reduce their benefits or make them ineligible for services altogether. Because PLWHA have blood test results from a medical provider verifying their HIV status, questions of fraud are less a part of the operating assumption within the HIV safety net. But it was also the culture, built by activists who shaped the terms by which bureaucrats would engage them, that powerfully set the tone. This created the space for what sociologist Dominique Adams-Santos defines as "intimate candor" to become the dominant ethos: the performative and rhetorical mechanism of publicly revealing highly personal life details in order to connect, teach, and share.[24] Intimate candor through storytelling serves as an act of resistance and healing, pushing against the tenets of respectability and breaking away from narrow and formulaic confines of who women living with HIV/AIDS might be and what they can do.

Nevertheless, for women who fear a loss of esteem as a result of intimate candor, the balance between disclosure and privacy as strategies for survival remains an enduring tension. HIV disclosure was likely palatable to women with few resources precisely because in some ways they perceived that they had nothing else to lose and complying with the expectations of the network of support was ultimately the better choice (even if it required them to engage in full disclosure). However, this approach had clear challenges for more affluent women, for whom disclosure was threatening and could have real consequences in terms of loss of status, employment, and possibly even health insurance.

All of these things suggest that while policies, institutions, services, and networks are vital, their cultural connective tissue promoting voice, agency, inclusion, intersectionality, an end to stigma, and a confrontation of trauma are what have made the HIV safety net so effective. These developments are very personal for WLWHA. Scientists predict that we will soon have injectable antiretrovirals on the market that can be taken monthly rather than daily. Researchers continue to make slow but steady progress in AIDS cure and vaccine research. "I've spent years after my diagnosis waiting for the other shoe to drop," Linda Scruggs commented during a discussion on HIV cure research. "It would be nice not to have the shoes." Naina Khanna echoed these sentiments: "My job is to work myself out of a job." In this biomedical era of AIDS care, in which the singular focus on "getting drugs into bodies" is gaining prominence, the ongoing importance of the HIV safety net and the multiple roles that it plays should not be overlooked.

WHEN (BLACK) WOMEN ENTER: INTERSECTIONAL POLITICS IN POLICY AND INSTITUTIONS

The cover image for this book is a stunning work by artist Sally Deng entitled *Another Struggle*. We see a black woman in movement—toward what/who/where, we can only speculate. She is traveling through a sea of people, mostly white men, as she swims her limbs through the masses to get to her destination. She could be an activist on her way to a demonstration, a congressional staffer shepherding an important piece of legislation through a complicated process, an advocate heading to a strategy meeting, or a woman living with HIV/AIDS traversing everyday life. The image, neither patronizing nor pitiful, symbolizes how black women are at once invisible and central in the AIDS epidemic and the global response.

Highlighting the experiences of black women within the AIDS epidemic and the organized response reveals what conventional modes of public policy analysis often overlook. Their stories don't end at trauma and victimhood, nor are they reducible to narratives of resilience and survival. What we witnessed is how black women became leaders in the fight against HIV/AIDS, active participants and key players in shaping public policy. Black women activists, advocates, and policy officials have been instrumental in pushing the AIDS response to be a truly intersectional social movement and policy formation. They have worked across lines of race, gender, sexuality, and class to confront the inequities driving the epidemic. Some are living with HIV; others are not. But what they have in common is a sentiment stated by Dázon Dixon Diallo as she reflected on the work: "The one thing that I want to be sure of is that black women, no matter where we live, get to the end of this epidemic at the same time as everybody else."

A new generation of HIV/AIDS leaders of color are explicitly drawing upon black feminist and black queer political frameworks in their work. As Charles Stephens of the Counter Narrative Project opined, "The intersectional social justice lens in the HIV movement has much, if not everything, to do with the efforts of black women and other women of color." This was reflected when, in July 2017, almost 20 years after the historic Palm Sunday meeting of black HIV/AIDS leaders at the CDC that led to the creation of the Minority AIDS Initiative, a new cadre of more than 20 leaders of color convened in New York City to begin articulating a racial justice analysis for the HIV field. Any response to the impact of the HIV, the collective argued, must be *rooted* (emphasis added) in a racial justice framework. By November of that year, the group had released "A Declaration of Liberation: Building a Racially Just and Strategic HIV Movement," which called for "an integration of racial justice into our organizations and political strategies; centering those communities most impacted by the epidemic in leadership and decision-making; rooting efforts to advance a racial justice lens in the HIV movement in accountability to the communities that we lead; ensuring equity around allocation of resources—human, material, and financial; and working to transform and, where necessary, dismantle institutions that uphold white supremacy and compromise the wellbeing of communities of color."[25]

Members of the group also explicitly committed to examining and eliminating anti-blackness "in our coalitions, our movements, and within ourselves." Chapter 5's Gina Brown of PWN-USA and PACHA also worked as a community organizer for the Southern AIDS Coalition and had this to say: "Anti-blackness ... you can see it everywhere—in care, in case management, among people living with HIV—in how black community members are judged, stereotyped, mocked, disregarded, in all kinds of large and small ways. We talk about stigma, but we don't talk about anti-blackness; we talk about institutional racism, but we don't talk about individual racism. That is always easiest, because you're not calling people out; but sometimes you have to call people out."[26]

Rather than allowing others to see them as problems to be solved, women applying an intersectional social justice framework to AIDS work see it as their role to push for more than incremental approaches to healing the injuries of inequality that their communities have suffered, "pressuring institutions from the clinic to the government, from funders to the courtroom" to not simply provide medications and services but to "act in the service of racial equity and justice, and to divest from the interests of white supremacy."[27] What these activists are calling for is critically important: rather than thinking of transformation exclusively in terms of the individual changes that specific people can make with adequate supports, they are calling for the larger structural transformations that might prevent people from finding themselves in a situation in which they have to "transform themselves" in order to shift from *dying to living* (with or without HIV).

In sum, in order for personal and political transformations to be successful, individuals must tap into the right networks and power structures to form effective alliances. As the subset of women most disproportionately impacted by HIV/AIDS, black women forged several partnerships to save their lives. They made up small but important numbers in ACT UP's caucuses for women and people of color.[28] They partnered with women across racial and class lines to challenge the case definition of AIDS, to create women- and family-centered HIV/AIDS services, and to build powerful networks of women working in the field of HIV/AIDS. They lobbied for the Ryan White CARE Act, finding their voice in an AIDS community largely dominated by white gay men who brought significant economic, cultural, and social capital to the policy-making process. They led efforts within black communities, partnering with black men to shape the Minority AIDS Initiative and other key policies that targeted the epidemic in black communities. And they joined with other activists of color to push for a racial justice framework to be adopted by the AIDS community. Even when the work was undercut and the resources were diminished compared to the need, black women forged cross-cultural alliances and played important roles in building the HIV safety net that exists today.

FUTURE DIRECTIONS IN THE HIV/AIDS RESPONSE

Perhaps the HIV safety net's most significant challenge derives from its success. Medical advances have transformed HIV/AIDS from a terminal to a chronic illness. Transmission rates have stabilized among certain populations. The highly visible AIDS political mobilization of the 1980s and 1990s has declined, and the LGBTQ community has expanded its political agenda to focus on a host of other issues. AIDS is no longer a crisis in the public imagination. Movies that depict HIV, such as *Dallas Buyers Club* and *The Normal Heart*, tend to historicize the epidemic, offering little perspective on the lives of those still grappling with the disease today. Some have even questioned why the HIV safety net should continue to exist and enjoy the specialized access to government resources that is currently legislated through the Ryan White CARE Act and other policies.

We must remember that there are about 1.1 million people who struggle daily with the virus in the United States and that there are more than 30 million PLWHA around the globe. We must acknowledge that the HIV safety net does not work equally for all populations and that gaps in services exist. We must repair the safety net where it is tattered and establish it where it is nonexistent. Geographic variations in the efficacy of the HIV safety net are particularly troubling. For the women in the Chicago study, access to resources was largely predicated on living in an urban center in the United States with a robust AIDS infrastructure that had historical roots in a politically mobilized gay community. The financial patchwork that many women weave together through AIDS services organizations is much more difficult to construct in the South and likely impossible to create in some rural areas. And increasingly, dollars are moving away from some community-driven services such as peer support, advocacy training, support groups, and case management.

Safety nets have been, throughout American history, consistently under political attack.[29] The public rhetoric that denigrates them has seemingly reached fever pitch as I write, and it has conditioned us to believe that every supportive service offered to a disadvantaged population is a hammock rather than a ladder, that every form of assistance encourages dependency and rewards those who evade the rules. But the story of the HIV safety net challenges those narratives. As we discovered, most of the women in this book didn't become dependent and stuck; they empowered themselves and moved forward with community support. Against the backdrop of the diminishing social safety net, the HIV safety net and the people, policies, and institutions that constitute it offer valuable lessons about aiding those in need of assistance. As we think about transformation and what it takes for people to achieve mobility, alter their status, or overcome incredible odds, we learn a valuable lesson: effective public policy and high-impact organizations can help to radically improve the lives of marginalized individuals.

As *Remaking a Life* goes to press, I am left with the question of whether the organizational and political power of the AIDS response will weaken, grow, or hold firm over the next decade. Will women have the right constellation of factors in the current sociopolitical environment to be able to transform their lives? What I find encouraging is that the long history of the national HIV/AIDS response, like other social movements before it, is rooted in its resolve. It has been very effective at wielding its political muscle, and my hope is that it continues to deploy those strategies and generate new ones, as the work clearly benefits the greater good. In order for us to continue to make the gains that will eradicate this devastating and costly epidemic, we must stay vigilant in the fight and continue to support the policies and institutions that have delivered results.

Acknowledgments

This book would not be possible without the support of the AIDS community. I want to thank all the women and men living with HIV/AIDS who shared their stories with me in an amazing show of generosity. You became a beacon of hope for me as I witnessed the strength, wisdom, and fierce intelligence that you bring to your lives and work. I also thank all the activists, advocates, service providers, and policy experts and officials who sat for interviews, opened doors of introduction, and worried less about the ego rush (or apprehension) of being featured in a book and more about getting the message out concerning the ongoing importance of the epidemic. Thank you for encouraging me; thank you for inspiring me.

Northwestern University has been a fantastic place to grow as a scholar. I've been incredibly fortunate to have colleagues who also happen to be preeminent scholars in their respective fields. By their presence, example, thoughtful critiques, and probing questions, they inspire me to even greater heights, while also being extremely fun to be around. E. Patrick Johnson read the entire manuscript and worked valiantly to help me think through that very difficult phase in the process when hard-fought words on the page have to be cut for the sake of word limits. I thank him and Stephen Lewis for housing me in their gorgeous home as I traveled between Chicago and Detroit for my almost weekly commute. Héctor Carrillo provided brilliant line-by-line edits of the manuscript drawing on his perspective as a scholar and a volunteer-activist in several AIDS organizations. Héctor was a mentor when I began conducting research on HIV/AIDS in 2004, and it was a wonderful full-circle moment to share the manuscript with him many years later. Special thanks to Mary Pattillo, who balances brilliance and life perspective in ways that kept me relaxed throughout the writing process. I also thank my fantastic colleagues Martha Biondi, Lindsay Chase-Lansdale, Steven Epstein, Carol Heimer, Aldon Morris, Jennifer Nash, Andrew Papachristos, kihana ross, Nitasha Sharma, Steven Thrasher, Tracy Vaughn, Kathleen Murphy, and Kathleen Bethel for their insights and advice on the project at various stages. In addition, I am very appreciative of my outstanding colleagues and the staffs in the Departments of African American Studies, Sociology, and the Institute for Policy Research at Northwestern. I also thank my dear friend Dwight McBride, whose mentorship during his time at Northwestern and now at Emory has been steadfast and strengthening for me.

I took on the role of associate vice president for research at Northwestern when this project was in its final stages. My new colleagues were extremely supportive as I worked to juggle competing demands. Special thanks to Jay Walsh, my associate vice president colleagues, Erin Wallace, and the first-rate and deeply committed members of the Office for Research at Northwestern. I also thank former dean Sarah Mangelsdorf and current dean Adrian Randolph for the support and resources necessary to take this project across the finish line.

I was very fortunate to receive fantastic feedback from several scholars from across the country who read the entire manuscript. I owe very special thanks to Scott Allard, Sandra Danziger, Mario Small, and Kathryn Edin for their excellent feedback and enthusiasm for this project. Thank you also to colleagues at Harvard, Columbia, Stanford, Duke, and the Universities of Chicago, Michigan, Washington, Maryland, Wisconsin, Illinois, North Carolina, California, and Texas who allowed me to test out the book's ideas during visits to their campuses. Portions of this book's arguments also appear in the journals *Social Science & Medicine* and *Annals of the American Academy of Political & Social Science*.

This project simply would not be what it is without the guidance of Judy Auerbach. Judy, both a scholar and longtime member of the AIDS advocacy community, beautifully and convincingly promotes the consideration of social dimensions of health and social science research as critical decisions are made at the highest echelons of the AIDS world. Not only did Judy read the manuscript twice, she was superb at brainstorming who I needed to speak with in the AIDS community and generously opened doors. Cynthia Tucker at the AIDS Foundation of Chicago was instrumental to my research, serving on my community advisory board, providing key introductions, and frequently inviting me to present my research in the Chicago AIDS community. I also would like to thank Olga Grinstead Reznick and the dedicated and brilliant scholars at the Center for AIDS Prevention Studies at the University of California San Francisco for being my first "HIV/AIDS teachers" when I participated in the HIV-Prevention Research in Minority Communities Collaborative Program and received a seed grant from which I built this project.

I am so fortunate to count as my most impactful mentors an illustrious group from my undergraduate alma mater Spelman College. I met Dr. Johnnetta B. Cole when I was a nineteen-year-old student at Spelman, and she has been my closest and longest-standing mentor. Dr. Cole never ceases to awe and amaze me with her love, wisdom, brilliance, and generosity. I want to thank Dr. Mary Schmidt Campbell, Rosalind Brewer, Dr. Beverly Daniel Tatum, and the board of trustees on which I had the pleasure of serving for over a decade for their constant encouragement, love, and support. Incomparable black feminist scholar and legendary Spelman professor Dr. Beverly Guy-Sheftall graced me by reading the entire manuscript, as I could not have imagined going to press without her trusted feedback. And I am very proud to say that four Spelman women served as research assistants on this project.

I was extremely fortunate to have a graduate school advisor at Harvard who told me that I could count on her to be a lifelong mentor, and I have taken Katherine Newman up on that. I want to thank her for her advice, strategic thinking, and encouragement through the years. I also want to thank William Julius Wilson, whom I also place in the category of lifelong mentor; I see this book as moving in the tradition of inequality and urban poverty scholarship for which he is known around the world. Special thanks to Barbara Reskin for lending her support as I developed a passion for studying organizations early in my career.

The research that led to this book allowed me to engage with students at various stages of their matriculation. They were among my most thoughtful and hardworking interlocutors, and the book is stronger because of their contributions. I hired Yondi Morris-Andrews, daughter of esteemed sociologist Aldon Morris, on the heels of her graduation from Spelman College. With her initiative, intelligence, and relationship skills, she was the perfect partner to help me launch this project in 2004. From there, several graduate students lent their brilliance and commitment to the work and have since gone on to outstanding careers. LaShawnDa Pittman and Jean Beaman took over for Yondi as extremely capable project coordinators at different stages of the work, and I thank them for coauthoring a paper with me that served as a crucial building block for this book. Elyse Kovalsky, Marisol Mastrangelo, Courtney Patterson, and Robert Vargas gathered many of the interviews for this project and brought smart analyses, excellent fieldwork skills, and deep empathy to every interaction that they had with study participants. Julian Kevon Glover joined the project as I was in the throes of drafting the manuscript, and he brought thoughtful and engaged critique and cutting-edge ideas as I developed my main theoretical arguments. I also thank Kenneth Pass for his fantastic suggestion that we meet regularly to discuss some of the latest research on the HIV/AIDS epidemic. Our conversations felt less like teacher-student interactions and more like colleagues growing together.

It is hard for me to imagine this project without the involvement of Dominique Adams-Santos. Dominique served as an indefatigable thought partner, tracked down information that would have stumped many students, and was there whenever I reached out with a random request. Her ideas and professionalism reflect a student mature beyond her years, and I am so grateful for her calm energy, unwavering excitement for the project, and constant willingness to roll up her sleeves as I dashed to the finish line. Elyse, Julian, Kenneth, and Dominique read drafts of the book, and their ideas, questions, and probes sharpened my thinking about the manuscript and inspired me to push the work even further. The students I have taught and advised throughout my years at Northwestern greatly contribute to the intellectual and cultural richness of the institution, and my scholarship is better because of my interactions with them.

I am very grateful to the undergraduate research assistants who worked on this project between 2005–2016: LaTisha Campbell, Jacqueline Coates, Diego Henriquez-Garcia, Marrion Johnson, Jasmyne McDonald, Joanne Ogundipe, Juliana Partridge, Bethany Polhamus, Kit Riehle, Jessica Schwalb, Alicia Sheares, Tiffany Tobias, Marcella Wagner, Shaquita Webster, Alexandra Woodson, Stephen Zajac, and Ivy Zhu. Special thanks to Amanda Armour and Amy Thom, who served as project coordinators when the project evolved from a small study of thirty women to a research operation with a team of students, a community advisory board, and over one hundred study participants.

I thank my fantastic editor Naomi Schneider, production editor Emilia Thiuri, editorial assistant Benjy Malings, and the entire team at the University of California Press for their extraordinary work, support, and encouragement. Jan Spauschus took such beautiful care with editing the manuscript to ensure that each word and punctuation mark on the page are presented well. Thanks are also due to the funders of this project, the National Science Foundation (award #0847809) and the Robert Wood Johnson Foundation, and I want to express special gratitude to longtime NSF program officer Patricia White. William Barnett has edited my work since my pre-tenure days, and he brought his usual fantastic skill to this project. Meggin McIntosh and Shari Caudron provided excellent guidance on how to see this project to completion, and they have my eternal gratitude.

My circle of friends is large and soul-nourishing, and it overwhelms me to think about just how many deep bonds I share with both friends on speed-dial and those with whom I can pick up where we left off after long periods apart. Jennifer Campbell and Johnita Mizelle read portions of the book, gave fantastic feedback, and affirmed the value and importance of having as wide an audience as possible. Laurel Beatty Blunt, Nicole and Andreas Buchanan, Lorri Pearson Grant, Eboni Creighton, Malene Dixon, Shari Hicks-Graham, and Stacey Abrams are just some of my dear friends who inspire me with their brilliance, passion, humor, and deep commitments to social justice. My Spelman connections have produced a loving and supportive network of sister-friends all over the country. My children's lives have also introduced me to some fantastic parents who have become new friends, and I'm appreciative of the well-wishes, support, and good humor that they've offered since we met. I also want to thank Darlynn Ford, Al Mitchell, and Heidi White for always lending an ear as I talked through my ideas and wondered aloud how I would balance my various commitments.

Words on a page cannot adequately express my love and gratitude to my family, and I dedicate this book to them. I thank my parents, Walter and Harriett Watkins, and my sister, Che' Watkins, for their love, encouragement, and yes, childcare, when I needed it the most. Special thanks to the Watkins, Drake, Hayes, and Stoute families. As a mother of young children, I could not have focused on the task of writing this book without safe, consistent, and nurturing child care. Marilyn Hunter and Sherry Martin, along with my husband and parents, make up the amazing village of love and support that surround my children so that mommy can have time to write. The joy and sense of security that my children enjoy is due in no small part to Marilyn and Sherry's labor and love. And to Hunter and Harper, thank you for your unconditional love, solicited and unsolicited visits to mommy's home office, and the hope that you represent by being in the world.

My husband Rejji Hayes had a difficult job. He was the one who lifted me up during some of the project's most difficult moments, when I was grappling with how best to express an idea or was overwhelmed by the responsibility of capturing the stories of people who had moved me so deeply and held great expectations for my ability to tell this story. For Rejji's love, partnership, sharp intellect, and contagious joy, laughter, and peace, I am eternally grateful.

APPENDIX A Methods of Research

There are 255 summits on the Appalachian Trail. Hiking the
trail is a great metaphor for life, because no day looks
exactly the way you expect it to, and every day you have to
climb a mountain, whether you want to or not. And sometimes it's more than one mountain. And many times it looks
like you're at the top of the mountain and you're not, and
you have to keep going. And every day you have to pick up
whatever it is you're carrying and put it on your back and
take it with you. So there's no hiding. And that process is
hard. I mean, I tell people that the physical challenge was
not insignificant, but it was nothing compared to the mental
challenge. . . . No matter what, every day you just had to
keep going. You had to put your pack on your back and keep
going. . . . There was a lot of really intense and hard stuff.
The good news and the bad news was that you couldn't hide
from it. And all you had was time. And space. To deal. So
that in and of itself was an enormous gift. To be able to say,
I'm going to have tea with my demons and here they are.

Dawn Averitt, Co-Founder of The Well Project

When Dawn Averitt told me this story of hiking the Appalachian Trail, it stopped
me in my tracks. As I described in chapter 5, Dawn had spent years working in the
world of HIV/AIDS treatment activism. Exhausted and carrying unprocessed grief
over the deaths of the many men and women who had succumbed to AIDS, she
decided it was time to pursue a lifelong dream of hiking the trail. While I in no way
want to equate the experience of living with HIV/AIDS with the challenges of writing a book, Dawn's description of her trek resonated with me. In the reflection below,
I comment on some of the key methodological issues that emerged in the work.

Table 2   The Health, Hardship, and Renewal Study

	Sister to Sister study	Snapshot study	HIV Safety Net study
Sample size	30	84	72
Time frame	2005–2018	2010–2012	2010–2017
One-time interviews		√	√
Recurring interviews and participant observation	√		

RESEARCH DESIGN

At the outset, the study on which this book is based was not intended to be a longitudinal project. But as my professional and personal life took various twists and turns, this project matured on the vine. The data presented were collected in three waves that amounted to one large research agenda: the Sister to Sister study, the snapshot study, and the HIV Safety Net study (see table 2). I call the umbrella project the Health, Hardship, and Renewal (HHR) study.

Wave 1: The Sister to Sister Study

In 2005, I began Sister to Sister (S2S), a qualitative study of 30 African American WLWHA in Chicago (see demographic details in table 5 in appendix B). By exploring a range of domains, such as social support, economic survival, child-bearing and childrearing, and intimate relationships, S2S sought to illustrate how HIV/AIDS affected women's everyday lives and social outcomes. My research assistant, Yondi Morris-Andrews, and I recruited women through physicians, AIDS service organizations, and word of mouth. We conducted at least three interviews with each woman, one of which included a participant-observation session during which we accompanied each respondent to a site where her HIV status was known and salient. We attended women's medical appointments and support group meetings, sat in the audience during speaking engagements as they told their stories, visited them in their homes, and were among the earliest visitors after the births of their children. The purpose was to observe women as they navigated social spaces related to their HIV status. In all locations, where appropriate, we obtained verbal consent from the other participants prior to sitting in. We did not obtain written consent to protect confidentiality and to minimize disruption in these settings. Yondi or I also debriefed each respondent after each observation session to understand how the respondent interpreted the event and to do a reliability check to discuss how the interaction was similar or different from her previous engagements with the setting and whether and how our presence as researchers may have shaped things.

The discoveries from the S2S study have been published in a variety of venues and, where appropriate, were revisited in this book.[1] Perhaps the most important finding emerging from that work, presented in an article that I coauthored with LaShawnDa Pittman and Jean Beaman, was the instrumental role of framing institutions in helping women move from *dying from* to *living with*.[2] We argued that certain organizations help positively or negatively frame what it means to live with HIV by offering critical information about HIV as a medical diagnosis and social status; language with which to talk about HIV and its implications for women's lives; and resources and networks that help or hinder women in restructuring post-diagnosis life. As institutional brokers, framing institutions are often invisible to those who do not rely on them but critically important to those who do.

Wave 2: The Snapshot Study

After S2S, I was left with additional questions. Could I paint a more expansive and comprehensive picture, drawing on the racial, ethnic, and class diversity among WLWHA to tell an even richer story about the transformation that we had previously identified as *dying from* to *living with?* In 2010, with funding from the National Science Foundation and the Robert Wood Johnson Foundation, I launched the follow-up to S2S. This was also a Chicago-based interview study of women of diverse socioeconomic backgrounds who were living with HIV, with an increased sample size and greater racial and ethnic diversity among the group members. I refer to it as the "snapshot" study because it provides data on a cross-section of women at a given moment in time. The snapshot study includes Latinas as well as black and white women, immigrants (English-speaking and Spanish only–speaking), and women who represent a wide age range (23 to 72 years; mean age 45.14). For the analysis of the significance of framing institutions as a critical piece of the transformative project, I felt it was important to include more women who did *not* have strong connections to the HIV/AIDS safety net, allowing me to test the validity of the arguments that we developed during the S2S study. I sought to recruit approximately 75 women for the study, providing large enough subgroups on the basis of race, socioeconomic status, and level of organizational connection, as these were my primary areas of interest in terms of sample variation. By the end, 84 women participated in the snapshot study. Demographic details about the women are presented in table 6 in appendix B.

The snapshot study employed a team approach to data collection. Research assistants Amanda Armour, Jean Beaman, Elyse Kovalsky, Marisol Mastrangelo, and Courtney Patterson conducted these interviews with me. We trained for months before we entered the field, reading previous literature about WLWHA, collectively revising the interview protocol, and talking about strategies to ensure the privacy, safety, and comfort of our respondents while eliciting rich and useful information. We had regular team meetings throughout the 24-month data collection process and made adjustments to our fieldwork strategies as needed to ensure a carefully collected dataset among a diverse group of women.

Nevertheless, as we launched the snapshot study, the stories of the S2S women stayed with me. Because of my ongoing participation in the HIV/AIDS community—as a board member of a local AIDS organization, presenting my research at various community meetings, and conducting the snapshot study—I continued to informally interact with some of the S2S women. The snapshot study had an early explicit focus on the economic survival strategies of WLWHA. But as we talked to more and more women in the snapshot study, the central idea that so many described was their journey of transformation, the same theme that had emerged in the S2S study. My interactions with the S2S women—during in-depth fieldwork and in later casual conversations—were converging with the data coming out of the snapshot study, and two key questions emerged: How did the *dying from* to *living with* coping process that Pittman, Beaman, and I described expand into other domains in the women's lives beyond HIV, and how did the process evolve and change over time?

While the snapshot study continued gleaning rich cross-sectional data about a diverse population of women, I invited a subset of seven S2S women to continue to participate in the larger HHR Study to deepen our longitudinal analysis. My interactions with these women were organic in nature, as I periodically checked in or requested that we meet for follow-up interviews. I visited them in their homes, invited them to my office, and traveled to meet with those who had moved out of town. Some called to share important news and agreed to allow me to capture the conversation in a fieldnote. Each woman provided me with her contact information (which usually included both a phone number and email address) as well as the contact information of a trusted friend or family member who would always know how to get in touch with her. Because of the nature of this fieldwork, the total number of interviews that I or a member of my team conducted with each member of this S2S subset varied from five to eight between 2005 and 2018. However, when I conducted follow-up interviews, I used roughly the same interview protocol, focusing on major changes in their health, economic strategies, social support networks, and political and civic engagement. I also asked about their use of AIDS service organizations and other framing institutions. Because of the longitudinal nature of this fieldwork, I was able to not only collect interview data, but also observe some life changes as they unfolded, such as Yvette's gradual movement toward disclosure of her HIV status to her son.

Wave 3: The HIV Safety Net Study

My research assistants and I supplemented the stories collected from the women with interviews conducted with 40 Chicago-based AIDS service providers in 2010. Robert Vargas and Marisol Mastrangelo conducted these interviews, bringing an organizational lens to our discussions with members of the HIV/AIDS community. We began by gathering the names of the 20 AIDS service organizations most frequently mentioned by the S2S and snapshot study respondents and approached each institution for interviews. In each organization, Robert and Marisol interviewed both a front-line staff member and a member of the leadership team. This helped us gain another perspective on some of the dynamics of settings Yondi and I observed in the S2S study and provided other insights into the organizational spaces that WLWHA were navigating.

During the process of analyzing data from both WLWHA and local AIDS organizations, the significance of the national HIV safety net in the everyday lives of women came into focus. In order to better understand the emergence and development of this piece of the story, I read several excellent AIDS histories that mined rich archival sources, but I wanted to hear firsthand from some of the women with whom I was now regularly interacting in various national HIV/AIDS meetings. I conducted snowball sampling, interviewing the first activists and advocates that I had gotten to know through attending these gatherings and then asking for additional names and introductions. Attending AIDS conferences, reading secondary material on AIDS history, and receiving feedback from reviewers of this manuscript also pointed me in the direction of the people with whom I should speak.

The original plan was to use these interviews to merely supplement what we were hearing about women's experiences in local organizations, but once it became clear that the institutional ties that women described were in fact connected to a larger national policy story, the HIV safety net study grew to include those working all over the country in this space. I personally interviewed 32 activists, advocates, and policy officials who were instrumental in the formation of, or who are currently staffing, the HIV/AIDS safety net across the United States. This allowed me to add a more historical and institutional dimension to what I was learning in Chicago from the WLWHA in the S2S and snapshot studies.[3]

ACCESS AND RECRUITMENT

The WLWHA in the HHR study were recruited through advertisements posted in Chicago-area hospitals and clinics, through HIV social service agencies, and by word of mouth. We also posted placards on city buses and in subway cars. In addition, I made presentations in various AIDS service organizations to advertise the study. Over the years, I made myself available to the AIDS community by doing presentations, sitting on various advisory boards for AIDS organizations, and attending events that both allowed me to learn the internal politics of the community and demonstrate my commitment to the issue and my willingness to give something in return for the generosity shown to me by making introductions, educating me about the issues, and inviting me into important conversations.

My team and I pursued trust-building with study participants from the earliest stages of the project, not just when we were in the interview room with respondents. Our efforts began with study design, as we pondered how we as researchers might collect information in a way that affirmed the rights, boundaries, and feelings of respondents. For example, an earlier design of our recruitment flyer presented the question, "Are you living with HIV/AIDS?" When we showed the flyer to one of our AIDS service provider partners, the physician pointed out that writing down our study's phone number, which was listed below the question, could be seen as an act of HIV-status disclosure. We subsequently changed the wording to read, "Do you know someone living with HIV/AIDS?" This is just one example of the care that had to be taken at recruitment in order to protect women's privacy.

The issue of privacy came up frequently as we tried to recruit our most elusive group: middle-class WLWHA. The reasons, I believe, are consistent with what I discuss in the book. Many of these women are not associated with AIDS service organizations, a main site from which we were recruiting. In order to attract this group to the project, we began recruiting from large private hospitals, contacting doctors and asking them to share information with their patients about the study. We also provided respondents with options for where we might conduct their interviews depending on their level of comfort, including reserved conference room space in a local AIDS service organization, a public library, or a nonprofit organization that did not offer HIV/AIDS-related services.

Building rapport quickly with respondents was an important part of our fieldwork given that our in-person interactions with a large subset of them only took place once. Again, this rapport-building process began with the study design, as we thought about what study activities would engender trust and comfort on the part of our respondents. We trained the undergraduate research assistants who were screening participants by phone to operate with the utmost care. Our level of preparation in entering the field—reading extant literature, talking to service providers working with the population to learn more, and investing significant time in fine-tuning our interview guide—all helped to set a tone with respondents.

But of course, the professionalism, intelligence, warmth, and comportment of the interviewers themselves were critical to the success of the project, and I selected graduate student interviewers in whom I had a great deal of trust. At the outset, we sought to match interviewers and interviewees by race, but this proved to be logistically challenging as the availability of our respondents did not always coincide with the availability of our interviewers, who were juggling graduate coursework alongside their fieldwork.[4] Spanish-language interviews were conducted by a member of the research team who was not of Latinx descent but who spoke fluent Spanish and had considerable experience conducting qualitative research in South America. Overall, we found that interviewers and interviewees found ways to connect and build rapport, and we did not observe major variation in the quantity, quality, or content of data collected through same-race or mixed-race pairings. When we began to see that the data we were collecting were similar across interviewers, we gained confidence that our multi-interviewer approach had validity and would produce analyzable information.

INTERVIEWING

This project relied on interviews as the primary source of data. "Through interviewing," Robert Weiss states in his classic *Learning from Strangers*, "we can learn about all the experiences, from joy through grief, that together constitute the human condition." Interviewing centers the voices of respondents in the analysis, allowing people to reflect on their social contexts and share the meaning-making that characterizes their experiences.[5] Interviews can reveal the emotional dimensions of social experience that are not always evident in behavior.

At the same time, faded memories, incorrect perceptions, or inaccurate information can all make their way into the interview. For example, Stevie (black, age 44) was one of the first women I interviewed during the S2S study. She passionately asserted that she "knew for sure" how she became HIV positive and pointed to her ex-boyfriend's infidelity. Delving deeper in our conversation, however, I quickly recognized that she had multiple experiences that potentially exposed her to the virus. But I could not ignore Stevie's narrative of "knowing for sure" and was obliged to think about the social significance of the assertion. "Interviews are social processes in themselves," Hanna Herzog writes; "They are an integral part of constructing individual subjectivity."[6] Perhaps "knowing for sure" was a way for Stevie to affirm her respectability and to safely situate herself in the pernicious dichotomy of those who were "innocent" versus "guilty" in the story of AIDS. I could then pursue a line of questioning in our interview and in my subsequent interviews with women that probed around these themes. I found that sometimes the most important data were not the statements themselves but how these statements fit into a broader social context and what it meant or signaled for women to adopt and assert particular narratives. In the writing process, I introduced women's assertions with language such as "she believes/recalls/reflects" in order to remind readers that data are based on respondents' accounts.

The interview itself can call forth a performance of respectability for some, in which the very act of being interviewed might encourage an interviewee to present a certain narrative or "neatly contained" story. In capturing women's trajectories of *dying from* to *living with*, we had to be careful not to push the data collection or analysis process in a way that ignored stories of non-transformation, "backsliding," non-linear routes, or that equated *dying from* with an embrace of non-normative behavior and *living with* as a strict adherence to normative behavior.

Some of this could be mitigated by an interviewer who was listening carefully and asking follow-up questions to clarify, verify, and gently push against what was being presented, as I did during my interview with Stevie. I attempted to train our interviewers to adopt a similar approach while being respectful of our respondents' presentation of information. In our interviews with activists and advocates, data could be checked against available documentation or the recollections of others. When we interviewed the S2S women whom we followed over time, we sometimes repeated a question or confirmed a response in a subsequent interview as a reliability check. We asked the interviewer to complete an ethnographic fieldnote after each interview, documenting the interview as event or interaction and capturing his/her impressions of what was shared. Coupling our interviews with participant-observation during waves 1 and 3 of the study was also helpful, although investigators have cautioned that even in ethnography, "One's lenses condition what can be seen."[7] Observing WLWHA traverse various spaces and watching activists and advocates debate and advocate for specific demands proved generative for my ideas as well. It also created moments of check-in where I could reconcile what we were hearing from women with what I was observing in various settings. I used these tools to try to ensure that the information presented in this book is as accurate as possible. But I also recognize both the significance and limitations of narrative accounts.

At the same time, we were also invested in ensuring that our interview process did not (re)traumatize our respondents. We were intentional about the execution of the interview. The team discussed the order of questions at length, experimenting with when in the interview to raise potentially sensitive topics such as histories of trauma, potentially illegal economic survival strategies, or experiences that could trigger HIV-related stigma. Attempting to reserve those topics until enough "warm-up" questions had been asked to build rapport and trust had to be balanced with the need to cover several topics within a 90-minute interview. While we revised the interview protocol several times before beginning fieldwork, we nevertheless used it as a guide rather than a script. Interviewers were free to ask open-ended questions and move around as the conversation progressed, based on their read of the comfort level of the interviewee, inserting planned questions into a conversation-style engagement. They then could check the protocol near the end of the interview to ensure that all of the topics had been addressed. The interview team discussed body language as well, building our skills around drawing out respondents by using a variety of techniques such as softening the tone of our voices, learning forward and offering nods of support as respondents shared intimate details, and being judicious about when and how we took notes as people spoke.

It is important to recognize the politics and risks of storytelling for respondents. A quote from Naina Khanna about WLWHA doing public speaking and telling their stories in various meetings with policy decision-makers applies to the research process as well:

> A lot of us were being invited to speak at places, but it was very clear that we were only being asked to come there to check a box: "Come tell your personal story on this panel. Here are all the 'experts,' and here's the 'community person.'" It's so disempowering. Our expertise is just as important, and our expertise matters because we've lived through the experience. And the very process of sharing our stories can be retraumatizing. One of the things we explicitly educate our folks on [at PWN-USA] is [that] we are not bound to share our stories in any type of way. If we are sharing our story, it's connected to a demand. There is always going to be to a demand. If I'm there to talk about [how] I asked to get tested twice and was denied HIV testing, the demand behind that is that testing should be available to everyone regardless of how [their] risk is perceived. It's not that people shouldn't share their stories, but our stories are political. It's important for us to understand that. Our stories are political and they are also tools for change, and we have the right to have boundaries around how we share them.

My team and I tried to be respectful and mindful of this, and we followed standard human subject research protocols. We reminded respondents that they could stop the interview at any time or choose not to answer any question without risking their research participant remuneration. For the protection of our respondents, we secured a Certificate of Confidentiality through the National Institutes of Health to protect identifiable research information from forced disclosure. Under the 21st Century Cures Act, any investigator or institution conducting research protected by such a certificate shall not, without the specific consent of the individual to whom the information pertains, disclose identifying information to any court or other person not connected with the research.[8] We also identified trained therapists working in the community to whom we could refer respondents in case the need arose.

We also viewed our respondents as co-creators of knowledge. It was not unusual during interviews for me to introduce either a preexisting sociological theory or to float one of my own to some of my most astute interviewees to hear their perspectives. Many times, that would lead to my best insights, as the women would remind me of contradictory examples, add a nuance that I had missed, or affirm that my thinking was heading in the right direction. This understanding of our respondents is an ethical matter given the susceptibility of WLWHA to exploitation and ethnography's (as a method) contentious history and habit of speaking *for* its research subjects rather than *with* or *alongside* them. Further, I believe that conceptualizing respondents as co-creators of knowledge facilitated the cultivation of the rapport our team enjoyed.[9]

DATA ANALYSIS

Interviews were tape-recorded and transcribed. We produced summaries for each transcript and entered key demographic data into spreadsheets in order to quickly see important trends. The interview transcripts were then coded by our undergraduate team members in two stages using Atlas data analysis software. Transcripts were first coded following themes identified in the interview guide. We later developed a set of codes that captured potential mechanisms of the transformative project and began trying to quantify how many of the women exhibited cognitive shifts, connections to the HIV safety net, connections to other institutions, and clear movement in terms of health, social support, economic, and political experiences. Through this data analysis, I developed and refined the concept of the transformative project. Coding was cross-checked across research assistants during the process to ensure reliability, and one undergraduate and a graduate assistant were later hired to check the reliability of the entire HHR dataset. This multi-staged coding process was inspired by a grounded theory approach that allowed categories to emerge from the data obtained, rather than imposing a theory on the data before research had begun, while maintaining connections with the extant literature to draw theoretical conclusions.[10] Finally, in the writing process, I engaged two new graduate research assistants who had not participated in the data collection process— Dominique Adams-Santos and Julian Glover—to read over the entire dataset and serve as interlocutors as I drafted and revised the manuscript. Having their perspective offered another useful check on my interpretation of the data and pushed my analysis even further.

During the writing phase, I selected four S2S women—Dawn Stevens, Beverly, Keisha, and Yvette—to feature as the central storytellers. Despite the volume of data we had collected by the end of project, coming back to a handful of individuals whose journeys readers could follow throughout the book felt like the best approach to explaining the transformative project. In my view, these central storytellers represent the diversity of the S2S group in terms of socioeconomic status, age, sexuality and sexual expression, histories of trauma, and organizational connectedness. I also wanted to ensure that I captured in depth at least one story of a woman who did not experience a transformation from *dying from* to *living with*, and readers had an opportunity to hear Tanya's story in chapter 5. I presented Trisha and Rosario's stories in depth in order to present a more racially diverse group of central storytellers, but I did not have the same level of multi-year interaction with them. I also did not include in-depth analyses of the other two S2S women I followed due to space constraints, but their stories shared several of the same themes with those of the central storytellers, and they offer shorter quotes throughout the book. While I made clear to the women that all of our interactions were part of my larger research project, I did not tell the central storytellers that they would occupy these roles in the book until we got very close to publication. I did not want women, upon realizing that they would be major figures in a book's narrative, to begin shaping their stories in particular ways toward that end. They were aware that I was writing a book, but because of the ways in which I moved in and out of their lives during my longitudinal fieldwork, I do not believe my project was at the front of their minds. My almost 15-year engagement with this group of women nevertheless provided me with a rich understanding of the depth of their stories, one that I believe helped illuminate the main theoretical offering of the book, the transformative project.

REPORTING BACK TO THE COMMUNITY

We had a community advisory board for the project that convened periodically in the early stages of the study. I then consulted members individually for advice, contacts, and feedback on developing tools such as the interview guide, recruitment materials, and drafts of this book. I received invitations from various members of the HIV/AIDS community to present my preliminary findings.

We also tried to be sensitive to the reality that WLWHA, especially in Chicago, with its thriving scientific community, are often asked to participate in research. This was driven home for me when, during my support group observations, I noticed that women routinely circulated flyers advertising the area's latest biomedical and social science research studies that were seeking participants. On the one hand, many women described their desire to help inform policy and scientific research, and women's increased participation in HIV treatment research was exactly the goal of activists like Dawn Averitt. On the other hand, we also must acknowledge the fraught history of the use of marginalized populations in scientific research and guard against research fatigue in women for whom every visit to a healthcare or social service provider becomes a moment in which they are pursued.[11] We tried to be mindful of all of these dynamics as we designed and carried out this research, exploring various options to reduce women's burdens along the way. We also financially compensated all S2S and snapshot study women for their participation in the research, with, on average, $40 for initial interviews and $60 for follow-up interviews. For better or for worse, it was evident that remuneration from research studies served as a component of some women's patchwork of economic survival strategies, raising ongoing and difficult questions about whether these resources serve as critically important acknowledgments of participants' time and labor, exploitation, or both.

Finally, each person whose story is presented at length in this book was either allowed to read or have read to them the sections in which they appear. This applied to the AIDS activists, advocates, and policy officials whose real names I use as well as the Chicago study women who appear under pseudonyms. This was important to ensure that I had not misrepresented or misinterpreted events. Further, I recognized the importance, particularly for the Chicago study women, who shared very intimate details about their lives, of giving them the opportunity to correct, to push back, to reflect, and to feel before others had access to their life stories. I wanted women to have an opportunity to process and come to terms with what would be shared with the world well before the book was released. The value of this approach was brought home to me when I received the following email from Yvette after she read the portions of the book in which she appears:

> My reaction to the excerpt of the book was not what I expected it to be. I started reading it on two occasions and each time I set it aside because it was painful, sad, and emotionally overwhelming to read. Thinking back on the young, vulnerable, and naïve woman I was is heart-breaking. Please accept my sincere apologies for the delayed response. After wrestling with my feelings, I was finally able to read the excerpt in its entirety. I loved it!!! You did a phenomenal job and I cannot wait to read the rest of the book. Thank you for allowing me to read it and provide comments. Also, thank you for caring enough to undertake this endeavor. I am eternally grateful that a part of my life story has been captured by the written word.

I was pleasantly surprised that no one attempted to significantly change her quotes or how she was presented. Instead, respondents offered corrections on dates, the sequence of events, and additional details, and in some instances edits to their quotes to improve clarity and readability. I appreciated these contributions and made the final decision about what feedback to include.

As the principle investigator for a research study of this size, I also felt a responsibility to the team to be intentional about our own self-care as researchers. We listened to many stories of trauma and injustice, and I tried to do regular check-ins with the graduate students and research staff who were gathering these stories in face-to-face interactions with the survivors, and with the undergraduate students who were sometimes spending hours reading truly difficult accounts. We tried to process some of this in research team meetings, and I encouraged team members to take regular breaks from the project to reflect and regroup. We also engaged in regular conversations about the motivations for our work: why we thought telling this story was important and what we hoped it would accomplish. Adopting an ethic of care for both our research participants and also for ourselves as investigators was absolutely necessary for sustaining the work.

REFLEXIVITY

My passion for social justice drew me to the topic of HIV/AIDS, but my belief in the power of rigorous scientific analysis equally contributed to the integrity and care taken to bring forth this book. I am an African American woman who grew up in a middle-class and later affluent household. After attending historically black colleges, my parents migrated to Michigan in the late 1960s from Nashville,

Tennessee, seeking opportunity in the wave of post–Civil Rights era initiatives designed to integrate the executive ranks working in the banking, automotive, and other industries of the north. When it became clear that the book's driving theme would be transformation, I had to be careful not to allow a narrative of black uplift through "respectable" means that had been so much a part of my own family's story to color my explication of the transformative project. My parents had long divorced me from any notion that there was "one right way" to exist in the world, and I similarly came to understand that there was no one right way to live before, during, or after an HIV diagnosis.

Therefore, I try to be careful throughout the book to demonstrate both the challenges that women faced even when they did "play by the rules," as well as to show women in all of their complexity, not only when they were *dying from* but also when they are *living with*. Rather than flatten their lives in later chapters or attempt to tie everything up in a neat bow, I sought to capture the ongoing conflicts and tensions and to include in my discussion behaviors that may fall outside of the confines of racial or sexual respectability. An opportunity for transformation should not require that women be saints, nor that they subscribe to a middle-class definition of success or failure. Part of the freedom that I sought to capture in this book was the way that women found strategies to live their lives on their own terms and in ways that were affirming and healthy for them.

During the course of working on this project, I also became a mother. Some of the ideas and experiences that respondents described related to motherhood were crystallized for me after becoming a parent myself. For example, learning how to assert myself as a patient and expectant mother while navigating a highly medicalized system brought in even sharper relief the magnitude of what Keisha was trying to navigate as a 19-year-old single expectant mother living with HIV. Both of us were operating in the shadow of a fraught medical system that did not always value our bodies, knowledge, or autonomy as black women, but we were bringing vastly different tools to guard against mistreatment. We were both fortunate enough to deliver our children in world-class hospitals, but I was also a middle-aged, married, tenured professor who brought additional support in the form of a hired doula. Hospital staff called me Dr. Watkins-Hayes and engaged me in conversation about my role as a Northwestern University professor in the delivery room, providing me with an additional layer of social status as I underwent the highly vulnerable process of giving birth.

During data analysis, when I came back to the story of Keisha's pregnancy and my visit to her in the hospital after her son's birth, I read the situation through a different lens. I better understood the duality of exuberance and frightful uncertainty that she was experiencing, and how it was exponentially compounded by her status as a woman living with HIV/AIDS. It complicated everything—from the potential health of her baby, to her social status in the delivery room, to the question of who would support her and the baby once she was discharged from the hospital. This is not to suggest that we must experience everything that our respondents experience in order to provide strong analysis. Of course a person who has not had a similar experience could no doubt come to the same conclusions that I did. But just as the charge to be reflexive in our research encourages us to examine our potential biases, so too does it reveal the tools we bring that might shape our understanding and interpretation of events. By being explicit about our vantage points and what they might mean for our analysis for others to see and assess, the work is enriched.

Returning to Dawn's quote at the beginning of this appendix, all of these debates and tensions, some resolved and others not, appear on the pages of *Remaking a Life*. There were several daunting peaks and seemingly endless valleys when the magnitude of what I was trying to capture in this book felt as though it would forever elude me. In those moments, I picked up whatever it was that I was carrying, put it on my back, and kept walking. I thank the people whose stories are captured in this book for doing the same.

Health, Hardship, and
Renewal Respondents

The following tables provide important information about the participants in the
Health, Hardship, and Renewal study. Table 3 provides information about Sister
to Sister and snapshot study participants whose quotes and stories appear in the
book. To preserve confidentiality, I use pseudonyms for all women in table 3.
Table 4 lists the names of all national AIDS activists, advocates, policy officials,
and service providers interviewed for this book, identified by their real names.

Table 3 Our Storytellers

Name	Race/ethnicity	Age at recruitment	Years since diagnosis
Barb	White	56	10+
Beverly Maxwell*	African American	41	10+
Charlene	Latina	47	10+
Dani	African American	44	10+
Dawn Stevens*	African American	48	20+
Estrella	Latina	31	<5
Eve	African American	31	5+
Gwen	African American	56	10+
Jacinda	African American	60	10+
Josie	African American	35	15+
June	Latina	48	10+
Katy	White	36	10+
Keisha Rainey*	African American	19	<5
Layla	White	41	10+
Lupe	Latina	56	10+
Maria	Latina	41	10+
Peggy	White	46	10+
Rochelle	African American	35	10+
Rosa	Latina	28	10+
Rosario Salazar*	African American & Latina	37	<5
Tanya	African American	40	<5
Tina	African American	28	10+
Trisha McIntosh*	White	55	10+
Yvette Simmons*	African American	38	10+

*Central storytellers

Name	Role and organizational affiliation	Race
Frances Ashe-Goins	Former Associate Director for Partnerships and Programs, HHS Office on Women's Health	Black
Dawn Averitt	Founder, The Well Project	White
Cornelius Baker	Chief Policy Advisor at US Department of State, Office of the US Global AIDS Coordinator and Health Diplomacy	Black
Alicia Beatty	Director (ret.), Circle of Care	Black
Gina Brown	Community Organizer, Southern AIDS Coalition	Black
Vignetta Charles	Chief Executive Officer, ETR	Black
Cecilia Chung	Founder, Positively Trans; Senior Director, Transgender Law Center	Asian
Rebecca Denison	Founder, Women Organized to Respond to Life-Threatening Diseases (WORLD)	White
Antigone Dempsey	Director, Division of Policy and Data, HIV/AIDS Bureau, HRSA	White
Dázon Dixon Diallo	Founder and President, SisterLove, Inc.	Black
Ingrid Floyd	Executive Director, Iris House	Black
Debra Frasier-Howze	Founding Executive Director (ret.), National Black Leadership Commission on AIDS; Senior Vice President of Government and External Affairs, OraSure Technologies (ret.)	Black
Helene Gayle	Former Director, National Center for HIV, STD, and TB Prevention, US CDC	Black
Bambi Gaddist	Executive Director, Joseph H. Neal Wellness Center	Black
Eric Goosby	Special Envoy on Tuberculosis (TB), United Nations; Professor of Medicine and Director of Global Health Delivery and Diplomacy, Institute for Global Health Sciences, University of California, San Francisco	Black
C. Virginia Fields	President and Chief Executive Officer, NBLCA	Black
David Harvey	Executive Director, National Coalition of STD Directors	White
Kathie Hiers	Chief Executive Officer, AIDS Alabama	White
David Holtgrave	Dean of the School of Public Health, University at Albany, State University of New York	White
Ernest Hopkins	Director of Legislative Affairs, San Francisco AIDS Foundation	Black
Jennifer Kates	Vice President and Director of Global Health and HIV Policy, Kaiser Family Foundation	White

Table 4   (continued)

Name	Role and organizational affiliation	Race
Naina Khanna	Executive Director, Positive Women's Network-USA	South Asian
Tiommi Luckett	Transgender Activist and HIV Awareness Advocate	Black
David Malebranche	Associate Professor of Medicine and Medical Director of Student and Employee Health, Morehouse School of Medicine	Black
Marsha Martin	Director/Coordinator, Global Network of Black People Working in HIV	Black
Terry McGovern	Founder, HIV Law Project	White
David Ernesto Munar	President and Chief Executive Officer, Howard Brown Health	Latinx
Pat Nalls	Founder and Executive Director, The Women's Collective	South Asian
Linda Scruggs	Co-Owner, Ribbon Consulting Group; Founding member, PWN-USA and the National Black Women's HIV/AIDS Network	Black
Charles Stephens	Founding Executive Director, The Counter Narrative Project	Black
Krishna Stone	Director of Community Relations, GMHC	Black
Carole Treston	Executive Director, Association of Nurses in AIDS Care	White
Ivy Turnbull	Deputy Executive Director, AIDS Alliance for Women, Infants, Children, Youth, and Families	Black
Phill Wilson	Founder and Former Chief Executive Officer, Black AIDS Institute	Black

Table 5   Sister to Sister Respondent Demographics

	Range	Mean	Mode
Age	19–60	37.9	41
Household income	< $15,000 – > $70,000	≈ $24,444	< $15,000
Years of education	8–17 years	12.6 years	14 years
Marital status	—	—	Single
Number of children	0–9	2.7	1

Table 6 Snapshot Study Respondent Demographics

	All (n = 84)	Black (n = 35)	White (n = 21)	Latina (n = 22)	Biracial (n = 6)
Age					
Mean	45.14	45.6	44.3	47.1	38
Median	46	46	46	49	39
Range	23–72	27–63	24–62	28–72	23–46
Birthplace					
Chicago Area	46 (55%)	27 (77%)	9 (43%)	6 (27%)	4 (66%)
Illinois (outside of Chicago Area)	7 (8%)	2 (6%)	5 (24%)	0	0
United States (outside of Illinois)	16 (19%)	6 (17%)	6 (29%)	2 (9%)	2 (33%)
Puerto Rico	2 (2%)	0	0	2 (9%)	0
Canada	1 (1%)	0	1 (4%)	0	0
Mexico	8 (9%)	0	0	8 (36%)	0
Latin America (outside of Mexico)	4 (5%)	0	0	4 (18%)	0
US citizen	71 (84%)	35 (100%)	20 (95%)	10 (45%)	6 (100%)
Time since diagnosis					
6 months–1 year	2 (2%)	1 (3%)	0	0	1 (17%)
2–4 years	6 (7%)	3 (9%)	1 (4%)	1 (4.5%)	1 (17%)
5–10 years	28 (33%)	11 (31%)	7 (33%)	8 (36%)	2 (33%)
11 or more years	48 (57%)	20 (57%)	13 (62%)	13 (59%)	2 (33%)
Number of children					
Mean	2.3	2.6	1.5	2.9	3.6
Median	4	2	1	3	4
Range	0–10	0–10	0–4	0–6	1–6
Marital status					
Single, never married	23 (27%)	13 (37%)	4 (19%)	4 (18%)	2 (33%)
Partnered	15 (18%)	5 (14%)	5 (24%)	3 (14%)	2 (33%)
Married	18 (21%)	7 (20%)	5 (24%)	5 (23%)	1 (17%)
Separated	10 (12%)	3 (9%)	1 (4%)	6 27%)	0
Divorced	15 (18%)	6 (17%)	4 (19%)	4 (18%)	1 (17%)
Widowed	3 (4%)	1 (3%)	2 (10%)	0	0

(continued)

Table 6 (continued)

	All *(n = 84)*	*Black* *(n = 35)*	*White* *(n = 21)*	*Latina* *(n = 22)*	*Biracial* *(n = 6)*
Education					
Less than high school	32 (38%)	9 (26%)	5 (24%)	15 (68%)	3 (50%)
GED	1 (1%)	1 (3%)	0	0	0
High school	21 (25%)	12 (34%)	4 (19%)	3 (14%)	2 (33%)
Some college	20 (24%)	9 (26%)	6 (29%)	4 (18%)	1 (17%)
College degree	7 (8%)	4 (11%)	3 (14%)	0	0
Graduate degree	3 (4%)	0	3 (14%)	0	0
Main income source					
Government subsidy	47 (56%)	24 (69%)	9 (43%)	11 (50%)	3 (50%)
Documented wages	20 (24%)	7 (20%)	7 (33%)	5 (23%)	1 (17%)
Undocumented wages	5 (6%)	1 (3%)	2 (10%)	2 (9%)	0
Gifts	4 (5%)	1 (3%)	1 (4%)	1 (4.5%)	1 (17%)
Unemployment	2 (2%)	1 (3%)	0	1 (4.5%)	0
Spouse's salary	3 (4%)	0	1 (4%)	2 (9%)	0
Savings	1 (1%)	0	1 (4%)	0	0
Multiple sources	2 (2%)	1 (3%)	0	0	1 (17%)
Annual personal income					
No income	3 (4%)	0	0	3 (14%)	0
Less than $20,000	68 (81%)	29 (83%)	16 (76%)	17 (77%)	6 (100%)
$20,001–40,000	6 (7%)	5 (14%)	0	1 (4.5%)	0
$40,001 or greater	7 (8%)	1 (3%)	5 (24%)	1 (4.5%)	0
Annual household income					
No income	1 (1%)	0	0	1 (4.5%)	0
Less than $20,000	59 (70%)	25 (71%)	13 (62%)	16 (73%)	5 (83%)
$20,001–40,000	13 (15%)	7 (20%)	1 (4%)	4 (18%)	1 (17%)
$40,001 or greater	11 (13%)	3 (9%)	7 (33%)	1 (4.5%)	0
Employment status					
Working full or part time	25 (30%)	9 (26%)	7 (33%)	7 (32%)	1 (17%)
Not working	59 (70%)	26 (74%)	14 (66%)	15 (68%)	5 (83%)
Public assistance history					
Present or past	31 (37%)	15 (43%)	6 (29%)	5 (23%)	5 (83%)
No history	53 (63%)	20 (57%)	15 (71%)	17 (77%)	1 (17%)

	All (n = 84)	*Black* (n = 35)	*White* (n = 21)	*Latina* (n = 22)	*Biracial* (n = 6)
Food stamp history					
Present or past	54 (64%)	26 (74%)	8 (38%)	14 (64%)	6 (100%)
No history	30 (36%)	9 (26%)	13 (62%)	8 (36%)	0
Medicaid / Medicare history					
Present or past	50 (60%)	25 (71%)	10 (48%)	10 (45%)	5 (83%)
No history	34 (40%)	10 (29%)	11 (52%)	12 (55%)	1 (17%)
Social Security history					
Present or past	43 (52%)	21 (60%)	9 (43%)	10 (45%)	3 (50%)
No history	41 (49%)	14 (.40)	12 (.57)	12 (55%)	3 (50%)

Notes

INTRODUCTION. INJURIES OF INEQUALITY AND THE
TRANSFORMATIVE PROJECT

1. Douglas S. Massey and Nancy A. Denton, *American Apartheid: Segregation and the Making of the Underclass* (Harvard University Press, 1993); Mary Pattillo, *Black Picket Fences: Privilege and Peril among the Black Middle Class* (University of Chicago Press, 2013); William Julius Wilson, *The Truly Disadvantaged: The Inner City, the Underclass, and Public Policy* (University of Chicago Press, 2012).

2. Michelle Alexander, *The New Jim Crow: Mass Incarceration in the Age of Colorblindness* (New Press, 2012); Todd R. Clear, *Imprisoning Communities: How Mass Incarceration Makes Disadvantaged Neighborhoods Worse* (Oxford University Press, 2007); Mary Pattillo, Bruce Western, and David Weiman, *Imprisoning America: The Social Effects of Mass Incarceration* (Russell Sage Foundation, 2004).

3. Routes of HIV transmission include sexual intercourse; exposure to blood (via transfusion of blood or blood products; sharing injection needles, syringes, or "works"; or an occupational needlestick); or perinatally (from mother to child during pregnancy or breast feeding).

4. CD4 cell counts below 200 cells per cubic millimeter of blood (200 cells /mm3) indicate that HIV has progressed to AIDS. Normal CD4 counts are between 500 and 1,600 cells/mm3. One can also be diagnosed with AIDS after

developing one or more opportunistic infections, regardless of CD4 count (see www.aids.gov).

5. AmfAR, "Statistics: Worldwide," www.amfar.org/worldwide-aids-stats/.

6. Cathy J. Cohen, *The Boundaries of Blackness: AIDS and the Breakdown of Black Politics* (University of Chicago Press, 1999); Robert Fullilove, "Mass Incarceration in the United States and HIV/AIDS: Cause and Effect," *Ohio State Journal of Criminal Law* 9 (2011): 353–61; Jacob Levenson, *The Secret Epidemic: The Story of AIDS and Black America* (Anchor, 2005).

7. Merrill Charles Singer et al., "Syndemics, Sex and the City: Understanding Sexually Transmitted Diseases in Social and Cultural Context," *Social Science & Medicine* 63, no. 8 (2006): 2010–21.

8. Kristine A. Johnson and Shannon M. Lynch, "Predictors of Maladaptive Coping in Incarcerated Women Who Are Survivors of Childhood Sexual Abuse," *Journal of Family Violence* 28, no. 1 (2013): 43–52.

9. Lawrence K. Altman, "AIDS Is Now the Leading Killer of Americans from 25 to 44," *New York Times*, January 31, 1995, C7.

10. Dawn was interviewed by three members of the study team over a decade. In 2005, the original project coordinator interviewed her twice and conducted an observation session with her. A graduate research assistant interviewed Dawn in 2010, and I conducted interviews with Dawn in 2014 and 2015. Having multiple interviewers allowed us to verify the consistency of Dawn's account and to follow her over a ten-year period.

11. Celeste Watkins-Hayes, LaShawnDa Pittman-Gay, and Jean Beaman, "'Dying from' to 'Living with': Framing Institutions and the Coping Processes of African American Women Living with HIV/AIDS," *Social Science & Medicine* 74, no. 12 (2012): 2028–36.

12. Jennifer Brier, *Infectious Ideas: US Political Responses to the AIDS Crisis* (University of North Carolina Press, 2009); Steven Epstein, *Impure Science: AIDS, Activism, and the Politics of Knowledge* (University of California Press, 1996); Patricia D. Siplon, *AIDS and the Policy Struggle in the United States* (Georgetown University Press, 2002); Raymond A. Smith and Patricia D. Siplon, *Drugs into Bodies: Global AIDS Treatment Activism* (Greenwood, 2006).

13. Anthropologist Laurence Ralph explores the depths and forms of injury in a west Chicago neighborhood, defining it as, "a vast spectrum . . . of encumbrances that followed [residents] through life, weighed them down, and affected their future prospects." Laurence Ralph, *Renegade Dreams: Living through Injury in Gangland Chicago* (University of Chicago Press, 2014), 5.

14. Mario Luis Small, *Unanticipated Gains: Origins of Network Inequality in Everyday Life* (Oxford University Press, 2009).

15. Scott W. Allard, *Out of Reach: Place, Poverty, and the New American Welfare State* (Yale University Press, 2009).

16. The Ryan White CARE Act is the largest federally funded program in the United States for PLWHA. The act provides funding to improve care availability for low-income, uninsured, and under-insured PLWHA and their families. I present more information about the history and implementation of the act in chapter 2.

17. Patrick Sharkey, *Stuck in Place: Urban Neighborhoods and the End of Progress toward Racial Equality* (University of Chicago Press, 2013); Wilson, *The Truly Disadvantaged;* William Julius Wilson, *When Work Disappears: The World of the New Urban Poor* (Vintage, 2011).

18. Edward Flores, *God's Gangs: Barrio Ministry, Masculinity, and Gang Recovery* (New York University Press, 2013); Sharon S. Oselin, *Leaving Prostitution: Getting Out and Staying Out of Sex Work* (New York University Press, 2014); Ralph, *Renegade Dreams;* Robert J. Sampson and John H. Laub, "Desistance from Crime over the Life Course," in *Handbook of the Life Course,* ed. Jeylan T. Mortimer and Michael J. Shanahan (Kluwer, 2003), 295–309. See also Shadd Maruna, *Making Good: How Ex-convicts Reform and Rebuild their Lives* (American Psychological Association, 2001); and David J. Brown, "The Professional Ex-: An Alternative for Exiting the Deviant Career," *Sociological Quarterly* 32, no. 2 (1991): 219–30.

19. Dexter R. Voisin, "The Relationship between Violence Exposure and HIV Sexual Risk Behaviors: Does Gender Matter?" *American Journal of Orthopsychiatry* 75, no. 4 (2005): 497–506.

20. Celeste Watkins-Hayes, "Intersectionality and the Sociology of HIV/ AIDS: Past, Present, and Future Research Directions," *Annual Review of Sociology* 40, no. 1 (2014): 431–57.

21. Frances Beal, "Double Jeopardy: To Be Black and Female," in *Words of Fire: An Anthology of African-American Feminist Thought,* ed. Beverly Guy-Sheftall (New Press, 1995), 146–55; Patricia Hill Collins, *Black Feminist Thought: Knowledge, Consciousness, and the Politics of Empowerment* (Routledge, 1990); Combahee River Collective, "A Black Feminist Statement," in *Home Girls: A Black Feminist Anthology,* ed. Barbara Smith (Rutgers University Press, 1983), 264–74; Anna Julia Cooper, *A Voice from the South* (Oxford University Press, 1988); Kimberlé Crenshaw, "Mapping the Margins: Intersectionality, Identity Politics, and Violence against Women of Color," *Stanford Law Review* 43, no. 6 (1991): 1241–99; and Deborah K. King, "Multiple Jeopardy, Multiple Consciousness: The Context of a Black Feminist Ideology," *Signs: Journal of Women in Culture & Society* 14, no. 1 (1988): 42–72.

22. Sumi Cho, Kimberlé Crenshaw, and Leslie McCall, "Toward a Field of Intersectionality Studies: Theory, Applications, and Praxis," *Signs: Journal of Women in Culture & Society* 38, no. 4 (2013): 785–810.

23. Hae Yeon Choo and Myra Marx Ferree, "Practicing Intersectionality in Sociological Research: A Critical Analysis of Inclusions, Interactions, and

Institutions in the Study of Inequalities," *Sociological Theory* 28, no. 2 (2010): 129–49; Brittney Cooper, "Intersectionality," in *The Oxford Handbook of Feminist Theory,* ed. Lisa Disch and Mary Hawkesworth (Oxford University Press, 2016); Leslie McCall, "The Complexity of Intersectionality," *Signs: Journal of Women in Culture & Society* 30 (2005): 1771–800.

24. Ange-Marie Hancock, "Intersectionality as a Normative and Empirical Paradigm," *Politics & Gender* 3, no. 2 (2007): 248–54; Jennifer Nash, *Black Feminism Reimagined: After Intersectionality* (Duke University Press, 2019).

25. amfAR, "Statistics: Women and HIV/AIDS," www.amfar.org/about-hiv-and-aids/facts-and-stats/statistics--women-and-hiv-aids/.

26. US CDC, "HIV/AIDS among Women."

27. Black Women's HIV/AIDS Network and National Black Gay Men's Advocacy Coalition, "Joint Statement from the Leadership Meeting of Black Women and Black Gay Men," 2007.

28. US CDC, WISQARS Leading Causes of Death Reports, 1999–2004; Demian Christiansen, Nanette Benbow, and Carrie Kempler, "The HIV/AIDS Epidemic in Chicago: Chicago HIV/AIDS Brief" (Office of AIDS Surveillance, Chicago Department of Public Health, 2006). All data for blacks and whites reflect non-Hispanic racial categories. All data are based on HIV/AIDS Reporting System (HARS) reports to the Chicago Department of Public Health as of September 30, 2006.

29. US CDC, "Leading Causes of Death in Females, United States."

30. I use the term *advocate* to refer to those who engage in "interventions such as speaking, writing or acting in favor of a particular issue or cause, policy or group of people. In the public health field, advocacy is assumed to be in the public interest, whereas lobbying by a special interest group may or may not be in the public interest." Activists can be thought of as those taking direct action to achieve a political or social goal. Public Health Agency of Canada, "Glossary of Terms," www.canada.ca/en/public-health/services/public-health-practice/skills-online/glossary-terms.html.

31. US CDC, "HIV among Transgender People."

32. Tonia Poteat, Danielle German, and Colin Flynn, "The Conflation of Gender and Sex: Gaps and Opportunities in HIV Data among Transgender Women and MSM," *Global Public Health* 11, no 7–8 (2016): 835–48.

33. Julian Kevon Glover, "Redefining Realness? On Janet Mock, Laverne Cox, T. S. Madison, and the Representation of Transgender Women of Color in Media," *Souls* 18, no. 2–4 (2016): 338–57.

34. Watkins-Hayes, Pittman-Gay, and Beaman, "'Dying from' to 'Living with.'"

35. "Ryan White 2016: Scientific and Programmatic Accomplishments," TargetHIV, https://targethiv.org/blog/ryan-white-2016-scientific-and-programmatic-accomplishments.

36. US CDC, "Dear Colleague: Information from the CDC's Division of HIV/ AIDS Prevention," September 27, 2017.

37. Johanna Crane, Kathleen Quirk, and Ariane Van Der Straten, "'Come Back When You're Dying': The Commodification of AIDS among California's Urban Poor," *Social Science & Medicine* 55, no. 7 (2002): 1115–27; Alyson O'Daniel, *Holding On: African American Women Surviving HIV/AIDS* (University of Nebraska Press, 2016); John A. Updegraff et al., "Positive and Negative Effects of HIV Infection in Women with Low Socioeconomic Resources," *Personality & Social Psychology Bulletin* 28, no. 3 (2002): 382–94.

CHAPTER 1. DYING FROM

1. Indiana Department of Health, "Scott County Public Health Emergency Declaration Extended," 2016, www.in.gov/isdh/files/May_2_2016_SCOTT_ COUNTY_PUBLIC_HEALTH_EMERGENCY_DECLARATION_ EXTENDED.pdf.

2. US CDC, "Community Outbreak of HIV Infection Linked to Injection Drug Use of Oxymorphone—Indiana, 2015," *Morbity and Mortality Weekly Report* 64 (2015): 443–44.

3. Jeffrey S. Crowley and Gregorio A. Millett, "Preventing HIV and Hepatitis Infections among People Who Inject Drugs: Leveraging an Indiana Outbreak Response to Break the Impasse," *AIDS & Behavior* 21, no. 4 (2017): 968–72; Colleen Nguyen, "HIV in Indiana: 81 Cases and Counting," *Health Map: The Disease Daily: Outbreak News* (blog), April 5, 2015, www.diseasedaily.org/diseasedaily /article/hiv-indiana-81-cases-and-counting-4515; Steffanie A. Strathdee and Chris Beyrer, "Threading the Needle: How to Stop the HIV Outbreak in Rural Indiana," *New England Journal of Medicine* 373, no. 5 (2015): 397–99.

4. Shari Rudavsky, "An Indiana Town Recovering from 190 HIV Cases," *IndyStar,* April 8, 2016.

5. US CDC, "Injection Drug Use and HIV Risk," 2018.

6. F. I. Bastos and S. A. Strathdee, "Evaluating Effectiveness of Syringe Exchange Programmes: Current Issues and Future Prospects," *Social Science & Medicine* 51, no. 12 (2000): 1771–82; Don C. Des Jarlais, "Research, Politics, and Needle Exchange," *American Journal of Public Health 90, no. 9* (2000): 1392–94; "HIV and AIDS Information: Injecting Drug Use—Why Is Injecting Drug Use a Risk for HIV Transmission?" *AIDSmap,* 2016; David Vlahov et al., "Needle Exchange Programs for the Prevention of Human Immunodeficiency Virus Infection: Epidemiology and Policy," *American Journal of Epidemiology* 154, no. 12 (2001): S70–S77; Alex Wodak and Annie Cooney, "Do Needle Syringe Programs Reduce HIV Infection among Injecting Drug Users: A Comprehensive Review of the International Evidence," *Substance Use & Misuse* 41, no. 6–7 (2006): 777–813.

7. Rudavsky, "An Indiana Town."

8. Sarah Parvini, "In Rural Indiana, Battling HIV, Drugs and Bleak Times," *Los Angeles Times*, April 1, 2015.

9. David Rutter, "Little Indiana Town Paid for War on Planned Parenthood,"*Post-Tribune*, June 6, 2015.

10. In many states, PLWHA can face felony charges for not disclosing their HIV status to their sexual or needle-sharing partners. It can be a felony for PLWHA to expose others to any bodily fluid, including those not known to transmit HIV such as saliva, sweat, and tears. It is a felony in some jurisdictions for PLWHA to donate or sell their semen, blood, or plasma, although those fluids are tested after collection. Trevor Hoppe, *Punishing Disease: HIV and the Criminalization of Sickness* (University of California Press, 2017); J. Stan Lehman et al., "Prevalence and Public Health Implications of State Laws That Criminalize Potential HIV Exposure in the United States," *AIDS & Behavior* 18, no. 6 (2014): 997–1006.

11. Danielle Paquette, "How an HIV Outbreak Hit Rural Indiana—and Why We Should Be Paying Attention," *Chicago Tribune*, March 30, 2015.

12. Judith D. Auerbach, Justin O. Parkhurst, and Carlos F. Cáceres, "Addressing Social Drivers of HIV/AIDS for the Long-Term Response: Conceptual and Methodological Considerations," *Global Public Health* 6, no. 3 (supp.; 2011): S293–309; Samuel R. Friedman et al., *Social Networks, Drug Injectors' Lives, and HIV/AIDS* (Springer Science and Business Media, 2006); Samuel R. Friedman and Sevgi Aral, "Social Networks, Risk-potential Networks, Health, and Disease," *Journal of Urban Health* 78, no. 3 (2001): 411–18; Andrew V. Papachristos, David M. Hureau, and Anthony A. Braga, "The Corner and the Crew: The Influence of Geography and Social Networks on Gang Violence," *American Sociological Review* 78, no. 3 (2013): 417–47.

13. Mark Granovetter, "The Strength of Weak Ties: A Network Theory Revisited," *Sociological Theory* (1983): 201–33.

14. Lisa Marie Cacho, *Social Death: Racialized Rightlessness and the Criminalization of the Unprotected* (New York University Press, 2012), 4.

15. US CDC, "Pneumocystis Pneumonia—Los Angeles," *Morbidity and Mortality Weekly Report* 30 (1981): 250–52.

16. Although the first known HIV cases were reported in 1981, the virus is thought to have existed in the United States since at least the mid- to late 1970s. In 1999, scientists mapped the origin of HIV to a subspecies of African chimpanzees. HIV is believed to have jumped from chimps to humans at some point, and recent research suggests that the virus most likely started circulating among humans in sub-Saharan Africa sometime between 1884 and 1924. One theory posits that hunters were likely exposed to the virus through infected chimpanzees, perhaps through contact with chimpanzee blood through cuts on the hands of hunters handling dead chimp carcasses, or by the consumption of chimp meat. Many theories attempt to explain HIV's global spread. Cases of the virus have

been found dating back as early as 1959, in the blood sample of a man from the Democratic Republic of Congo. From the Congo, the virus potentially spread to Europe, through channels dating back to colonialism, and to North America, perhaps through channels between the Congo and Haiti. Other theories have posited the potential spread of the virus through the administration of vaccines and unsafe needle practices by Europeans operating in sub-Saharan Africa in the early twentieth century or through the blood plasma trade between the US and Haiti. Other transmission channels were likely expanded during rapid urbanization in west-central Africa. Victoria A. Harden and Anthony Fauci, *AIDS at 30: A History* (Potomac Books, 2012); "What Is HIV/AIDS?" www.aids.gov; "HIV/AIDS Emerged as Early as 1880s," *The AIDS Reader,* November 2, 2008.

17. US CDC, "Kaposi's Sarcoma and Pneumocystis Pneumonia among Homosexual Men—New York City and California," *Morbidity and Mortality Weekly Report* 30 (1981): 305–8.

18. Lawrence K. Altman, "Rare Cancer Seen in 41 Homosexuals," *New York Times,* July 3, 1981.

19. For more on this history, see Jennifer Brier, *Infectious Ideas: US Political Responses to the AIDS Crisis* (University of North Carolina Press, 2009); Gena Corea, *The Invisible Epidemic: The Story of Women and AIDS* (Harper Collins, 1992); Steven Epstein, *Impure Science: AIDS, Activism, and the Politics of Knowledge* (University of California Press, 1996); Patricia D. Siplon, *AIDS and the Policy Struggle in the United States* (Georgetown University Press, 2002).

20. Cathy J. Cohen, *The Boundaries of Blackness: AIDS and the Breakdown of Black Politics* (University of Chicago Press, 1999).

21. Congress enacted a ban on federal funding for syringe services programs in 1988, lifting it briefly during fiscal year 2010–2011 before reinstating the ban in 2012. In 2016, in response to the Scott County outbreak and the opioid crisis, congressional leaders modified the law to allow federal funding to pay for the operation of these programs but not the syringes themselves. Nevertheless, in 2015, 23 states had laws that criminalized the distribution or possession of syringes for illegal drug use, and only 16 states had laws that explicitly authorized needle- and syringe-exchange programs.

For more on the political history of needle-exchange programs, see Ethan Nadelmann and Lindsay LaSalle, "Two Steps Forward, One Step Back: Current Harm Reduction Policy and Politics in the United States," *Harm Reduction Journal* 14, no. 1 (2017): 37–43; Josiah D. Rich and Eli Y. Adashi, "Ideological Anachronism Involving Needle and Syringe Exchange Programs: Lessons from the Indiana HIV Outbreak," *JAMA* 314, no. 1 (2015): 23–24; Richard Weinmeyer, "Needle Exchange Programs' Status in US Politics," *American Medical Association Journal of Ethics* 18, no. 3 (2016): 252–57.

22. David Vlahov and Benjamin Junge, "The Role of Needle Exchange Programs in HIV Prevention," *Public Health Reports* 113, supp. 1 (1998): 75.

23. US CDC, "HIV in the United States," 2016.

24. Alfredo Nicolosi et al., "The Efficiency of Male-to-Female and Female-to-Male Sexual Transmission of the Human Immunodeficiency Virus: A Study of 730 Stable Couples," *Epidemiology* 5, no. 6 (1994): 570–75.

25. US CDC, "Sexual Violence: Facts at a Glance," 2012.

26. Also see Georgia Walton et al., "High Prevalence of Childhood Emotional, Physical and Sexual Trauma among a Canadian Cohort of HIV-Seropositive Illicit Drug Users," *AIDS Care* 23, no. 6 (2011): 714–21.

27. Michele Tracy Berger, *Workable Sisterhood: The Political Journey of Stigmatized Women with HIV/AIDS* (Princeton University Press, 2010); Darlene Clark Hine, "Rape and the Inner Lives of Black Women in the Middle West," *Signs* 14, no. 4 (1989): 912–20; Danielle L. McGuire, *At the Dark End of the Street: Black Women, Rape, and Resistance—a New History of the Civil Rights Movement from Rosa Parks to the Rise of Black Power* (Vintage, 2011); Beth Richie, *Arrested Justice: Black Women, Violence, and America's Prison Nation* (New York University Press, 2012).

28. Evelynn Hammonds, "Missing Persons: African American Women, AIDS, and the History of Disease," in *Words of Fire: An Anthology of African-American Feminist Thought*, ed. Beverly Guy-Sheftall (New Press, 1995), 440.

29. Saidiya V. Hartman, *Scenes of Subjection: Terror, Slavery, and Self-Making in Nineteenth-Century America* (Oxford University Press, 1997).

30. Patricia Hill Collins, *Black Feminist Thought: Knowledge, Consciousness, and the Politics of Empowerment* (London: Routledge, 2000); Ange-Marie Hancock, *The Politics of Disgust: The Public Identity of the Welfare Queen* (New York University Press, 2004); Evelyn Brooks Higginbotham, *Righteous Discontent: The Women's Movement in the Black Baptist Church, 1880–1920* (Harvard University Press, 1993).

31. Bryana H. French, "More than Jezebels and Freaks: Exploring How Black Girls Navigate Sexual Coercion and Sexual Scripts," *Journal of African American Studies* 17, no. 1 (2013): 35–50; Monique Morris, *Pushout: The Criminalization of Black Girls in Schools* (New Press, 2016).

32. Evelynn M. Hammonds, "Seeing AIDS: Race, Gender, and Representation," in *The Gender Politics of HIV/AIDS in Women: Perspectives on the Pandemic in the United States*, ed. Nancy Goldstein and Jennifer L. Manlowe (New York University Press, 1997), 113–26.

33. Marlon T. Riggs, *Tongues Untied: Black Men Loving Black Men*, Frameline's Lesbian and Gay Cinema, 1989.

34. Shanta R. Dube et al., "Childhood Abuse, Neglect, and Household Dysfunction and the Risk of Illicit Drug Use: The Adverse Childhood Experiences Study," *Pediatrics* 111, no. 3 (2003): 564–72; Dexter R. Voisin, "The Relationship between Violence Exposure and HIV Sexual Risk Behaviors: Does Gender Matter?" *American Journal of Orthopsychiatry* 75, no. 4 (2005): 497–506; Helen W.

Wilson and Cathy Spatz Widom, "An Examination of Risky Sexual Behavior and HIV in Victims of Child Abuse and Neglect: A 30-Year Follow-Up," *Health Psychology* 27, no. 2 (2008): 149.

35. Gail E. Wyatt et al., "Does a History of Trauma Contribute to HIV Risk for Women of Color? Implications for Prevention and Policy," *American Journal of Public Health* 92, no. 4 (2002): 660–65.

36. These patterns are not limited to women. In a study of gay men, Allers and Benjack found that a majority of their HIV-positive participants had experienced some type of sexual abuse during childhood. Christopher T. Allers and Karen J. Benjack, "Connections between Childhood Abuse and HIV Infection," *Journal of Counseling & Development* 70, no. 2 (1991): 309–13. Also see Sheldon D. Fields, David Malebranche, and Sonja Feist-Price, "Childhood Sexual Abuse in Black Men Who Have Sex with Men: Results from Three Qualitative Studies," *Cultural Diversity & Ethnic Minority Psychology* 14, no. 4 (2008): 385.

37. UNAIDS, *AIDS Epidemic Update: December 2004* (UNAIDS, 2004), 9–10.

38. Geeta Rao Gupta, "Globalization, Women and the HIV/AIDS Epidemic," *Peace Review* 16, no. 1 (2004): 79–83.

39. Paul Farmer, Margaret Connors, and Janie Simmons, *Women, Poverty, and AIDS: Sex, Drugs, and Structural Violence* (Common Courage Press, 1996).

40. US CDC, "New CDC Analysis Reveals Strong Link between Poverty and HIV Infection," press release, 2010.

41. US CDC, "New CDC Analysis Reveals Strong Link."

42. Douglas Massey and Nancy Denton, *American Apartheid: Segregation and the Making of the Underclass* (Harvard University Press, 1993); William Julius Wilson, *The Truly Disadvantaged: The Inner City, the Underclass, and Public Policy* (University of Chicago Press, 1987).

43. Waverly Duck, *No Way Out: Precarious Living in the Shadow of Poverty and Drug Dealing* (University of Chicago Press, 2015); Sonja Mackenzie, *Structural Intimacies: Sexual Stories in the Black AIDS Epidemic* (Rutgers University Press, 2013).

44. Tim Rhodes et al., "The Social Structural Production of HIV Risk among Injecting Drug Users," *Social Science & Medicine* 61, no. 5 (2005): 1026–44.

45. Elizabeth Bernstein, *Temporarily Yours: Intimacy, Authenticity, and the Commerce of Sex* (University of Chicago Press, 2007).

46. Victor M. Rios, *Punished: Policing the Lives of Black and Latino Boys* (New York University Press, 2011).

47. Michelle Alexander, *The New Jim Crow: Mass Incarceration in the Age of Colorblindness* (New Press, 2012); Nicole Gonzalez Van Cleve, *Crook County: Racism and Injustice in America's Largest Criminal Court* (Stanford University Press, 2016).

48. Robert Vargas, *Wounded City: Violent Turf Wars in a Chicago Barrio* (Oxford University Press, 2016); Sudhir Alladi Venkatesh, *American Project: The Rise and Fall of a Modern Ghetto* (Harvard University Press, 2009).

49. Scott Burris and Edwin Cameron, "The Case against Criminalization of HIV Transmission," *JAMA* 300, no. 5 (2008): 578–81; Trevor Hoppe, *Punishing Disease: HIV and the Criminalization of Sickness* (University of California Press, 2017).

50. Steven Thrasher, "A Black Body on Trial: The Conviction Of HIV-Positive 'Tiger Mandingo,'" *BuzzFeed*, November 30, 2015.

51. Shannon L. Hader et al., "HIV Infection in Women in the United States: Status at the Millennium," *JAMA* 285, no. 9 (2001): 1186–92.

52. US CDC, "HIV/AIDS among African Americans," 2016.

53. US CDC, "Epidemiologic Notes and Reports Acquired Immunodeficiency Syndrome (AIDS) among Blacks and Hispanics—United States," *Morbidity and Mortality Weekly Report* 35, no. 42 (1986): 655–58, 663–66.

54. US CDC, "30 Years of HIV in African American Communities: A Timeline," 2016.

55. US CDC, "Lifetime Risk of HIV Diagnosis: Half of Black Gay Men and a Quarter of Latino Gay Men Projected to Be Diagnosed within Their Lifetime," 2016.

56. Benoit Denizet-Lewis, "Double Lives on the Down Low," *New York Times*, August 3, 2003, www.nytimes.com/2003/08/03/magazine/double-lives-on-the-down-low.html; J. L. King and Karen Hunter, *On the Down Low: A Journey into the Lives of "Straight" Black Men Who Sleep with Men* (Harmony, 2004).

57. For excellent scholarly cultural critiques of the "down-low" discussion, see Jeffrey Q. McCune Jr., *Sexual Discretion: Black Masculinity and the Politics of Passing* (University of Chicago Press, 2014); David J. Malebranche, "Bisexually Active Black Men in the United States and HIV: Acknowledging More than the 'Down Low,'" *Archives of Sexual Behavior* 37, no. 5 (2008): 810–16; G. Millett et al., "Focusing 'Down Low': Bisexual Black Men, HIV Risk and Heterosexual Transmission," *Journal of the National Medical Association* 97, no. 7 (2005): 52S–59S; Maureen Miller, Malin Serner, and Meghan Wagner, "Sexual Diversity among Black Men Who Have Sex with Men in an Inner-City Community," *Journal of Urban Health* 82, no. 1 (2005): i26–i34; G. Millett et al., "Greater Risk for HIV Infection of Black Men Who Have Sex with Men," *American Journal of Public Health* 96, no. 6 (2006): 1007–19; C. Riley Snorton, *Nobody Is Supposed to Know: Black Sexuality on the Down Low* (University of Minnesota Press, 2014).

58. US CDC, "HIV in the United States and Dependent Areas," 2019.

59. Millett et al., "Greater Risk for HIV Infection."

60. Matt G. Mutchler et al., "Psychosocial Correlates of Unprotected Sex without Disclosure of HIV-Positivity among African-American, Latino, and White Men Who Have Sex with Men and Women," *Archives of Sexual Behavior* 37, no. 5 (2008): 736–47.

61. Marcus Anthony Hunter, "All the Gays Are White and All the Blacks Are Straight: Black Gay Men, Identity, and Community," *Sexuality Research & Social Policy* 7, no. 2 (2010): 81–92; E. Patrick Johnson, *Sweet Tea: Black Gay Men of the South* (University of North Carolina Press, 2011).

62. Cohen, *The Boundaries of Blackness*.

63. Cohen, *The Boundaries of Blackness;* Adam Geary, *Antiblack Racism and the AIDS Epidemic: State Intimacies* (Springer, 2014).

64. US CDC, "HIV Transmission at Each Stage of Care," press release, 2015.

65. Michael Arnold et al., "Race, Place and AIDS: The Role of Socioeconomic Context on Racial Disparities in Treatment and Survival in San Francisco," *Social Science & Medicine* 69, no. 1 (2009): 121–28.

66. In an analysis of data from four nationally representative US surveys, Morris and colleagues find consistent support for the hypothesis that higher levels of concurrent sexual partnerships among blacks, coupled with lower rates of interracial dating, may help to explain the disproportionately high prevalence of HIV and other STIs in predominantly black communities. Martina Morris et al., "Concurrent Partnerships and HIV Prevalence Disparities by Race: Linking Science and Public Health Practice," *American Journal of Public Health* 99, no. 6 (2009): 1023–31. Also see Edward O. Laumann and Yoosik Youm, "Racial/Ethnic Group Differences in the Prevalence of Sexually Transmitted Diseases in the United States: A Network Explanation," *Sexually Transmitted Diseases* 26, no. 5 (1999): 250–61.

67. Evelynn M. Hammonds, "Toward a Genealogy of Black Female Sexuality: The Problematic of Silence," in *Feminist Theory and the Body: A Reader,* ed. Janet Price and Margrit Shildrick (Routledge, 1999), 93–104.

68. Ryan P. Westergaard, Anne C. Spaulding, and Timothy P. Flanigan, "HIV among Persons Incarcerated in the US: A Review of Evolving Concepts in Testing, Treatment and Linkage to Community Care," *Current Opinion in Infectious Diseases* 26, no. 1 (2013): 10.

69. Ronald L. Braithwaite and Kimberly R.J. Arriola, "Male Prisoners and HIV Prevention: A Call for Action Ignored," *American Journal of Public Health* 93, no. 5 (2003): 759–63; US CDC, "HIV Transmission among Male Inmates in a State Prison System—Georgia, 1992–2005," *Morbidity and Mortality Weekly Report* 55, no. 15 (2006): 421.

70. Kim M. Blankenship et al., "Black-White Disparities in HIV/AIDS: The Role of Drug Policy and the Corrections System," *Journal of Health Care for the Poor & Underserved* 16, no. 4, supp. B (2005): 140.

71. Adaora A. Adimora and Victor J. Schoenbach, "Social Context, Sexual Networks, and Racial Disparities in Rates of Sexually Transmitted Infections," *Journal of Infectious Diseases* 191, supp. 1 (2005): S119; Andrea Kim et al., "Vulnerability to HIV among Women Formerly Incarcerated and Women with Incarcerated Sexual Partners," *AIDS & Behavior* 6, no. 4 (2002): 331–38.

72. Westergaard, Spaulding, and Flanigan, "HIV among Persons Incarcerated in the US."

73. Jason Schnittker, Michael Massoglia, and Christopher Uggen, "Incarceration and the Health of the African American Community," *Du Bois Review: Social Science Research on Race* 8, no. 1 (2011): 133–41.

74. Rucker C. Johnson and Steven Raphael, "The Effects of Male Incarceration Dynamics on Acquired Immune Deficiency Syndrome Infection Rates among African American Women and Men," *Journal of Law & Economics* 52, no. 2 (2009): 251–93; Seijeoung Kim, "Incarcerated Women in Life Context," *Women's Studies International Forum* 26, no. 3 (2003): 95–100; Schnittker, Massoglia, and Uggen, "Incarceration and the Health of the African American Community"; Loic Wacquant, "Deadly Symbiosis When Ghetto and Prison Meet and Mesh," *Punishment & Society* 3, no. 1 (2001): 95–133; Nicholas Freudenberg and Megha Ramaswamy, "The Impact of Incarceration on the Health of African Americans," *Health Issues in the Black Community*, 2009, 209–29.

75. Cohen, *The Boundaries of Blackness;* Ernest Quimby and Samuel R. Friedman, "Dynamics of Black Mobilization against AIDS in New York City," *Social Problems* 36, no. 4 (1989): 403–415.

76. Higginbotham, *Righteous Discontent*, 198.

77. Sanyu A. Mojola, *Love, Money, and HIV: Becoming a Modern African Woman in the Age of AIDS* (University of California Press, 2014).

78. Adimora and Schoenbach, "Social Context, Sexual Networks," S118; Wilson, *The Truly Disadvantaged.*

79. Shari L. Dworkin, *Men at Risk: Masculinity, Heterosexuality and HIV Prevention* (New York University Press, 2015).

80. Lisa Bowleg and Anita Raj, "Shared Communities, Structural Contexts, and HIV Risk: Prioritizing the HIV Risk and Prevention Needs of Black Heterosexual Men," *American Journal of Public Health* 102, no. S2 (2012): S173.

81. Carole A. Campbell, *Women, Families and HIV/AIDS: A Sociological Perspective on the Epidemic in America* (Cambridge University Press, 1999); US CDC, "HIV Risk among Persons Who Exchange Sex for Money or Nonmonetary Items"; James M. McMahon et al., "Contextual Determinants of Condom Use among Female Sex Exchangers in East Harlem, NYC: An Event Analysis," *AIDS & Behavior* 10, no. 6 (2006): 731–41.

82. Alexis C. Dennis et al., "'You're in a World of Chaos': Experiences Accessing HIV Care and Adhering to Medications after Incarceration," *Journal of the Association of Nurses in AIDS Care* 26, no. 5 (2015): 542–55; Perry N. Halkitis et al., "Characteristics of HIV Antiretroviral Treatments, Access and Adherence in an Ethnically Diverse Sample of Men Who Have Sex with Men," *AIDS Care: Psychological & Socio-medical Aspects of AIDS/HIV* 15, no. 1 (2003): 89–102.

83. Elisa Janine Sobo, *Choosing Unsafe Sex: AIDS-Risk Denial among Disadvantaged Women* (University of Pennsylvania Press, 1995).

84. Sobo, *Choosing Unsafe Sex*, 1; Kathryn Edin and Maria Kefalas, *Promises I Can Keep: Why Poor Women Put Motherhood before Marriage* (University of California Press, 2011).

85. Orlando Patterson, *Slavery and Social Death* (Harvard University Press, 1982).

86. Valerie Sacks, "Women and AIDS: An Analysis of Media Misrepresentations," *Social Science & Medicine* 42, no. 1 (1996): 59–73; Sonia Lawless, Susan Kippax, and June Crawford, "Dirty, Diseased and Undeserving: The Positioning of HIV Positive Women," *Social Science & Medicine* 43, no. 9 (1996): 1371–77.

87. Evelynn Hammonds, "Black (W)holes and the Geometry of Black Female Sexuality," *Differences: A Journal of Feminist Cultural Studies* 6, no. 2–3 (1994): 126–45.

88. Stuart Hall, "The Spectacle of the Other," in *Discourse Theory and Practice: A Reader*, ed. Margaret Wetherell, Stephanie Taylor, and Simeon J. Yates (SAGE Publications, 2001), 324–44.

89. Jeffrey S. Crowley and Gregorio A. Millett, "Preventing HIV and Hepatitis Infections among People Who Inject Drugs: Leveraging an Indiana Outbreak Response to Break the Impasse," *AIDS & Behavior* 21, no. 4 (2017): 968–72.

90. Michele Tracy Berger, *Workable Sisterhood: The Political Journey of Stigmatized Women with HIV/AIDS* (Princeton University Press, 2010).

91. Collins, *Black Feminist Thought;* Dorie J. Gilbert and Ednita M. Wright, *African American Women and HIV/AIDS: Critical Responses* (Greenwood, 2003); Hammonds, "Missing Persons."

92. Melissa Harris-Perry, *Sister Citizen: Shame, Stereotypes, and Black Women in America* (Yale University Press, 2011).

93. Auerbach, Parkhurst, and Cáceres, "Addressing Social Drivers of HIV/AIDS"; Celeste Watkins-Hayes, "Intersectionality and the Sociology of HIV/AIDS: Past, Present, and Future Research Directions," *Annual Review of Sociology* 40, no. 1 (2014): 431–57.

94. Crowley and Millett, "Preventing HIV and Hepatitis Infections."

CHAPTER 2. THE SAFETY NET THAT AIDS
ACTIVISM BUILT

1. Cathy J. Cohen, *The Boundaries of Blackness: AIDS and the Breakdown of Black Politics* (University of Chicago Press, 1999); Steven Epstein, *Impure Science: AIDS, Activism, and the Politics of Knowledge* (University of California Press, 1996); Joshua Gamson, "Silence, Death, and the Invisible Enemy: AIDS Activism and Social Movement 'Newness,'" *Social Problems* 36, no. 4 (October 1, 1989): 351–67; Deborah B. Gould, *Moving Politics: Emotion and ACT UP's Fight against AIDS* (University of Chicago Press, 2009); Benita Roth, *The Life and Death of ACT*

UP/LA: Anti-AIDS Activism in Los Angeles from the 1980s to the 2000s (Cambridge University Press, 2017); Brett C. Stockdill, *Activism against AIDS: At the Intersection of Sexuality, Race, Gender, and Class* (Lynne Rienner, 2003).

2. Ange-Marie Hancock, *The Politics of Disgust* (New York University Press, 2004).

3. Susan Sontag, *Illness as Metaphor and AIDS and Its Metaphors* (Macmillan, 2001); Barry D. Adam, "The State, Public Policy, and AIDS Discourse," *Crime, Law & Social Change* 13, no. 1 (1989): 1–14.

4. Adam, "The State, Public Policy, and AIDS Discourse"; Jennifer Brier, *Infectious Ideas: US Political Responses to the AIDS Crisis* (University of North Carolina Press, 2009); Epstein, *Impure Science*; Mary Irvine, "From 'Social Evil' to Public Health Menace: The Justifications and Implications of Strict Approaches to Prostitutes in the HIV Epidemic," *Berkeley Journal of Sociology*, 1998, 63–96; Bruce D. Johnson, Lisa Maher, and Samuel R. Friedman, "What Public Policies Affect Heroin Users," *Journal of Applied Sociology* 18, no. 1 (2001): 14–49; Evan S. Lieberman, *Boundaries of Contagion: How Ethnic Politics Have Shaped Government Responses to AIDS* (Princeton University Press, 2009).

5. Jonathan Bell et al., "Interchange: HIV/AIDS and US History," *Journal of American History* 104, no. 2 (2017): 433.

6. Epstein, *Impure Science*.

7. Lewis Katoff and Richard Dunne, "Supporting People with AIDS: The Gay Men's Health Crisis Model," *Journal of Palliative Care* 4, no. 4 (1988): 88–95; Philip M. Kayal, *Bearing Witness: Gay Men's Health Crisis and the Politics of AIDS* (Westview Press, 1993).

8. Kayal, *Bearing Witness*, 109.

9. Katoff and Dunne, "Supporting People with AIDS."

10. Howard Lune and Hillary Oberstein, "Embedded Systems: The Case of HIV/AIDS Nonprofit Organizations in New York City," *Voluntas: International Journal of Voluntary & Nonprofit Organizations* 12, no. 1 (2001): 17–33.

11. Lune and Oberstein, "Embedded Systems," 24.

12. Lune and Oberstein, "Embedded Systems," 24.

13. Lillian Faderman, *The Gay Revolution: The Story of the Struggle* (Simon and Schuster, 2015), 441.

14. Epstein, *Impure Science*, 8.

15. Jacquelyn Dowd Hall, "The Long Civil Rights Movement and the Political Uses of the Past," in *The Best American History Essays 2007*, ed. Jacqueline Jones (Palgrave Macmillan, 2007), 235–71; Aldon D. Morris, *The Origins of the Civil Rights Movement* (Simon and Schuster, 1986).

16. Evelynn Hammonds, "Missing Persons: African American Women, AIDS, and the History of Disease," in *Words of Fire: An Anthology of African-American Feminist Thought*, ed. Beverly Guy-Sheftall (New Press, 1995), 438.

17. Candice Marie Jenkins, *Private Lives, Proper Relations: Regulating Black Intimacy* (University of Minnesota Press, 2007), 5.

18. Hammonds, "Missing Persons," 438.

19. Alexis Shotwell, "'Women Don't Get AIDS, They Just Die from It': Memory, Classification, and the Campaign to Change the Definition of AIDS," *Hypatia* 29, no. 2 (March 1, 2014): 509–25.

20. Louis Sullivan was Secretary of HHS at the time and therefore named as the defendant.

21. Gena Corea, *The Invisible Epidemic: The Story of Women and AIDS* (HarperCollins, 1992).

22. Judy Clark and Kathy Boudin, "Community of Women Organize Themselves to Cope with the AIDS Crisis: A Case Study from Bedford Hills Correctional Facility," *Social Justice* 17, no. 2 (1990): 90–109.

23. Clark and Boudin, "Community of Women Organize Themselves."

24. Kathy Boudin, "The Resilience of the Written Off: Women in Prison as Women of Change," *Women's Rights Law Reporter* 29, no. 1 (2007): 18.

25. E.g., see the interview with Jean Carlomusto conducted by Sarah Schulman, December 19, 2002, interview no. 005, ACT UP Oral History Project; the interview with Maxine Wolfe conducted by Jim Hubbard, February 19, 2004, interview no. 043, ACT UP Oral History Project; Corea, *The Invisible Epidemic*.

26. US CDC, "HIV/AIDS Surveillance Report, 1994."

27. In 1988, the Abandoned Infants Assistance Act became law and supported moving so-called boarder babies into safe living arrangements. Many of the babies were exposed to drugs or HIV while in utero.

28. Evenlyn Brooks Higginbotham, *Righteous Discontent: The Women's Movement in the Black Baptist Church, 1880–1920* (Harvard University Press, 1993); Evelynn M. Hammonds, "Seeing AIDS: Race, Gender, and Representation," in *The Gender Politics of HIV/AIDS in Women: Perspectives on the Pandemic in the United States,* ed. Nancy Goldstein and Jennifer L. Manlowe (New York University Press, 1997), 94.

29. Hancock, *The Politics of Disgust.*

30. Valerie Purdie-Vaughns, "Intersectional Invisibility: The Distinctive Advantages and Disadvantages of Multiple Subordinate-Group Identities," *Sex Roles* 59, no. 5–6 (2008): 377–91.

31. Dorothy E. Roberts, *Killing the Black Body: Race, Reproduction, and the Meaning of Liberty* (Vintage Books, 1999).

32. Vicki Lens, "Confronting Government after Welfare Reform: Moralists, Reformers, and Narratives of (Ir)Responsibility at Administrative Fair Hearings," *Law & Society Review* 43, no. 3 (2009): 563–92.

33. Dorothy Roberts, *Shattered Bonds: The Color of Child Welfare* (Civitas Books, 2009).

34. Cathy J. Cohen, "Punks, Bulldaggers, and Welfare Queens: The Radical Potential of Queer Politics," *GLQ: A Journal of Lesbian & Gay Studies* 3 (1997): 437–65.

35. Stockdill, *Activism against AIDS;* Michele Tracy Berger, *Workable Sisterhood: The Political Journey of Stigmatized Women with HIV/AIDS* (Princeton University Press, 2010); Cohen, *The Boundaries of Blackness.*

36. There was also one cosponsor who was a registered Independent and one who was an Independent Democrat.

37. Prior to the Ryan White CARE Act, Congress had approved $30 million in emergency funding to states for AZT.

38. Epstein, *Impure Science.*

39. Berger, *Workable Sisterhood.*

40. Ashe-Goins's career also included stints as policy analyst and public liaison at the National Commission on AIDS and senior policy analyst with the White House Office on National AIDS Policy.

41. John Weiser et al., "Service Delivery and Patient Outcomes in Ryan White HIV/AIDS Program–Funded and –Nonfunded Health Care Facilities in the United States," *JAMA Internal Medicine* 175, no. 10 (October 1, 2015): 1650–59; Heather Bradley et al., "Ryan White HIV/AIDS Program Assistance and HIV Treatment Outcomes," *Clinical Infectious Diseases* 62, no. 1 (January 1, 2016): 90–98; Rupali Kotwal Doshi et al., "High Rates of Retention and Viral Suppression in the US HIV Safety Net System: HIV Care Continuum in the Ryan White HIV/AIDS Program, 2011," *Clinical Infectious Diseases* 60, no. 1 (January 1, 2015): 117–25.

42. "A Timeline of HIV/AIDS," www.aids.gov/hiv-aids-basics/hiv-aids-101 /aids-timeline/.

43. "A Timeline of HIV/AIDS."

44. Amy Goldstein, "U.S. to Begin Minority AIDS Initiative," *Washington Post,* October 29, 1998, www.washingtonpost.com/archive/politics/1998/10/29 /us-to-begin-minority-aids-initiative/d0299ac3-a51e-48a7-be11–9695ae77db23/?utm_term=.aa6977ddd993.

45. David Carter, *Stonewall: The Riots That Sparked the Gay Revolution* (Macmillan, 2004); Lillian Faderman and Stuart Timmons, *Gay LA: A History of Sexual Outlaws, Power Politics, and Lipstick Lesbians* (University of California Press, 2009).

46. Eileen Boris, Stephanie Gilmore, and Rhacel Parrenas, "Sexual Labors: Interdisciplinary Perspectives toward Sex as Work," *Sexualities* 13, no. 2 (2010): 131–37.

47. Stefan D. Baral et al., "Worldwide Burden of HIV in Transgender Women: A Systematic Review and Meta-analysis," *The Lancet Infectious Diseases* 13, no. 3 (2013): 214–22; Don Operario, Toho Soma, and Kristen Underhill, "Sex Work and HIV Status among Transgender Women: Systematic Review and

Meta-analysis," *Journal of Acquired Immune Deficiency Syndromes* 48, no. 1 (2008): 97–103.

48. Tonia Poteat, Danielle German, and Colin Flynn, "The Conflation of Gender and Sex: Gaps and Opportunities in HIV Data among Transgender Women and MSM," *Global Public Health* 11, no. 7–8 (2016): 835–48.

49. Combahee River Collective, "A Black Feminist Statement," in *Home Girls: A Black Feminist Anthology,* ed. Barbara Smith (Rutgers University Press, 1983), 272.

50. Gould, *Moving Politics,* 45; Epstein, *Impure Science.*

CHAPTER 3. LIVING WITH

1. Because Josie was scheduled to facilitate the meeting, I asked her beforehand if I needed permission from anyone else to attend (to which she replied "no"). My agreement with the IRB was to verbally solicit consent during observations in support groups and other gatherings of PLWHA. However, per my agreement with the IRB, I did not ask participants to document that consent by signing paperwork to protect their confidentiality. Names and key identifying characteristics of group participants have therefore been altered.

2. Michele Tracy Berger, *Workable Sisterhood: The Political Journey of Stigmatized Women with HIV/AIDS* (Princeton University Press, 2010).

3. Celeste Watkins-Hayes, LaShawnDa Pittman-Gay, and Jean Beaman, "'Dying from' to 'Living with': Framing Institutions and the Coping Processes of African American Women Living with HIV/AIDS," *Social Science & Medicine* 74, no. 12 (2012): 2028–36.

4. Malin Berghammer, Mikael Dellborg, and Inger Ekman, "Young Adults Experiences of Living with Congenital Heart Disease," *International Journal of Cardiology* 110, no. 3 (2006): 340–47; Janine Pierret, "The Illness Experience: State of Knowledge and Perspectives for Research," *Sociology of Health & Illness* 25, no. 3 (2003): 4–22; Karolynn Siegel and Beatrice J. Krauss, "Living with HIV Infection: Adaptive Tasks of Seropositive Gay Men," *Journal of Health & Social Behavior,* 1991, 17–32.

5. Michael Bury, "The Sociology of Chronic Illness: A Review of Research and Prospects," *Sociology of Health & Illness* 13, no. 4 (1991): 451–68; Kathy Charmaz, "Experiencing Chronic Illness," in *The SAGE Handbook of Social Studies in Health and Medicine,* ed. Gary Albrecht, Ray Fitzpatrick, and Susan C. Scrimshaw (SAGE Publications, 2000), 277–92.

6. Pierret, "The Illness Experience"; Siegel and Krauss, "Living with HIV Infection."

7. Silje Marie Haga, Pål Kraft, and Emma-Kate Corby, "Emotion Regulation: Antecedents and Well-Being Outcomes of Cognitive Reappraisal and Expressive

Suppression in Cross-Cultural Samples," *Journal of Happiness Studies* 10, no. 3 (2009): 271–91.

8. Jody Miller, *Getting Played: African American Girls, Urban Inequality, and Gendered Violence* (New York University Press, 2008).

9. Christine Dunkel-Schetter et al., "Patterns of Coping with Cancer," *Health Psychology* 11, no. 2 (1992): 79–87.

10. Erving Goffman, *Frame Analysis: An Essay on the Organization of Experience* (Harvard University Press, 1974); Robert D. Benford and David A. Snow, "Framing Processes and Social Movements: An Overview and Assessment," *Annual Review of Sociology*, 2000, 611–39.

11. Erving Goffman, *Stigma: Notes on the Management of Spoiled Identity* (Simon and Schuster, 1963).

12. Laura D. Stanley, "Transforming AIDS: The Moral Management of Stigmatized Identity," *Anthropology & Medicine* 6, no. 1 (1999): 103–20.

13. Steven Epstein, *Impure Science: AIDS, Activism, and the Politics of Knowledge* (University of California Press, 1996).

14. Jennifer Brier, *Infectious Ideas: US Political Responses to the AIDS Crisis* (Chapel Hill: University of North Carolina Press, 2009); Epstein, *Impure Science;* Deborah B. Gould, *Moving Politics: Emotion and ACT UP's Fight against AIDS* (Chicago: University of Chicago Press, 2009).

15. Edward Flores, *God's Gangs: Barrio Ministry, Masculinity, and Gang Recovery* (New York University Press, 2013).

16. Cathy J. Cohen, "Deviance as Resistance: A New Research Agenda for the Study of Black Politics," *Du Bois Review: Social Science Research on Race* 1, no. 1 (2004): 27–45.

17. Mustafa Emirbayer and Ann Mische, "What Is Agency?" *American Journal of Sociology* 103, no. 4 (1998): 963.

18. Lisa Marie Cacho, *Social Death: Racialized Rightlessness and the Criminalization of the Unprotected* (New York University Press, 2012); Orlando Patterson, *Slavery and Social Death* (Harvard University Press, 1982).

19. Pamela Y. Collins, Hella von Unger, and Adria Armbrister, "Church Ladies, Good Girls, and Locas: Stigma and the Intersection of Gender, Ethnicity, Mental Illness, and Sexuality in Relation to HIV Risk," *Social Science & Medicine* 67, no. 3 (2008): 389–97; Johanna Crane, Kathleen Quirk, and Ariane Van Der Straten, "'Come Back When You're Dying': The Commodification of AIDS among California's Urban Poor," *Social Science & Medicine* 55, no. 7 (2002): 1115–27; Julia Dickson-Gomez et al., "Access to Housing Subsidies, Housing Status, Drug Use and HIV Risk among Low-Income US Urban Residents," *Substance Abuse Treatment, Prevention, & Policy* 6, no. 1 (2011): 1; Celeste Watkins-Hayes, "The Micro Dynamics of Support Seeking: The Social and Economic Utility of Institutional Ties for HIV-Positive Women," *Annals of the American Academy of Political & Social Science* 647, no. 1 (2013): 83–101.

20. Daniel P. Kidder et al., "Access to Housing as a Structural Intervention for Homeless and Unstably Housed People Living with HIV: Rationale, Methods, and Implementation of the Housing and Health Study," *AIDS & Behavior* 11, no. 2 (2007): 149–61; Richard J. Wolitski et al., "Randomized Trial of the Effects of Housing Assistance on the Health and Risk Behaviors of Homeless and Unstably Housed People Living with HIV," *AIDS & Behavior* 14, no. 3 (2010): 493–503; David R. Holtgrave et al., "Cost-Utility Analysis of the Housing and Health Intervention for Homeless and Unstably Housed Persons Living with HIV," *AIDS & Behavior* 17, no. 5 (2013): 1626–31; Virginia Shubert and Nancy Bernstine, "Moving from Fact to Policy: Housing Is HIV Prevention and Health Care," *AIDS & Behavior* 11, no. 2 (2007): 172–81.

21. Dickson-Gomez et al., "Access to Housing Subsidies"; Suzanne Leclerc-Madlala, "'We Will Eat When I Get the Grant': Negotiating AIDS, Poverty and Antiretroviral Treatment in South Africa," *African Journal of AIDS Research* 5, no. 3 (2006): 249–56; Crane, Quirk, and Van Der Straten, "'Come Back When You're Dying.'"

22. Crane, Quirk, and Van Der Straten, "'Come Back When You're Dying,'" 1116.

23. Matthew Desmond, "Disposable Ties and the Urban Poor," *American Journal of Sociology* 117, no. 5 (2012): 1295–1335; Joan Maya Mazelis, *Surviving Poverty: Creating Sustainable Ties among the Poor* (New York University Press, 2017).

24. For more on the frequency and dynamics of evictions, see Matthew Desmond, *Evicted: Poverty and Profit in the American City* (Broadway Books, 2016).

25. Bich N. Dang, Thomas P. Giordano, and Jennifer H. Kim, "Sociocultural and Structural Barriers to Care among Undocumented Latino Immigrants with HIV Infection," *Journal of Immigrant & Minority Health* 14, no. 1 (2012): 124–31; Sherry Deren et al., "Research Challenges to the Study of HIV/AIDS among Migrant and Immigrant Hispanic Populations in the United States," *Journal of Urban Health* 82, no. 3 (2005): iii13–25; Claudia L. Moreno, "The Relationship between Culture, Gender, Structural Factors, Abuse, Trauma, and HIV/AIDS for Latinas," *Qualitative Health Research* 17, no. 3 (2007): 340–52.

26. Peggy A. Thoits, "Mechanisms Linking Social Ties and Support to Physical and Mental Health," *Journal of Health & Social Behavior* 52, no. 2 (2011): 153.

27. Annette Lareau, *Unequal Childhoods: Class, Race, and Family Life* (University of California Press, 2011).

28. Kathryn Edin and Laura Lein, *Making Ends Meet: How Single Mothers Survive Welfare and Low-Wage Work* (Russell Sage Foundation, 1997); Michael Lipsky, *Street-Level Bureaucracy: Dilemmas of the Individual in Public Service* (Russell Sage Foundation, 1980); Celeste Watkins-Hayes, *The New Welfare Bureaucrats: Entanglements of Race, Class, and Policy Reform* (University of Chicago Press, 2009).

29. Patrice Rosenthal and Riccardo Peccei, "The Social Construction of Clients by Service Agents in Reformed Welfare Administration," *Human Relations* 59, no. 12 (2006): 1633–58.

30. Mary Pattillo, *Black on the Block: The Politics of Race and Class in the City* (University of Chicago Press, 2008).

31. Jason Schnittker, Michael Massoglia, and Christopher Uggen, "Incarceration and the Health of the African American Community," *Du Bois Review: Social Science Research on Race* 8, no. 1 (2011): 133–41.

32. Michelle Alexander, *The New Jim Crow: Mass Incarceration in the Age of Colorblindness* (New Press, 2012); Mary Pattillo, Bruce Western, and David Weiman, *Imprisoning America: The Social Effects of Mass Incarceration* (Russell Sage Foundation, 2004).

CHAPTER 4. THE HIV SAFETY NET MEETS
THE TEST-AND-TREAT REVOLUTION

1. When to Start Consortium, "Timing of Initiation of Antiretroviral Therapy in AIDS-Free HIV-1-Infected Patients: A Collaborative Analysis of 18 HIV Cohort Studies," *The Lancet* 373, no. 9672 (n.d.): 1352–63.

2. Myron S. Cohen et al., "Prevention of HIV-1 Infection with Early Antiretroviral Therapy," *New England Journal of Medicine* 365, no. 6 (2011): 493–505.

3. US CDC, "HIV Transmission at Each Stage of Care," press release, 2015.

4. Steve Epstein, *Impure Science: AIDS, Activism, and the Politics of Knowledge* (University of California Press, 1996).

5. US CDC, "NCHHSTP Social Determinants of Health," 2014.

6. Judith Auerbach, "Transforming Social Structures and Environments to Help in HIV Prevention," *Health Affairs* 28, no. 6 (2009): 1655–65; Judith D. Auerbach, Justin O. Parkhurst, and Carlos F. Cáceres, "Addressing Social Drivers of HIV/AIDS for the Long-Term Response: Conceptual and Methodological Considerations," *Global Public Health* 6, supp. 3 (2011): S293–S309; Adaora A. Adimora and Judith D. Auerbach, "Structural Interventions for HIV Prevention in the United States," *Journal of Acquired Immune Deficiency Syndromes* 55, supp. 2 (2010): S132; Sarita K. Davis and Aisha Tucker-Brown, "The Effects of Social Determinants on Black Women's HIV Risk: HIV Is Bigger Than Biology," *Journal of Black Studies* 44, no. 3 (April 1, 2013).

7. Eric Mykhalovskiy and Marsha Rosengarten, "Commentaries on the Nature of Social and Cultural Research: Interviews on HIV/AIDS with Judy Auerbach, Susan Kippax, Steven Epstein, Didier Fassin, Barry Adam and Dennis Altman," *Social Theory & Health* 7, no. 3 (2009): 284–304.

8. US CDC, "Vital Signs: HIV Diagnosis, Care, and Treatment Among Persons Living with HIV—United States, 2011," *Morbidity and Mortality Weekly Report* 63, no. 47 (2014): 1113–17.

9. Chicago Department of Public Health, "HIV/STI Surveillance Report," 2018.

10. Barry D. Adam, "Epistemic Fault Lines in Biomedical and Social Approaches to HIV Prevention," *Journal of the International AIDS Society* 14, no. 2 (2011): S6. Also see Judith Auerbach and Trevor A. Hoppe, "Beyond 'Getting Drugs into Bodies': Social Science Perspectives on Pre-Exposure Prophylaxis for HIV," *Journal of the International AIDS Society* 18 (2015): 19983–87.

11. This story is taken from a fieldnote written by the author on March 12, 2007. The names of all participants in the story, including the physicians, have been changed to protect confidentiality.

12. Pamela Y. Collins, Hella von Unger, and Adria Armbrister, "Church Ladies, Good Girls, and Locas: Stigma and the Intersection of Gender, Ethnicity, Mental Illness, and Sexuality in Relation to HIV Risk," *Social Science & Medicine* 67, no. 3 (2008): 389–97; Christina S. Meade and Kathleen J. Sikkema, "HIV Risk Behavior among Adults with Severe Mental Illness: A Systematic Review," *Clinical Psychology Review* 25, no. 4 (2005): 433–57.

13. Alyson O'Daniel, *Holding On: African American Women Surviving HIV/AIDS* (University of Nebraska Press, 2016); Stephen Inrig, *North Carolina and the Problem of AIDS: Advocacy, Politics, and Race in the South* (University of North Carolina Press, 2011).

CHAPTER 5. THRIVING DESPITE

1. Sara Ahmed, *Living a Feminist Life* (Duke University Press, 2017); Audre Lorde, *A Burst of Light: Essays* (Firebrand Books, 1988); Audre Lorde, *Sister Outsider: Essays and Speeches* (Crossing Press, 2012).

2. Tamara Winfrey Harris, *The Sisters Are Alright: Changing the Broken Narrative of Black Women in America* (Berrett-Koehler, 2015); Melissa Harris-Perry, *Sister Citizen: Shame, Stereotypes, and Black Women in America* (Yale University Press, 2011).

3. Darlene Clark Hine, "Rape and the Inner Lives of Black Women in the Middle West," *Signs* 14, no. 4 (1989): 912–20.

4. Evelynn Hammonds, "Black (W)holes and the Geometry of Black Female Sexuality," *Differences: A Journal of Feminist Cultural Studies* 6, no. 2–3 (1994): 126–45.

5. Jenny A. Higgins, Susie Hoffman, and Shari L. Dworkin, "Rethinking Gender, Heterosexual Men, and Women's Vulnerability to HIV/AIDS," *American Journal of Public Health* 100, no. 3 (2010): 435–45.

6. See for example Evelyn Brooks Higginbotham, "African-American Women's History and the Metalanguage of Race," *Signs: Journal of Women in Culture & Society* 17, no. 2 (1992): 251–74; Audre Lorde, "The Uses of the Erotic: The Erotic as Power," *Lesbian & Gay Studies Reader* (1993): 339–43; Jennifer Nash, "Theorizing Pleasure: New Directions in Black Feminist Studies," *Feminist Studies* (2012): 507–15; Tricia Rose, *Longing to Tell: Black Women Talk about Sexuality and Intimacy* (Farrar, Straus and Giroux, 2004).

7. Evelynn M. Hammonds, "Toward a Genealogy of Black Female Sexuality: The Problematic of Silence," in *Feminist Theory and the Body: A Reader,* ed. Janet Price and Margrit Shildrick (Routledge, 1999), 93–104.

8. Douglas Ezzy, Richard De Visser, and Michael Bartos, "Poverty, Disease Progression and Employment among People Living with HIV/AIDS in Australia," *AIDS Care* 11, no. 4 (1999): 405–14; Michael P. Massagli et al., "Correlates of Employment after AIDS Diagnosis in the Boston Health Study," *American Journal of Public Health* 84, no. 12 (1994): 1976–81; Edward Yelin, "The Myth of Malingering: Why Individuals Withdraw from Work in the Presence of Illness," *Milbank Quarterly,* 1986, 622–49; Edward H. Yelin et al., "The Impact of HIV-Related Illness on Employment," *American Journal of Public Health* 81, no. 1 (1991): 79–84.

9. Amin Ghaziani, "Anticipatory and Actualized Identities: A Cultural Analysis of the Transition from AIDS Disability to Work," *Sociological Quarterly* 45, no. 2 (2004): 273–301; Ronald A. Brooks et al., "Perceived Barriers to Employment among Persons Living with HIV/AIDS," *AIDS Care* 16, no. 6 (2004): 756–66; Sue E. Ferrier and J. N. Lavis, "With Health Comes Work? People Living with HIV/AIDS Consider Returning to Work," *AIDS Care* 15, no. 3 (2003): 423–35; Stephanie Nixon and Rebecca Renwick, "Experiences of Contemplating Returning to Work for People Living with HIV/AIDS," *Qualitative Health Research* 13, no. 9 (2003): 1272–90; Jaimie Ciulla Timmons and Sheila Lynch Fesko, "The Impact, Meaning, and Challenges of Work: Perspectives of Individuals with HIV/AIDS," *Health & Social Work* 29, no. 2 (2004): 137–44.

10. For further discussion of institutions as resource brokers, see Mario Luis Small, *Unanticipated Gains: Origins of Network Inequality in Everyday Life* (Oxford University Press, 2009).

11. Alondra Nelson, *Body and Soul: The Black Panther Party and the Fight against Medical Discrimination* (University of Minnesota Press, 2011).

CONCLUSION. INEQUALITY FLOWS
THROUGH THE VEINS

1. Elizabeth Bernstein, *Temporarily Yours: Intimacy, Authenticity, and the Commerce of Sex* (University of Chicago Press, 2007); Eileen Boris, Stephanie

Gilmore, and Rhacel Parreñas, "Sexual Labors: Interdisciplinary Perspectives Toward Sex as Work," *Sexualities* (2010): 131–37.

2. Kathryn J. Edin and H. Luke Shaefer, *$2.00 a Day: Living on Almost Nothing in America* (Houghton Mifflin Harcourt, 2015).

3. US CDC, "HIV in the United States: Statistics Overview."

4. US CDC, "HIV among Women."

5. UNAIDS, "Global Statistics," November 20, 2017, www.hiv.gov/hiv-basics /overview/data-and-trends/global-statistics.

6. John Weiser et al., "Service Delivery and Patient Outcomes in Ryan White HIV/AIDS Program–Funded and –Nonfunded Health Care Facilities in the United States," *JAMA Internal Medicine* 175, no. 10 (October 1, 2015): 1650–59.

7. "Hatch Speaks at White House on 25th Anniversary of Ryan White CARE Act to Fight HIV/AIDS," www.hatch.senate.gov/public/index.cfm/2015/9 /hatch-speaks-at-white-house-on-25th-anniversary-of-ryan-white-care-act-to-fight-hiv-aids.

8. "Treat the Opioid Crisis like the HIV/AIDS Epidemic: Elizabeth Warren and Elijah Cummings," *USA Today,* March 29, 2018, www.usatoday.com/story /opinion/2018/03/29/new-legislation-treat-opioid-crisis-hiv-aids-epidemic-congressman-cummings-senator-warren-column/459036002/.

9. Kelly A. Gebo et al., "Contemporary Costs of HIV Health Care in the HAART Era," *AIDS* 24, no. 17 (2010): 2705–15; Bruce R. Schackman et al., "The Lifetime Cost of Current Human Immunodeficiency Virus Care in the United States," *Medical Care* 44, no. 11 (2006): 990–97; Madeline Vann, "Can You Afford Your HIV Treatment?" EverydayHealth.com, 2009.

10. Claire Laurier Decoteau, *Ancestors and Antiretrovirals: The Biopolitics of HIV/AIDS in Post-Apartheid South Africa* (University of Chicago Press, 2013); Paul Farmer, Margaret Connors, and Janie Simmons, eds., *Women, Poverty, and AIDS: Sex, Drugs, and Structural Violence* (Common Courage, 1996); Carol A. Heimer, "Old Inequalities, New Disease: HIV/AIDS in Sub-Saharan Africa," *Annual Review of Sociology* 33 (2007): 551–77; Evan Lieberman, *Boundaries of Contagion: How Ethnic Politics Have Shaped Government Responses to AIDS* (Princeton University Press, 2009).

11. Sanyu A. Mojola, *Love, Money, and HIV: Becoming a Modern African Woman in the Age of AIDS* (University of California Press, 2014), 202.

12. Shari Rudavsky, "An Indiana Town Recovering from 190 HIV Cases," *IndyStar,* April 8, 2016.

13. Partly in response to the HIV outbreak in Indiana, in 2015 Congress modified restrictions that prevented states and localities from spending federal funds for needle-exchange programs.

14. Eric Mykhalovskiy and Marsha Rosengarten, "Commentaries on the Nature of Social and Cultural Research: Interviews on HIV/AIDS with Judy

Auerbach, Susan Kippax, Steven Epstein, Didier Fassin, Barry Adam and Dennis Altman," *Social Theory & Health* 7, no. 3 (2009): 291.

15. Racial Justice Framework Group, "A Declaration of Liberation: Building a Racially Just and Strategic Domestic HIV Movement," November 9, 2017, 7.

16. Kimberlé Crenshaw, "Mapping the Margins: Intersectionality, Identity Politics, and Violence against Women of Color," *Stanford Law Review* 43, no. 6 (1991): 1299.

17. Celeste Watkins-Hayes, *The New Welfare Bureaucrats: Entanglements of Race, Class, and Policy Reform* (University of Chicago Press, 2009).

18. Steve Epstein, *Impure Science: AIDS, Activism, and the Politics of Knowledge* (University of California Press, 1996); Nancy Goldstein and Jennifer L. Manlowe, eds., *The Gender Politics of HIV/AIDS in Women: Perspectives on the Pandemic in the United States* (New York University Press, 1997); Beth E. Schneider and Nancy E. Stoller, eds., *Women Resisting AIDS: Feminist Strategies of Empowerment* (Temple University Press, 1995); Patricia D. Siplon, *AIDS and the Policy Struggle in the United States* (Georgetown University Press, 2002).

19. Patricia Hill Collins, *Black Feminist Thought: Knowledge, Consciousness, and the Politics of Empowerment* (Routledge, 2002).

20. Trevor Hoppe, *Punishing Disease: HIV and the Criminalization of Sickness* (University of California Press, 2017).

21. Barry D. Adam, "The State, Public Policy, and AIDS Discourse," *Crime, Law & Social Change* 13, no. 1 (1989): 2.

22. Edward L. Machtinger et al., "From Treatment to Healing: The Promise of Trauma-Informed Primary Care," *Women's Health Issues* 25, no. 3 (May 1, 2015): 193–97.

23. Elizabeth K. Hopper, Ellen L. Bassuk, and Jeffrey Olivet, "Shelter from the Storm: Trauma-Informed Care in Homelessness Services Settings," *Open Health Services & Policy Journal* 3, no. 1 (2010): 82. Also see Denise E. Elliott et al., "Trauma-Informed or Trauma-Denied: Principles and Implementation of Trauma-Informed Services for Women," *Journal of Community Psychology* 33, no. 4 (2005): 461–77.

24. Dominique Adams-Santos, "Something a Bit More Personal: Digital Storytelling and Intimacy among Queer Black Women." Master's thesis, Northwestern University, 2017.

25. Racial Justice Framework Group, "A Declaration of Liberation," 3–4.

26. Racial Justice Framework Group, "A Declaration of Liberation," 5.

27. Racial Justice Framework Group, "A Declaration of Liberation," 6.

28. Tamar W. Carroll, *Mobilizing New York: AIDS, Antipoverty, and Feminist Activism* (University of North Carolina Press, 2015); Benita Roth, *Life and Death of ACT UP/LA: Anti-AIDS Activism in Los Angeles from the 1980s to the 2000s* (Cambridge University Press, 2017).

29. Ange-Marie Hancock, *The Politics of Disgust: The Public Identity of the Welfare Queen* (New York University Press, 2004); Michael B. Katz, *The Undeserving Poor: America's Enduring Confrontation with Poverty* (Oxford University Press, 2013); Celeste Watkins-Hayes and Elyse Kovalsky, "The Discourse of Deservingness: Morality and the Dilemmas of Poverty Relief in Debate and Practice," in *Oxford Handbook of the Social Science of Poverty*, ed. David Brady and Linda M. Burton (Oxford University Press, 2016), 193.

APPENDIX A. METHODS OF RESEARCH

1. Celeste Watkins-Hayes, LaShawnDa Pittman-Gay, and Jean Beaman, "'Dying from' to 'Living with': Framing Institutions and the Coping Processes of African American Women Living with HIV/AIDS," *Social Science & Medicine* 74, no. 12 (2012): 2028–36; Celeste Watkins-Hayes, "The Micro Dynamics of Support Seeking: The Social and Economic Utility of Institutional Ties for HIV-Positive Women," *Annals of the American Academy of Political & Social Science* 647, no. 1 (2013): 83–101; Celeste Watkins-Hayes, "Intersectionality and the Sociology of HIV/AIDS: Past, Present, and Future Research Directions," *Annual Review of Sociology* 40, no. 1 (2014): 431–57.

2. Watkins-Hayes, Pittman-Gay, and Beaman, "'Dying from' to 'Living with.'"

3. Michèle Lamont and Ann Swidler, "Methodological Pluralism and the Possibilities and Limits of Interviewing," *Qualitative Sociology* 37, no. 2 (2014): 153–71.

4. For discussions of the advantages, disadvantages, and complexities of this approach, see Marjorie DeVault, *Liberating Method: Feminism and Social Research* (Temple University Press, 1999); Reuben A. Buford May, "When the Methodological Shoe Is on the Other Foot: African American Interviewer and White Interviewees," *Qualitative Sociology* 37, no. 1 (2014): 117–36; Alford A. Young Jr., "White Ethnographers on the Experience of African American Men: Then and Now," in *White Logic, White Methods*, ed. Tufuku Zuberi and Eduardo Bonilla-Silva (Rowman and Littlefield, 2008), 179–200.

5. Robert S. Weiss, *Learning from Strangers: The Art and Method of Qualitative Interview Studies* (Simon and Schuster, 1995), 1.

6. Hanna Herzog, "Interview Location and Its Social Meaning," in *The SAGE Handbook of Interview Research: The Complexity of the Craft*, 2nd ed., ed. Jaber F. Gubrium et al. (SAGE Publications, 2012), 208.

7. Lamont and Swidler, "Methodological Pluralism," 155.

8. See www.niehs.nih.gov/research/clinical/patientprotections/coc/index.cfm.

9. D. Soyini Madison, *Critical Ethnography: Method, Ethics, and Performance* (SAGE Publications, 2011).

10. Juliet M. Corbin and Anselm Strauss, "Grounded Theory Research: Procedures, Canons, and Evaluative Criteria," *Qualitative Sociology* 13, no. 1 (1990): 3–21.

11. Harriet A. Washington, *Medical Apartheid: The Dark History of Medical Experimentation on Black Americans from Colonial Times to the Present* (Doubleday, 2006).

Index

diagnoses of HIV/AIDS *(continued)*
of HIV, 286–87n16; of Health, Hardship,
and Renewal Study participants, 234, 274
diagnoses of HIV/AIDS *(continued)*
table; as respectability crisis, 73–75;
return to risky behavior following, 63–69;
secrecy of, as injury of persistent inequality, 37, 55–63. *See also* risk factors of HIV/
AIDS; test-and-treat approach
Diallo, Dázon Dixon, 108–9, 113–14, 201, 248
Dickson-Gomez, Julia, 298n19, 299n21
Dinkins, David, 102
Disch, Lisa, 284n23
disclosure, 213–14, 247
"disposable ties," 161
Doshi, Rupali Kotwal, 296n41
down low (DL) discourse, 57–60
drug addiction. *See* sexualized drug economy;
substance abuse
Dube, Shanta R., 288n34
Duck, Waverly, 289n43
Dunkel-Schetter, Christine, 298n9
Dunne, Richard, 294n7, 294n9
Dworkin, Shari L., 292n79, 301n5
dying from: and agency of women with HIV,
77–79; and confronting inequality, 232–
34, 237, 239, 249; defined, 15; and denial,
188; diagnosis of HIV as, 64, 69–73; as
existential struggle, 232; HIV safety net
for *living with*, 87–89, 91–92, 97, 107, 110,
117–18, 122, 127, 130–34; to *living with*
and *thriving despite* HIV, 11, 15, 228, 233;
regression to, 224; and risks of contracting HIV, 37; self-acceptance as transformation indicator, 209–12; stress and
mental health issues of, 200

economic factors: and confronting inequality,
231; and disclosure, 247; and food security, 159, 161–62; framing institutions and
isolating factors of, 162–67; HIV safety
net and significance of, 167–75; household
incomes of Snapshot Study participants,
206 *fig.*, 207–8; and intersectionality with
race and gender, 102–4; and need for HIV
safety net, 18; as risk factor for HIV, 47;
as transformation indicator, 206 *fig.*, 207–
8; of transformative projects and sustainability, 221–24. *See also* health insurance;
HIV safety net
Edin, Kathryn J., 233, 293n84, 299n28, 303n2
Ekman, Inger, 297n4
Elliott, Denise E., 304n23

Emirbayer, Mustafa, 156, 298n17
epidemics, collision of. *See* risk factors of
HIV/AIDS
Epstein, Steven, 82, 84, 240, 254, 282n12,
287n19, 293n1, 294n4, 294n6, 294n14,
296n38, 297n50, 298nn13–14, 300n4,
304n14, 304n18
ESSENCE (magazine), on HIV/AIDS risk factors, 63
Ezzy, Douglas, 302n8

Faderman, Lillian, 294n13, 296n45
Family Planning Council, 98–99
Farmer, Paul, 289n39, 303n10
Fauci, Anthony, 287n16
Feist-Price, Sonja, 289n36
Feminist Women's Health Center, 108–9
Ferree, Myra Marx, 283n23
Ferrier, Sue E., 302n9
Fesko, Sheila Lynch, 302n9
Fields, C. Virginia, 114
Fields, Sheldon D., 289n36
Fisher, Mary, 39, 110
Fitzpatrick, Ray, 297n5
Flanigan, Timothy P., 291n68, 292n72
Flores, Edward, 283n18, 298n15
Floyd, Ingrid, 159–61
Flynn, Colin, 284n32, 297n48
Food and Drug Administration (FDA), 84
food security, 159, 161–62
Ford Foundation, 104
framing institutions: and conflicting mes-
sages about HIV, 152–54; and confronting
inequality, 230, 233; and effect of class
on, 167–75; and engagement with HIV
safety net, 142–43; framing agents of,
189; HIV education and institutional fail-
ings, 6, 19; isolating factors of, 162–67;
language and discourse of transformative
projects, 154–57; limitations of, 29; negative framing institutions and perverse
safety nets of, 175–76, 197; for support of
transformative projects, 149–52, 151 *table*.
See also transformative projects
Fraser-Howze, Debra, 124
French, Bryana H., 288n31
Freudenberg, Nicholas, 292n74
Friedman, Samuel R., 286n12, 292n75, 294n4
Fullilove, Robert, 282n6

Gaddist, Bambi, 170–71, 231
Gamson, Joshua, 293n1
gangs, and injuries of inequality, 20–21

Founded in 1893,
UNIVERSITY OF CALIFORNIA PRESS
publishes bold, progressive books and journals
on topics in the arts, humanities, social sciences,
and natural sciences—with a focus on social
justice issues—that inspire thought and action
among readers worldwide.

The UC PRESS FOUNDATION
raises funds to uphold the press's vital role
as an independent, nonprofit publisher, and
receives philanthropic support from a wide
range of individuals and institutions—and from
committed readers like you. To learn more, visit
ucpress.edu/supportus.